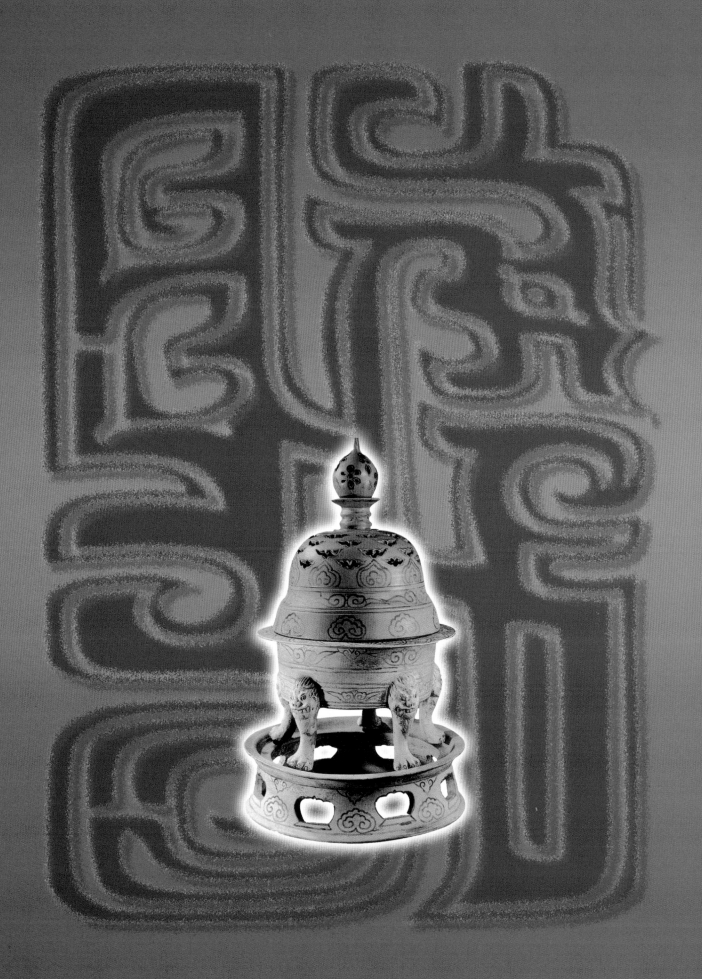

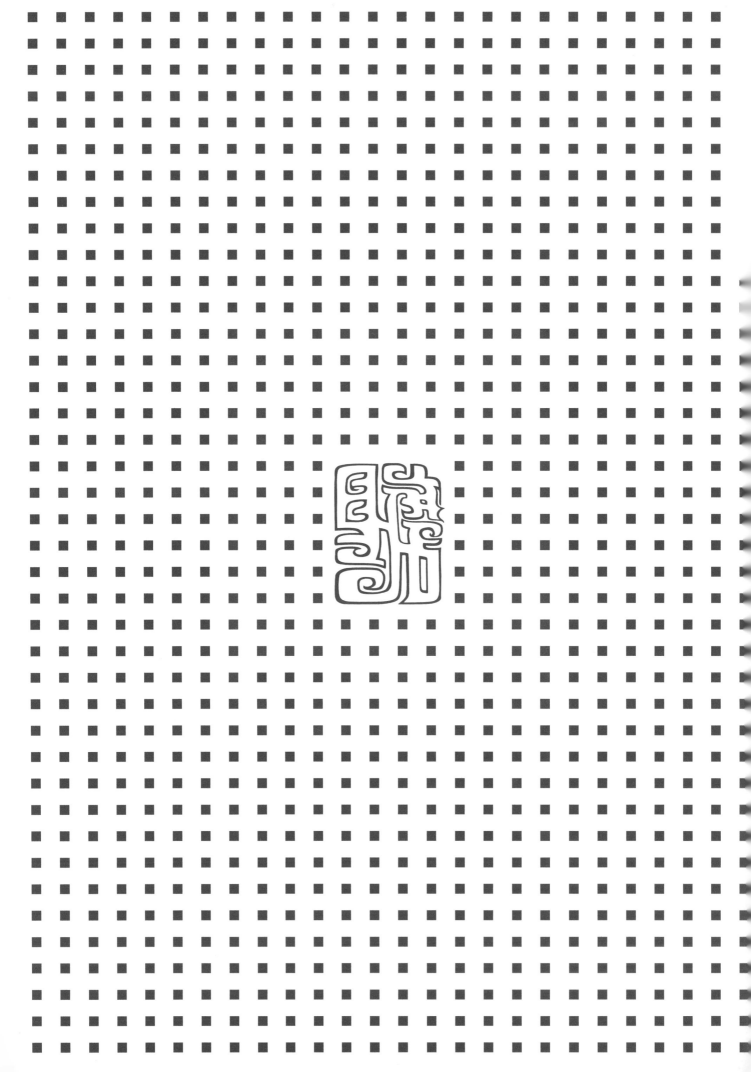

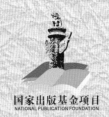

国家出版基金项目
NATIONAL PUBLICATION FOUNDATION

中华医药卫生

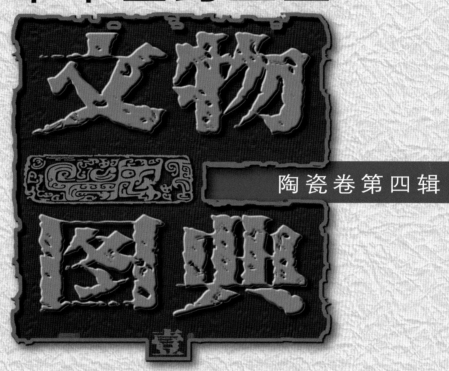

陶瓷卷第四辑

主　编　李经纬　梁　峻　刘学春
总主译　白永权
主　译　陈向京

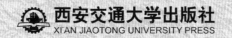
西安交通大学出版社
XI'AN JIAOTONG UNIVERSITY PRESS

图书在版编目 (CIP) 数据

中华医药卫生文物图典 . 1. 陶瓷卷 . 第 4 辑 . / 李经纬，
梁峻，刘学春主编 . — 西安：西安交通大学出版社，2016.12

ISBN 978-7-5605-7031-0

Ⅰ . ①中… Ⅱ . ①李… ②梁… ③刘… Ⅲ . ①中国医药学—
古代陶瓷—中国—图录 Ⅳ . ① R-092 ② K870.2

中国版本图书馆 CIP 数据核字（2015）第 013553 号

书　　名	中华医药卫生文物图典（一）陶瓷卷第四辑
主　　编	李经纬　梁　峻　刘学春
责任编辑	王　磊　李　晶

出版发行	西安交通大学出版社
	（西安市兴庆南路 10 号　邮政编码 710049）
网　　址	http://www.xjtupress.com
电　　话	（029）82668805　82668502（医学分社）
	（029）82668315（总编办）
传　　真	（029）82668280
印　　刷	中煤地西安地图制印有限公司

开　　本	889mm×1194mm　1/16　　**印张** 40.25　**字数** 648 千字
版次印次	2017 年 12 月第 1 版　2017 年 12 月第 1 次印刷
书　　号	ISBN 978-7-5605-7031-0
定　　价	1180.00 元

读者购书、书店添货、如发现印装质量问题，请通过以下方式联系、调换。

订购热线：（029）82665248　（029）82665249

投稿热线：（029）82668805　（029）82668502

读者信箱：medpress@126.com

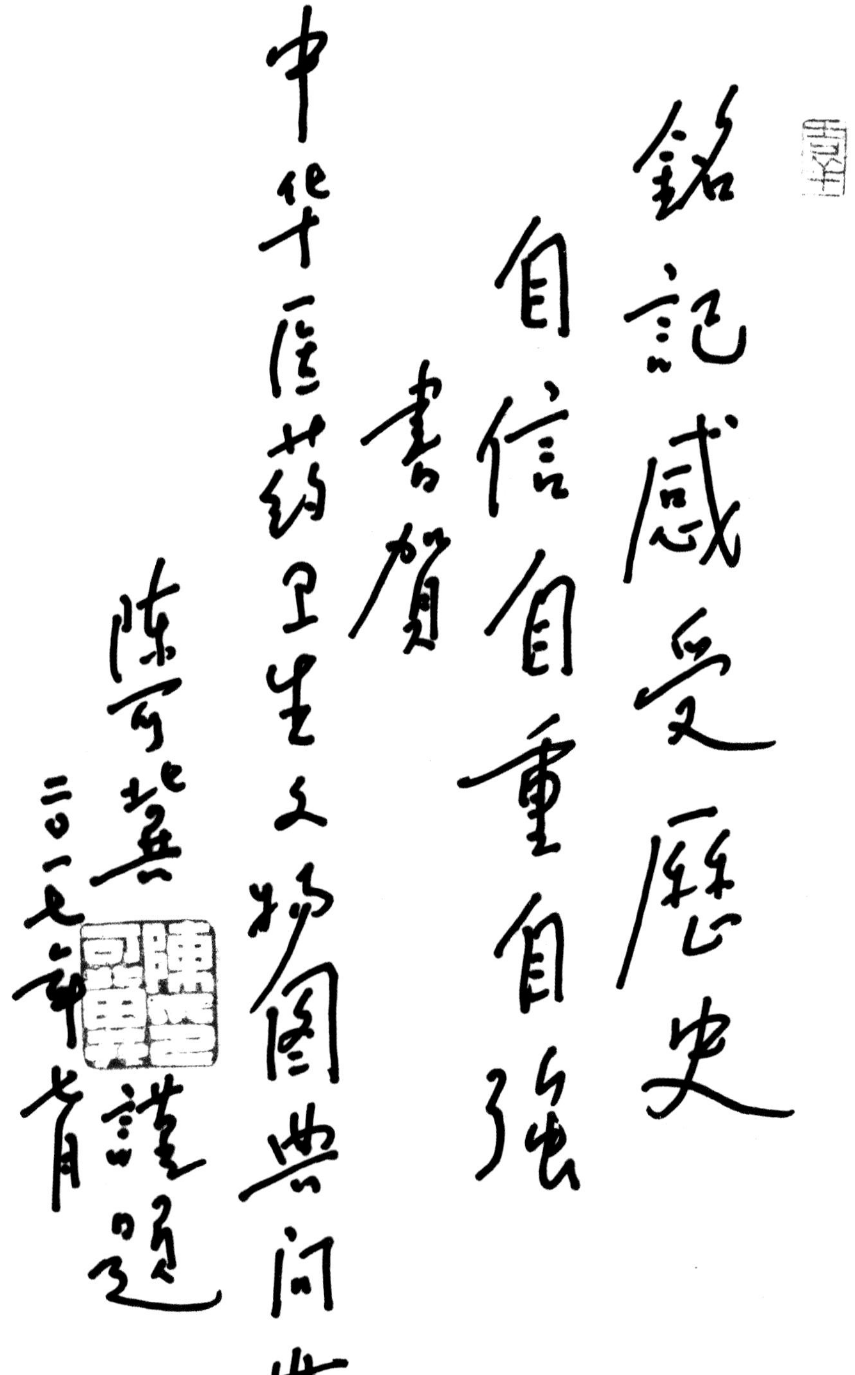

铭记感受历史

自信自重自强

书贺

中华医药卫生文物图典问世

陈可冀 谨题

二〇一七年秋

陈可冀　中国科学院院士、国医大师

精修醫藥衛生文物

圖典功著當代

深究岐黃學術思想

淵源惠澤千秋

中華醫藥衛生文物圖典出版誌慶

丁酉孟秋　孫光榮　敬題於北京

孫光荣　国医大师

中華醫藥衛生文物圖典出版

彰顯中醫藥
文化精神

体现中醫药
历史价值

歲次丁酉夏 王琦

王琦　国医大师

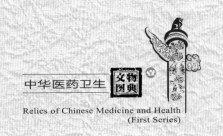

中华医药卫生

Relics of Chinese Medicine and Health
(First Series)

中华医药卫生文物图典（一）
丛书编撰委员会

主　编　李经纬　梁　峻　刘学春

副主编　廖　果　吴鸿洲　康兴军　和中浚　刘小斌　杨金生

　　　　　郑怀林　徐江雁　白建疆　黄　煌

编　委　李洪晓　梁永宣　王强虎　董树平　马　健　王　霞

　　　　　张雅宗　朱德明　包哈申　张建青　郑　蓉　庄乾竹

　　　　　李宏红　刘哲峰　王宏才　陈润东

总主译　白永权

主　译　陈向京　聂文信　范晓晖　温　睿　赵永生　杜彦龙

　　　　　吉　乐　李小棉　郭　梦　陈　曦

副主译（按姓氏音序排列）

　　　　　董艳云　姜雨孜　李建西　刘　慧　马　健　任宝磊

　　　　　任　萌　任　莹　王　颇　习通源　谢皖吉　徐素云

　　　　　许崇钰　许　梅　詹菊红　赵　菲　邹郝晶

译　者（按姓氏音序排列）

迟征宇　邓　甜　付一豪　高　琛　高　媛　郭　宁

韩　蕾　何宗昌　胡勇强　黄　鋆　蒋新蕾　康晓薇

李静波　刘雅恬　刘妍萌　鲁显生　马　月　牛笑语

唐云鹏　唐臻娜　田　多　铁红玲　佟健一　王　晨

王　丹　王　栋　王　丽　王　媛　王慧敏　王梦杰

王仙先　吴耀均　席　慧　肖国强　许子洋　闫红贤

杨姣姣　姚　晔　张　阳　张　鋆　张继飞　张梦原

张晓谦　赵　欣　赵亚力　郑　青　郑艳华　朱江嵩

朱瑛培

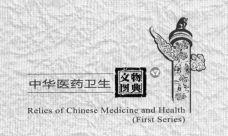

中华医药卫生文物图典

Relics of Chinese Medicine and Health
(First Series)

本册编撰委员会

主　编　李经纬　梁　峻　刘学春

副主编　廖　果　吴鸿洲　康兴军　和中浚　刘小斌　杨金生

　　　　　郑怀林　徐江雁　白建疆　黄　煌

编　委　李洪晓　梁永宣　王强虎　董树平　马　健　王　霞

　　　　　张雅宗　朱德明　包哈申　张建青　郑　蓉　庄乾竹

　　　　　李宏红　刘哲峰　王宏才　陈润东

总主译　白永权

主　译　陈向京

副主译　董艳云

译　者　许　梅　邹郝晶　张晓谦　王　丽　许子洋

　　　　　刘妍萌　高　媛　王　晨　郑艳华　王梦杰

丛书策划委员会

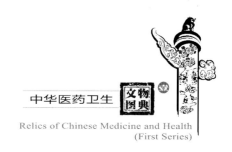

序 言

　　探索天、地、人运动变化规律以及"气化物生"过程的相互关系，是人类永恒的课题。宇宙不可逆，地球不可逆，人生不可逆业已成为共识。天地造化形成自然，人类活动构成文化。文物既是文化的载体，又是物化的历史，还是文明的见证。

　　追求健康长寿是人类共同的夙愿。中华民族之所以繁衍昌盛，健康文化起了巨大的推动作用。由于古人谋求生存发展、应对环境变化产生的智慧，大多反映在以医药卫生为核心的健康文化之中，所以，习总书记说："中医药学是中国古代科学的瑰宝，也是打开中华文明宝库的钥匙"。

　　秉持文化大发展、大繁荣理念，中国中医科学院李经纬、梁峻等为负责人的科研团队在完成科技部"国家重点医药卫生文物收集调研和保护"课题获 2005 年度中华中医药学会科技二等奖基础上，又资鉴"夏商周断代工程""中华文明探源工程"等相关考古成果，用有重要价值的新出土文物置换原拍摄质量较差的文物，适当补充民族医药文物，共精选收载 5000 余件。经西安交通大学出版社申报，《中华医药卫生文物图典（一）》（以下简称《图典》）于 2013 年获得了国家出版基金的资助，并经专业翻译团队翻译，使《图典》得以面世。

　　文物承载的信息多元丰富，发掘解读其中蕴藏的智慧并非易事。　医药卫生文物更具有特殊性，除文物的一般属性外，还承载着传统医学发展史迹与促进健康的信息。运用历史唯物主义观察发掘文物信息，善于从生活文物中领悟卫生信息，才能准确解读其功能，也才能诠释其在民生健康中的历史作用，收到以古鉴今之效果。"历史是现实的根源"，任何一个民族都不能割断历史，史料都包含在文化中。"文化是民族的血脉，是人民的精神家园"，文化繁荣才能实现中华民族的伟大复兴。值本《图典》付梓之际，用"梳理文化之脉，必获健康之果"作为序言并和作者、读者共勉！

中央文史研究馆馆员
中国工程院院士　　王永炎
丁酉年仲夏

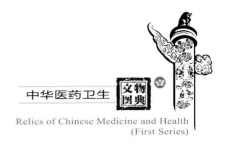

中华医药卫生 文物图典

Relics of Chinese Medicine and Health
(First Series)

前 言

　　文化是相对自然的概念，是考古界常用词汇。文物是文化的重要组成部分，既是文明的物证，又是物化的历史。狭义医药卫生文物是疾病防治模式语境下的解读，而广义医药卫生文物则是躯体、心态、环境适应三维健康模式下的诠释。中华民族是56个民族组成的多元一体大家庭，中华医药卫生文物当然包括各民族的健康文化遗存。

　　天地造化如造山、板块漂移、气候变迁、生物起源进化等形成自然。气化物生莫贵于人，即整个生物进化的最高成果是人类自身。广义而言，人类生存思维留下的痕迹即物质财富和精神财富总和构成文化，其一般的物化形式是视觉感知的文物、文献、胜迹等。其中质变标志明晰的文化如文字、文物、城市、礼仪等可称作文明。从唯物史观视角观察，狭义文化即精神财富，尤其体现人类精、气、神状态的事项，其本质也具有特殊物质属性，如量子也具有波粒二相性，这种粒子也是物质，无非运动方式特殊而已。现代所谓可重复验证的"科学"，事实上也是从文化中分离出来的事项，因此也是一种特殊文化形式。追求健康长寿是人类共同的夙愿。中华民族之所以繁衍昌盛，是因为健康文化异彩纷呈。中华优秀传统医药文化之所以博大精深，是因为其原创思维博大、格物致知精深，所以，习总书记说："中医药学是中国古代科学的瑰宝，也是打开中华文明宝库的钥匙"。

文化既反映时代、地域、民族分布、生产资料来源、技术水平等信息，又反映人类认知水平和生存智慧。发掘解读文物、文献中蕴藏的健康知识和灵动智慧，首先是从事健康工作者的责任和义务。《易经》设有"观"卦，人类作为观察者，不仅要积极收藏展陈文物，而且要善于捕捉文物倾诉的信息，汲取养分，启迪思维，收到古为今用之效果。墨子三表法，首先一表即"本之于古者圣王之事"，也是强调古代史实的重要性。"历史是现实的根源"，现实是未来的基础。任何一个国家、地区、民族都不能割断历史、忽略基础，这个基础就是文化。"文化是民族的血脉，是人民的精神家园"。文化繁荣才能驱动各项事业发展，才能实现中华民族的伟大复兴。

人类从类人猿分化出来。"禄丰古猿禄丰种"是云南禄丰发现的类人猿化石，距今七八百万年。距今200万年前人类进入旧石器时代，直立行走，打制石器产生工具意识，管理火种，是所谓"燧人氏"时代。中国留存有更新世早、中期的元谋、蓝田、北京人等遗址。距今10万—5万年前，人类进入旧石器时代中期，即早期智人阶段，脑容量增加，和欧洲、非洲人种相比，原始蒙古人种颧骨前突等，是所谓"伏羲氏"时代。中国发现的马坝、长阳、丁村人等较典型。距今5万—1万年前，人类进入旧石器时代晚期，即晚期智人阶段，细石器、骨角器等遍布全国，山顶洞、柳江、资阳人等较典型。

中石器时代距今约1万年，是旧石器时代向新石器时代的短暂过渡期，弓箭发明，狗被驯化。河南灵井、陕西沙苑遗址等作为代表。距今1万—公元前2600年前后，人类进入新石器时代，磨光石器、烧制陶器，出现农业村落并饲养家畜，是所谓"神农氏"时代。公元前7000年以来，在甲、骨、陶、石等载体上出现契刻符号、七音阶骨笛乐器等，反映出人文气息趋浓。公元前6000—公元前3500年的老官台、裴李岗、河姆渡、马家浜、仰韶等文化遗址，彰显出先民围绕生存健康问题所做的各种努力。

公元前4800年以来，以关中、晋南、豫西为中心形成的仰韶文化，是中原史前文化的重要标志。以半坡、庙底沟类型为典型，自公元前3500年走向繁荣，属于锄耕粟黍稻兼营渔猎饲养猪鸡经济方式，彩陶尤其发达。公元前4400—公元前3300年，长江中游的大溪文化，薄胎彩陶和白陶发达。公元前4300—公元前2500年山东半岛的大汶口文化，红陶为主。公元前3500年前后，辽东的红山文化原始宗教发展。公元前 3300 年以来，长江下游由河姆渡、马家浜文化衍续的良渚文化和陇西的马家窑文化、江淮间的薛家岗文化时趋发达。

公元前 2600—公元前 2000 年，黄河中下游龙山文化群形成，冶铸铜器，制作玉器，土坯、石灰、夯筑技术开始应用。公元前 2697 年，轩辕战败炎帝（有说其后裔）、蚩尤而为黄帝纪元元年。黄帝西巡访贤，"至岐见岐伯，引载而归，访于治道"。其引归地"溱洧襟带于前，梅泰环拱于后"，即今河南新密市古城寨。岐黄答问，构建《黄帝内经》健康知识体系，中华文明从关注民生健康起步。颛顼改革宗教，神职人员出现；帝喾修身节用，帝尧和合百国，舜同律度量衡，大禹疏导治水，中华民族不断繁衍昌盛。

公元前 2070 年，禹之子启以豫西晋南为中心建立夏王朝，二里头青铜文化为其特征，半地穴、窑洞、地面建筑并存。饮食卫生器具、酒器增多。朱砂安神作用在宫殿应用。公元前 1600 年，商灭夏。偃师商城设有铸铜作坊。公元前 1300 年，盘庚迁殷，使用甲骨文。武丁时期青铜浑铸、分铸并存。公元前 1056 年，相传周"文王被殷纣拘于羑里，演《周易》，成六十四卦"。公元前 1046 年，武王克商建周，定都镐京。青铜器始铸长篇铭文，周原发掘出微型甲骨文字。公元前 770 年，平王东迁。虢国铸铜柄铁剑。公元前 753 年，秦国设置史官。公元前 707 年出现蝗灾、公元前 613 年出现"哈雷彗星"，均被孔子载入《春秋》。公元前 221 年，秦始皇统一中国，多元一体民族大家庭形成，中华医药卫生文物异彩纷呈。

中国是治史大国，历来重视发展文化博物事业，1955 年成立卫生部中医研究院时就设置医史研究室，1982 年中国医史文献研究所成立时复建中国医史博物馆研究收藏展陈文物。2000—2003 年，经王永炎院士、姚乃礼院长等呼吁，科技部批准立项，由李经纬、梁峻为负责人的团队完成"国家重点医药卫生文物收集调研和保护"项目任务，受到科技部项目验收组专家的高度评价，获中华中医药学会科技进步二等奖。2013 年，在国家出版基金资助下，课题组对部分文物重新拍摄或必要置换、充实民族医药文物后，由西安交通大学出版社编辑、组聘国内一流翻译团队英译说明文字付梓，受到国家中医药博物馆筹备工作领导小组和办公室的高度重视。

"物以类聚"，《图典》主要依据文物质地、种类分为 9 卷，计有陶瓷，金属，纸质，竹木，玉石、织品及标本，壁画石刻及遗址，少数民族文物，其他，备考等卷。同卷下主要根据历史年代或小类分册设章。每卷下的历史时段不求统一。遵循上述规则将《图典》划分为21册，总计收载文物5000余件。对每件文物的描述，除质地、规格、馆藏等基本要素外，重点描述其在民生健康中的作用。对少数暂不明确的事项在括号中注明待考。对引自各博物馆的材料除在文物后列出馆藏外，还在书后再次统一列出馆名或参考书目，以充分尊重其馆藏权，也同时维护本典作者的引用权。

21世纪，围绕人类健康的生命科学将飞速发展，但科学离不开文化，文化离不开文物。发掘文物承载的信息为现实服务，谨引用横渠先生四言之两语："为天地立心，为生民立命"，既作为编撰本《图典》之宗旨，也是我们践行国家"一带一路"倡议的具体努力。希冀通过本《图典》的出版发行，教育国人，提振中华民族精神；走向世界，为人类健康事业贡献力量。

李经纬　梁峻　刘学春

2017 年 6 月于北京

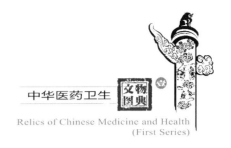

中华医药卫生 文物图典

Relics of Chinese Medicine and Health
(First Series)

目 录

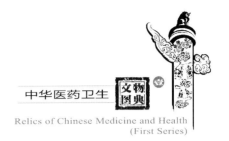

Contents

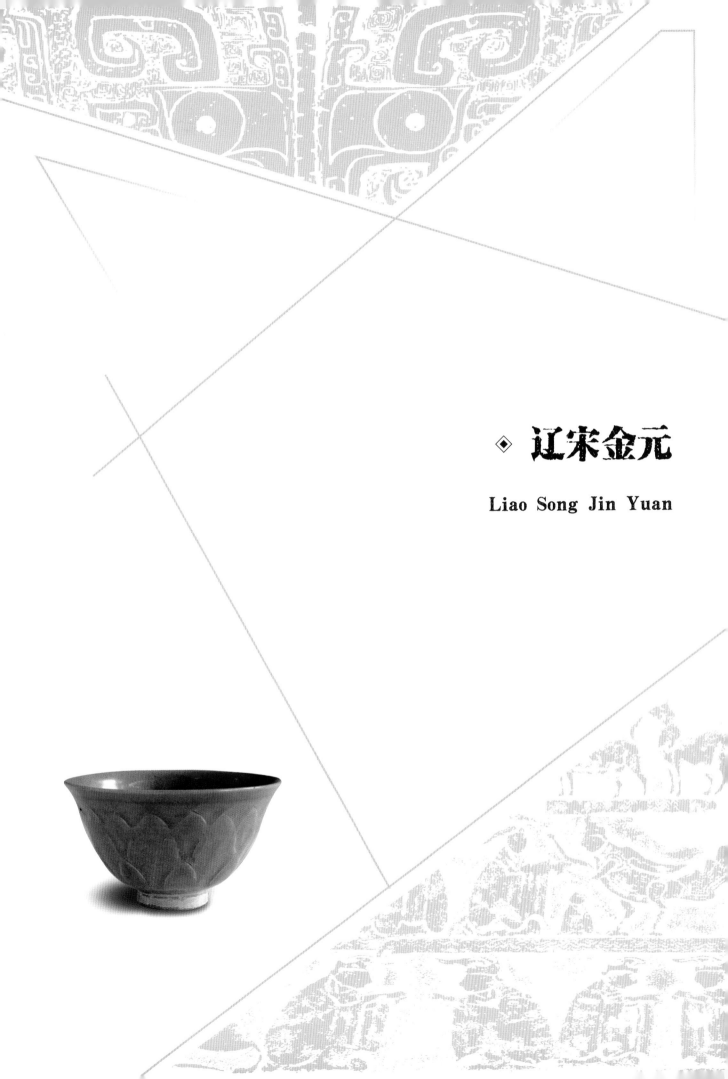

◇ 辽宋金元

Liao Song Jin Yuan

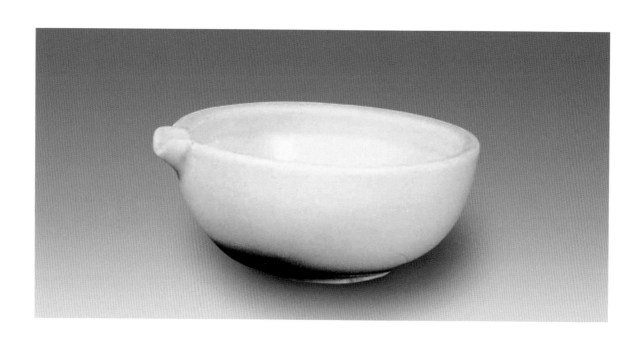

龙泉窑乳钵

宋

瓷质

口径 12.5 厘米，底径 5 厘米，高 5 厘米

整器外施以绿釉，带流。

上海中医药博物馆藏

Mortar, Longquan Kiln Ware

Song Dynasty

Porcelain

Mouth Diameter 12.5 cm/ Bottom Diameter 5cm/ Height 5 cm

Green glaze is applied to the exterior of the mortar, which is equipped with a spout.

Preserved in Shanghai Museum of Traditional Chinese Medicine

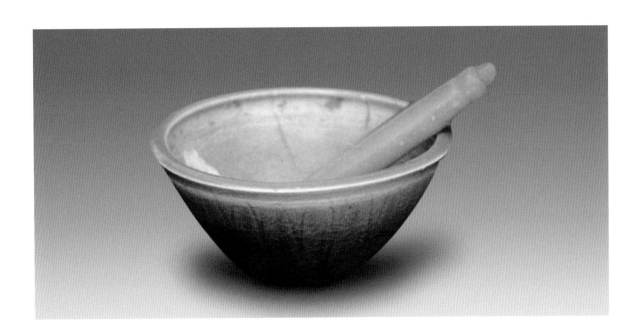

研钵

宋

青瓷质

口径 20 厘米，高 6.5 厘米

敞口，器壁和底都较厚，与棒状的杵配合使用。研杵圆柱形，一头略大，圆头，一头略小。

广东中医药博物馆藏

Mortar

Song Dynasty

Celadon

Mouth Diameter 20 cm/ Height 6.5 cm

This mortar has a flared mouth. Its wall and bottom are thick. A cylinder-shaped pestle with a thick round end is used together with it.

Preserved in Guangdong Chinese Medicine Museum

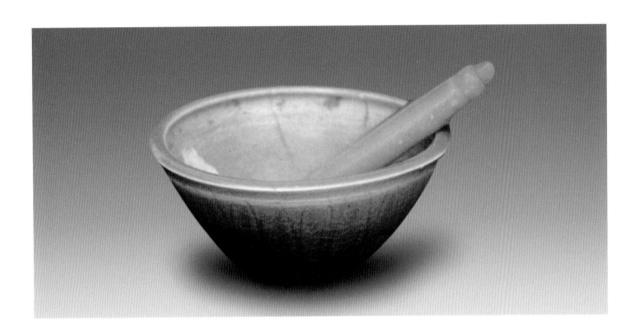

研钵

宋

青瓷质

口径 20 厘米，高 6.5 厘米

敞口，器壁和底都较厚，与棒状的杵配合使用。研杵圆柱形，一头略大，圆头，一头略小。

广东中医药博物馆藏

Mortar

Song Dynasty

Celadon

Mouth Diameter 20 cm/ Height 6.5 cm

This mortar has a flared mouth. Its wall and bottom are thick. A cylinder-shaped pestle with a thick round end is used together with it.

Preserved in Guangdong Chinese Medicine Museum

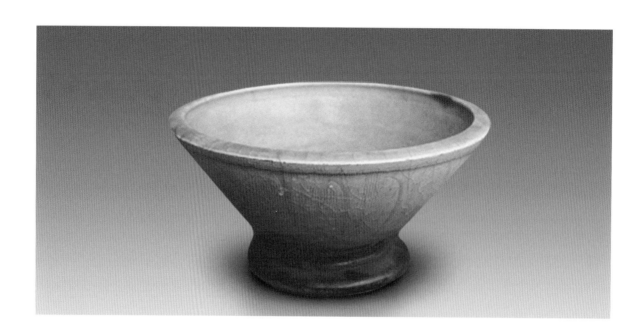

龙泉研钵

宋

瓷质

口外径 16.7 厘米，底径 5.27 厘米，通高 6.5 厘米，腹深 5.5 厘米，重 545 克

白胎，钵口及钵背面饰有瓜裂纹。用于研碎药物。

广东中医药博物馆藏

Mortar, Longquan Kiln Ware

Song Dynasty

Porcelain

Outer Mouth Diameter 16.7 cm/ Bottom Diameter 5.27 cm/ Height 6.5 cm/ Depth 5.5 cm/ Weight 545 g

This porcelain mortar has a white body with netted melon patterns at the mouth and on the outside wall of the mortar. It was utilized for grinding drugs.

Preserved in Guangdong Chinese Medicine Museum

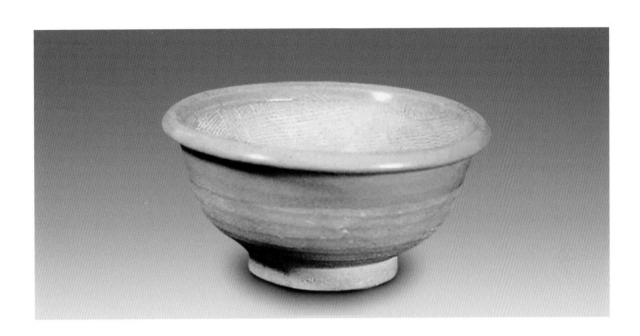

研钵

宋

瓷质

口径 14.5 厘米，底径 6.5 厘米，高 7 厘米

外层涂以薄层炒米黄色釉，腰以下露出灰白色胎体，腹内划有不规则线槽，便于研药。

上海中医药博物馆藏

Mortar

Song Dynasty

Porcelain

Mouth Diameter 14.5 cm/ Bottom Diameter 6.5 cm/ Height 7 cm

The exterior of the mortar is coated with a thin beige glaze. The pale grey body is shown below the waist.

There are irregular line-shaped grooves carved on the inside belly, making it convenient to grind drugs.

Preserved in Shanghai Museum of Traditional Chinese Medicine

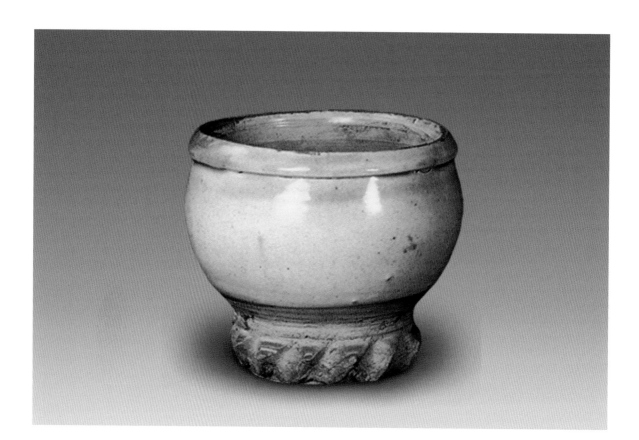

研钵

宋

瓷质

口径 8 厘米，底径 6 厘米，高 14 厘米

Mortar

Song Dynasty

Porcelain

Mouth Diameter 8 cm/ Bottom Diameter 6 cm/ Height 14 cm

鼓腹，敞口，绳纹圈足，器内及底部玄纹明显，器体厚重，胎质粗糙，外施黄釉，钵底无釉，无杵。

上海中医药博物馆藏

This mortar has a swelling belly, a flared mouth and a string-patterned ring foot. There are clear string patterns both in the inside and on the bottom. Its body is thick, heavy and rough, coated with yellow glaze, its bottom having no coat. There is no pestle.

Preserved in Shanghai Museum of Traditional Chinese Medicine

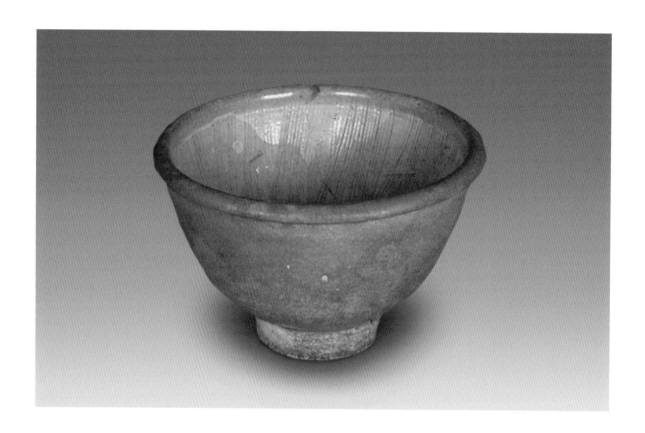

研钵

宋

陶质

Mortar

Song Dynasty

Pottery

圆钵形。该藏为土黄釉，敞口，平底，假圈足，底、足均无釉，钵内有放射状条纹，工艺粗糙，体量厚重，便于研磨，缺杵。制药工具。1956 年入藏。保存基本完好。

中华医学会 / 上海中医药大学医史博物馆藏

Coated with yellowish brown glaze, the mortar is in the shape of a round bowl. It has a flat bottom, a flared mouth and a false ring foot which is unglazed. Inside of the mortar are incised radial stripes. Though rough in workmanship, the mortar is strong and robust in form making it convenient to grind drugs. The pestle is missing. The mortar was utilized as an early pharmaceutical tool. It was collected in 1956 and still remains intact.

Preserved in Chinese Medical Association/ Museum of Chinese Medicine, Shanghai University of Traditional Chinese Medicine

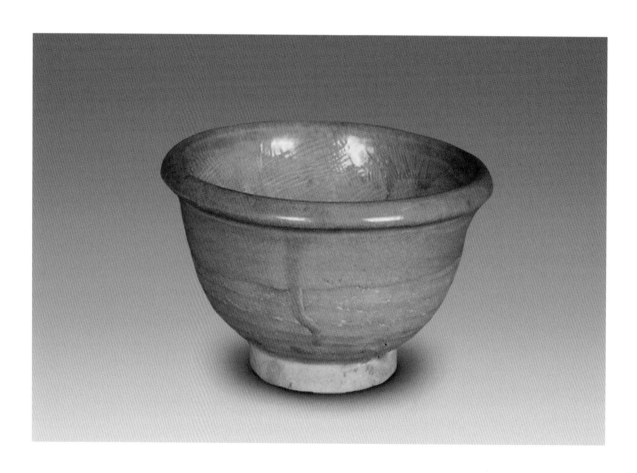

瓷研钵

宋

瓷质

口外径 14.55 厘米，高 7.5 厘米

Porcelain Mortar

Song Dynasty

Porcelain

Mouth Outer Diameter 14.55 cm/ Height 7.5 cm

圆钵形。该藏口沿及外上部施土黄色釉，钵

内有锉纹，外部玄纹明显，假圈足，底无款，

缺杵。制药工具。工艺较好。1955 年入藏。

保存基本完好。

中华医学会 / 上海中医药大学医史博物馆藏

The mortar, in the shape of a round bowl, is
coated with yellowish brown glaze on the
upper part of exterior wall and the rim. Inside
of the mortar are some rough cut files, while
on the exterior are clear spiral patterns. It has a
false ring foot and a base without inscription.
The pestle is missing. The mortar was used
as an early pharmaceutical tool with fine
workmanship. It was collected in the year 1955
and still remains intact.

Preserved in Chinese Medical Association/
Museum of Chinese Medicine, Shanghai
University of Traditional Chinese Medicine

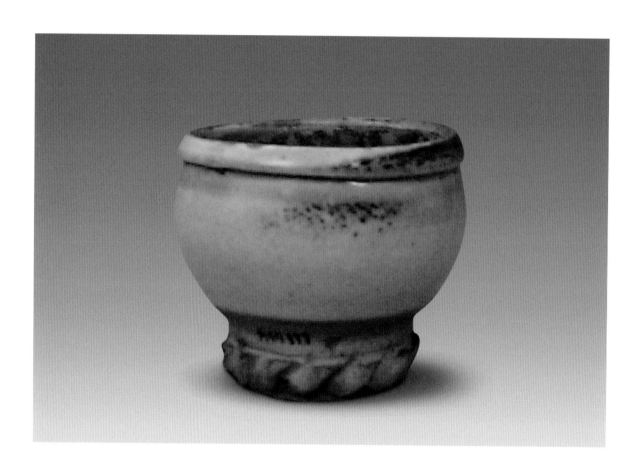

研钵

宋

瓷质

口径 11 厘米，腹径 11.6 厘米，底径 7.1 厘米，通高 10 厘米

Mortar

Song Dynasty

Porcelain

Mouth Diameter 11 cm/ Belly Diameter 11.6 cm/ Bottom Diameter 7.1 cm/ Height 10 cm

钵形。该藏由瓷制成，施土黄釉，敞口，绳
纹圈足，钵体厚重，便于研磨。制药用具。
1955 年入藏。保存基本完好。

中华医学会 / 上海中医药大学医史博物馆藏

The yellowish brown glazed porcelain mortar
is in the shape of a bowl. It has a flared mouth
and a ring foot decorated with twisted rope
patterns. The body of the mortar is thick, which
is suitable for grinding drugs. It served as a
pharmaceutical tool. It was collected in 1955
and still remains intact.

Preserved in Chinese Medical Association/
Museum of Chinese Medicine, Shanghai
University of Traditional Chinese Medicine

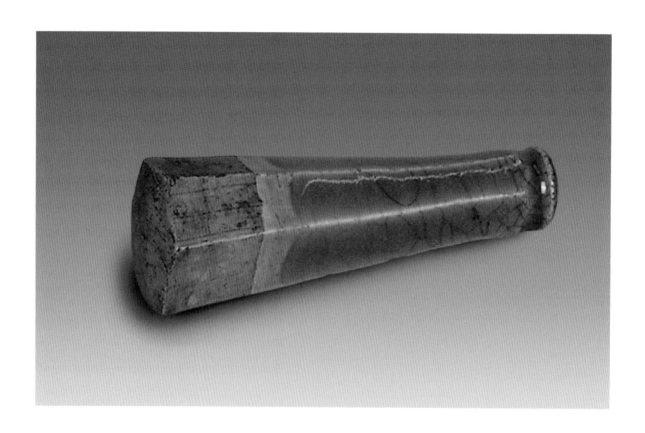

青瓷研杵

宋

瓷质

通长 12.2 厘米，杵径 34.5 厘米

Celadon Pestle

Song Dynasty

Porcelain

Length 12.2 cm/ Diameter 34.5 cm

杵状。该藏为宋龙泉窑瓷杵，呈不规则六棱柱形，下粗上细收敛为圆形钮，杵头无釉，有使用痕迹，杵柄施灰绿釉，有开片，工艺一般。制药工具。1959年入藏。保存基本完好。

中华医学会／上海中医药大学医史博物馆藏

The porcelain pestle was made in Longquan kiln. It is in the shape of an irregular hexagonal prism, with one end narrowing down to a round knob. The pestle head is unglazed, which shows signs of actual use. The stem of the pestle is celadon glazed with crackles. The pestle of ordinary workmanship was a tool for pharmaceutical use. It was collected in 1959, and it is still in good shape.

Preserved in Chinese Medical Association/ Museum of Chinese Medicine, Shanghai University of Traditional Chinese Medicine

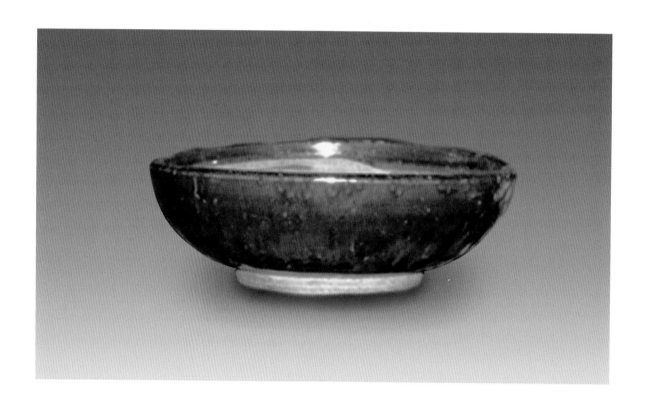

黑釉瓷研钵

元

瓷质

口径 18 厘米，底径 9.6 厘米，通高 6 厘米，重 700 克

Black-glazed Porcelain Mortar

Yuan Dynasty

Porcelain

Mouth Diameter 18 cm/ Bottom Diameter 9.6 cm/ Height 6 cm/ Weight 700 g

敞口，扁腹，圈足，钵内及底无釉。医药器具。
完整无损。陕西省咸阳市秦都区征集。

陕西医史博物馆藏

The mortar is designed with a flared mouth, a
flattened belly and a ring foot, with its bottom
and the interior wall unglazed. It was utilized
as a pharmaceutical tool, and is still in good
shape. It was collected from Qindu District of
Xianyang, Shaanxi Province.

Preserved in Shaanxi Museum of Medical History

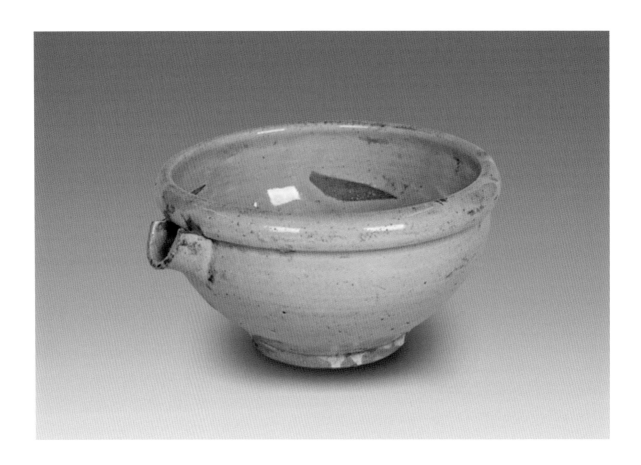

带流药钵

元

瓷质

口外径 14.3 厘米，口内径 12.7 厘米，通高 7.1 厘米

Mortar with a Spout

Yuan Dynasty

Porcelain

Mouth Outer Diameter 14.3 cm/ Mouth Inner Diameter 12.7 cm/ Height 7.1 cm

碗形。该药钵施黄绿釉，口沿下伸出一流，内外旋纹明显，施釉不匀，圈足和底均无釉，底无款识，工艺较粗糙。制药工具。1957 年入藏。保存基本完好。

中华医学会 / 上海中医药大学医史博物馆藏

Yellowish green glaze is unevenly applied to the bowl-shaped mortar. With clear spiral patterns incised inside and outside, the mortar has a spout stretching out below the rim, an unglazed ring foot and a bottom without inscription. The mortar of rough workmanship, collected in 1975, was a pharmaceutical tool and is still in good condition.

Preserved in Chinese Medical Association/ Museum of Chinese Medicine, Shanghai University of Traditional Chinese Medicine

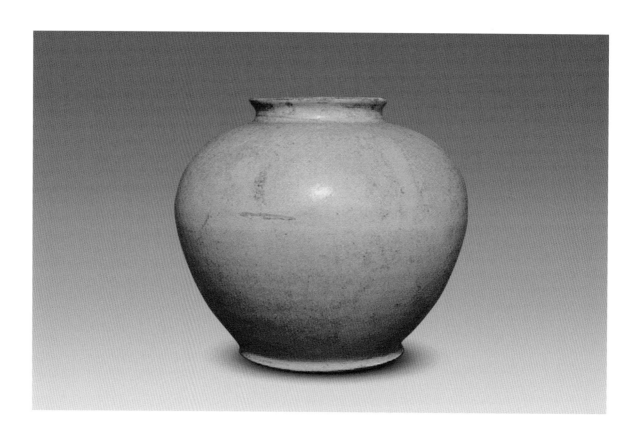

瓷坛

宋

瓷质

口外径 8.2 厘米，腹径 18 厘米，底径 10.2 厘米，通高 15.3 厘米，腹深 14.8 厘米，重 1350 克

Porcelain Jar

Song Dynasty

Porcelain

Mouth Outer Diameter 8.2 cm/ Belly Diameter 18 cm/ Bottom Diameter 10.2 cm/ Height 15.3 cm/ Depth 14.8 cm/ Weight 1,350 g

大口若悬河，口唇外侈，鼓腹，圈足。用于
盛药。

广东中医药博物馆藏

The jar, a drug container, has a wide mouth with
a flared rim, a globular body and a ring foot.
Preserved in Guangdong Chinese Medicine
Museum

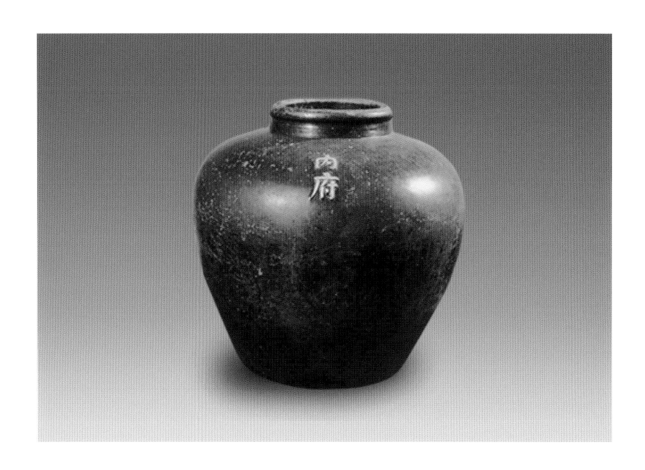

"内府"黑釉大药坛

宋

瓷质

口径 29 厘米，底径 42 厘米，高 57 厘米

Black-glazed Medicine Jar with "Nei Fu" Inscription

Song Dynasty

Porcelain

Mouth Diameter 29 cm/ Bottom Diameter 42 cm/ Height 57 cm

胎体为灰黑色，釉色不露极光。外壁有"内府"二字并涂以白釉。宫内贮药容器。

上海中医药博物馆藏

The roughcast of the jar is in ash black, coated with black luster glaze. This jar is inscribed with two Chinese characters "Nei Fu" (For use in the Inner Palace) on the exterior wall with white glaze. It was used as a drug container for the imperial court.

Preserved in Shanghai Museum of Traditional Chinese Medicine

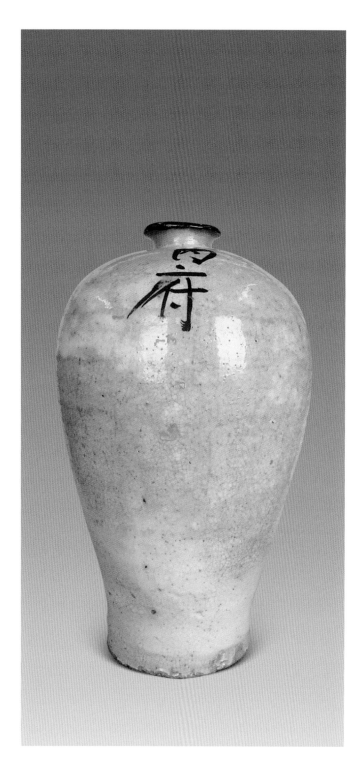

内府瓷药瓶

元

瓷质

腹围 63.5 厘米，通高 33.5 厘米

Porcelain Medicine Bottle with "Nei Fu" Inscription

Yuan Dynasty

Porcelain

Belly Diameter 63.5 cm/ Height 33.5 cm

圆形。该瓶通身施乳白釉，小开片，釉面光亮，瓶口施棕色釉，圈足，底面无釉、无款识，肩部书有"内府"二字，是该馆仅藏不多的元代盛药陶瓷器之一。盛药器具。1960 年入藏。保存基本完好，口沿有残。

中华医学会 / 上海中医药大学医学博物馆藏

The globular vase is fully coated with cream glaze, lustering with little crackles. With the rim glazed brown, the bottle has a ring foot, an unglazed bottom without inscription, a shoulder on which are inscribed two Chinese characters "Nei Fu" (For use in the Inner Palace). It is one of the few porcelain drug containers in the Yuan dynasty that has been preserved in this museum. The vase was collected in 1960 and is kept intact with just the rim cracked.

Preserved in Chinese Medical Association/ Museum of Chinese Medicine, Shanghai University of Traditional Chinese Medicine

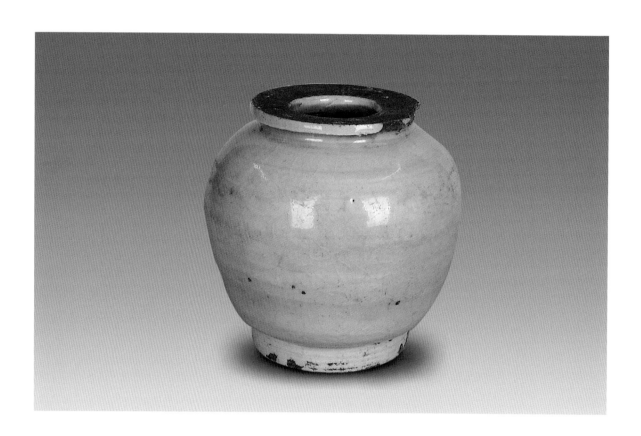

青瓷药罐

宋

瓷质

口外径 7.25 厘米，口内径 3.7 厘米，腹径 11.1 厘米，底径 7.05 厘米，通高 15 厘米

Porcelain Medicine Jar

Song Dynasty

Porcelain

Mouth Outer Diameter 7.25 cm/ Mouth Inner Diameter 3.7 cm/ Belly Diameter 11.1 cm/ Bottom Diameter 7.05 cm/ Height 15 cm

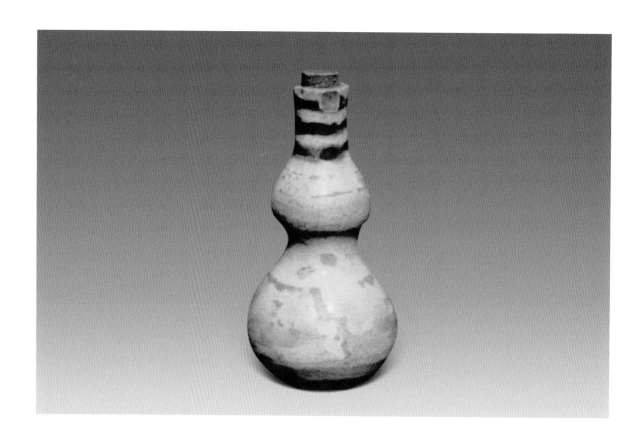

磁州窑小瓶

宋

瓷质

上葫芦直径 2.0 厘米，高 1.41 厘米；下葫芦直径 3.1 厘米，高 2.74 厘米，通高 6.1 厘米，重 20 克

Small Vase, Cizhou Kiln Ware

Song Dynasty

Porcelain

Upper gourd: Diameter 2.0 cm/ Height 1.41 cm; Lower gourd: Diameter 3.1 cm/ Height 2.74 cm;Total Height 6.1 cm/ Weight 20 g

瓷质葫芦形，平口，直颈，束腰，平底。盛
药或酒用。

广东中医药博物馆藏

This vase, in the shape of a gourd, has a flat
mouth, a straight neck, a contracted waist
and a flat bottom. It served as a drug or wine
container.
Preserved in Guangdong Chinese Medicine
Museum

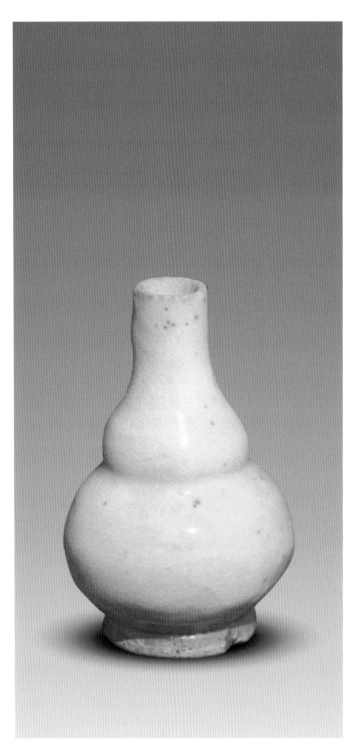

磁州窑小瓶

宋

瓷质

上葫芦直径2.4厘米，下葫芦直径3.8厘米，通高5.7厘米，重25克

葫芦形，平口，颈长直，圈足。可用于装细药或酒。

广东中医药博物馆藏

Small Vase, Cizhou Kiln Ware

Song Dynasty

Porcelain

Upper gourd: Diameter 2.4 cm/ Lower gourd: Diameter 3.8 cm/ Total Height 5.7 cm/ Weight 25 g

The gourd-shaped vase has a flat mouth, a long and straight neck and a ring foot. It was used for holding liquor or drugs of fine powder.

Preserved in Guangdong Chinese Medicine Museum

磁州窑小瓶

宋

瓷质

上葫芦直径 2.65 厘米，高 2.05 厘米；
下葫芦直径 3.57 厘米，高 2.8 厘米；通
高 7.97 厘米，重 30 克

葫芦形，平口，束腰，葫芦身呈瓜棱形，
平底。盛药用。

广东中医药博物馆藏

Small Vase, Cizhou Kiln Ware

Song Dynasty

Porcelain

Upper gourd: Diameter 2.65 cm/ Height
2.05 cm;Lower gourd: Diameter 3.57 cm/
Height 2.8 cm; Total Height 7.97 cm/
Weight 30 g

The gourd-shaped vase has a flat mouth,
a contracted waist and a flat bottom. The
gourd-shaped body is designed in the
form of a ribbed pumpkin. It was used for
holding drugs.

Preserved in Guangdong Chinese Medicine
Museum

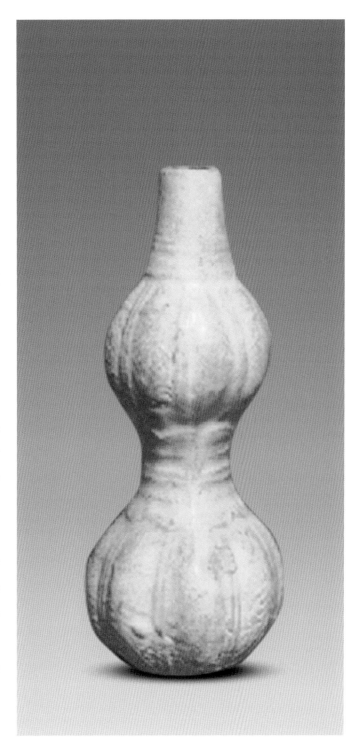

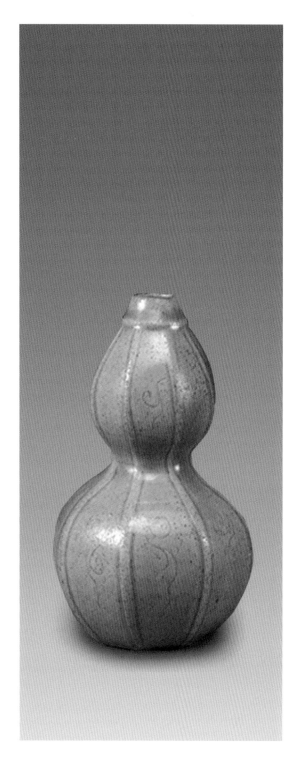

越窑青釉暗花花草纹八棱葫芦瓶

北宋

瓷质

口径 1 厘米，底径 2.4 厘米，高 7.7 厘米

八棱葫芦形。每面均装饰花卷草纹，线条纤细清晰。全器施青釉，釉色略泛灰，釉质清亮。瓶底无釉，胎色灰白。

常州博物馆藏

Octagonal Gourd-shaped Celadon Vase with Veiled Floral and Grass Motif

Northern Song Dynasty

Porcelain

Mouth Diameter 1 cm/ Bottom Diameter 2.4 cm/ Height 7.7 cm

The vase is shaped into an octagonal gourd. On each facet are incised floral scrolls and curling tendril designs with thin and clear lines. The entire vessel, except the outside bottom, is covered with clear and lustrous celadon glaze with a tinge of grey. The body of the pottery is in greyish white.

Preserved in Changzhou Museum

黑釉葫芦瓶

宋

瓷质

口径 2.5 厘米，底径 6 厘米，高 16.5 厘米

曾两次上釉，首为黑釉，次为透明釉。陕西西安出土。

陕西医史博物馆藏

Gourd-shaped Vase with Black Glaze

Song Dynasty

Porcelain

Mouth Diameter 2.5 cm/ Bottom Diameter 6 cm/ Height
16.5 cm

This bottle was glazed twice, with the first layer of glaze
black, and the second transparent. It was unearthed from
Xi'an, Shaanxi Province.

Preserved in Shaanxi Museum of Medical History

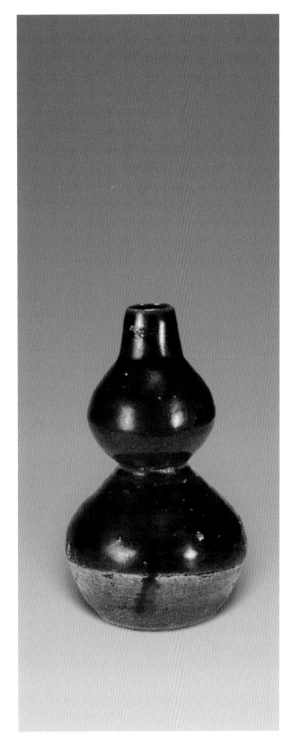

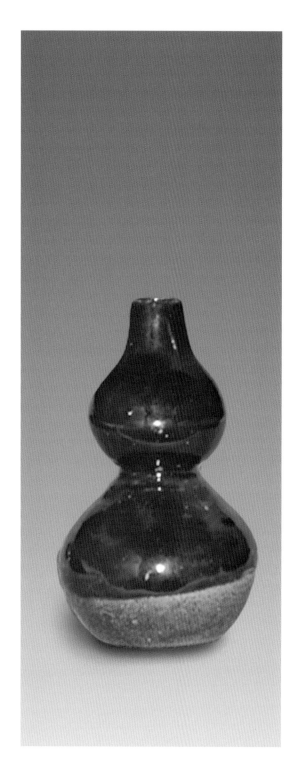

黑瓷葫芦瓶

宋

瓷质

口径 2 厘米，底径 6 厘米，通高 15.5 厘米，重 200 克

Gourd-shaped Vase with Black Glaze

Song Dynasty

Porcelain

Mouth Diameter 2 cm/ Bottom Diameter 6 cm/ Height 15.5 cm/ Weight 200 g

葫芦状。小口，浅圈足，黑瓷，接近底处无釉。

盛贮器。完整无损。陕西历史博物馆调拨。

陕西医史博物馆藏

The gourd-shaped vase, a storage container, is
designed with a small mouth and a shallow ring
foot. The bottle is covered with black glaze,
ending above the unglazed foot. It is kept intact.
It was allocated from Shaanxi History Museum.
Preserved in Shaanxi Museum of Medical History

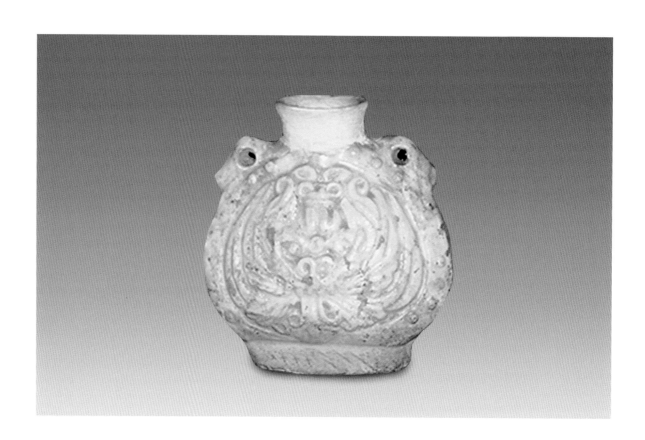

白瓷扁瓶

元

白瓷质

口径 2.6 厘米，底长 4.5 厘米，底宽 2.4 厘米，通高 7.1 厘米，重 50 克

Oblate White Porcelain Vase

Yuan Dynasty

White Porcelain

Mouth Diameter 2.6 cm/ Bottom Length 4.5 cm/ Bottom Width 2.4 cm/ Height 7.1 cm/ Weight 50 g

直口,扁腹,扁足,肩上有双耳,腹有浮雕白瓷,印花兽面纹。贮药器具。三级资料,口沿有修补。陕西省咸阳市征集。

陕西医史博物馆藏

The vase has a straight mouth, an oblate abdomen and an oblate foot with two ears on the shoulder. The belly is incised with floral motifs in relief and beast-face veins. The vase, classified as the third-class relic, was used as a drug container. The mouth rim appears to have been restored. It was collected from Xianyang, Shaanxi Province.

Preserved in Shaanxi Museum of Medical History

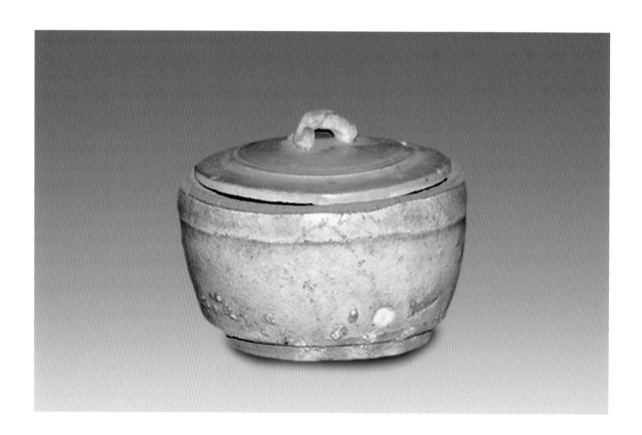

青瓷小药盒

宋

瓷质

口径 7 厘米，底径 5.3 厘米，通高 5.6 厘米，高 4 厘米，重 100 克

Porcelain Drug Case

Song Dynasty

Porcelain

Mouth Diameter 7 cm/ Bottom Diameter 5.3 cm/ Height (including lid) 5.6 cm/ Height 4 cm/ Weight 100 g

子母口，直腹，假圈足，带一盖，盖上有一
麻式化纽，并有一道弦纹和小孔。豆青釉，
碗内和底无釉。医药器具。完整。陕西省西
安市鼓楼文物市场征集。

陕西医史博物馆藏

The case is designed with a straight belly, a
false ring foot and a buckle lid, on which can be
found a twisted knob, a band of string patterns
and a small hole. The case is glazed pea green
except the interior surface and the bottom. It is
a well-kept case for pharmaceutical purposes.
It was collected from Drum Tower Antique
Market of Xi'an in Shaanxi Province.
Preserved in Shaanxi Museum of Medical History

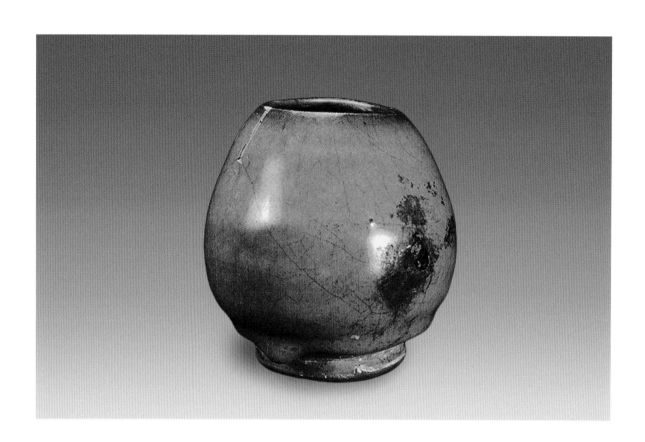

钧瓷拔火罐

元

瓷质

口径 5.5 厘米，腹围 30.5 厘米，底径 6 厘米，

高 10.4 厘米

灰釉。口沿有烧痕。内蒙古托县出土。

陕西医史博物馆藏

Porcelain Cupping Cup, Jun Kiln Ware

Yuan Dynasty

Porcelain

Mouth Diameter 5.5 cm/ Belly Diameter 30.5 cm/

Bottom Diameter 6 cm/ Height 10.4 cm

There are burn marks on the rim of the grey glazed cup.

It was unearthed from Tuoxian County, Inner Mongolia

Autonomous Region.

Preserved in Shaanxi Museum of Medical History

瓷仓

宋

瓷质

高 32cm

着青褐色釉，釉多脱落。器上部为双层圆塔形。覆两坡顶，下部作罐状，干腹部刻出一对斗拱图，斗拱之间有用数字加以标识的楼层象征图案。由此可见当时的建筑技艺。

南京博物院藏

Porcelain Storehouse

Song Dynasty

Height 32 cm

Most of the greenish brown glaze on the storehouse has peeled off. On the top of the object is a double-decked round tower covered with a duo-pitched roof. The lower part is in the shape of a pot. On the stem is carved a pair of Dou-Gong brackets, between which are numbers marking the floor. This storehouse represents the architectural techniques at that time.

Preserved in Nanjing Museum

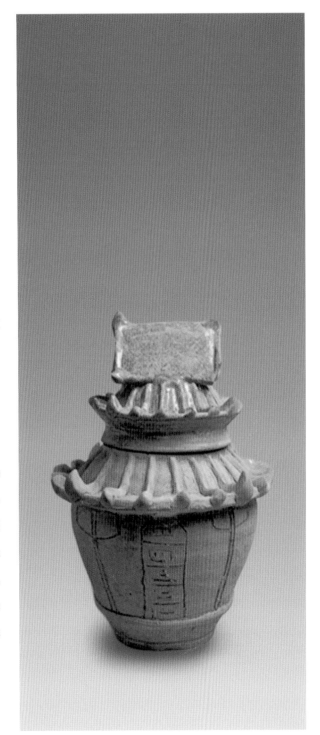

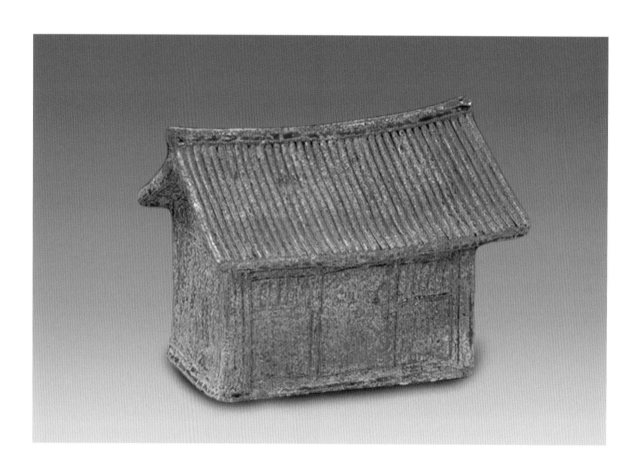

黄釉陶仓

宋

瓷质

面宽 24 厘米，进深 16.8 厘米，通高 24 厘米

Yellow-glazed Pottery Storehouse

Song Dynasty

Pottery

Facet Width 24 cm/ Depth 16.8 cm/ Height 24 cm

整体长方形，屋顶、房身施黄褐色釉，四面墙体用阴线条横直划出柱、檩、枋、窗的结构，前后墙可分出堂间和左右边间。正面堂间檐口之下处，有一长方形门孔，左右边间、后墙堂间封闭，其柱、枋、窗与正面对称。高淳区三中工地出土。

高淳博物馆藏

The roof and the body of the rectangular storehouse are glazed yellowish brown. The construction of the beams, purlins, square-columns and windows are expressed by the concave lines carved on the walls. From the front and the back wall, the image of the main hall and the lateral rooms at the both sides can be identified. A rectangular door opening is made under the cornice of the front hall, while the lateral rooms and the rear are inaccessible. The rear beams, square-columns and windows are symmetrical to those of the front hall. It was excavated from the construction site of No. 3 Middle School of Gaochun County, Jiangsu Province.

Preserved in Gaochun Museum

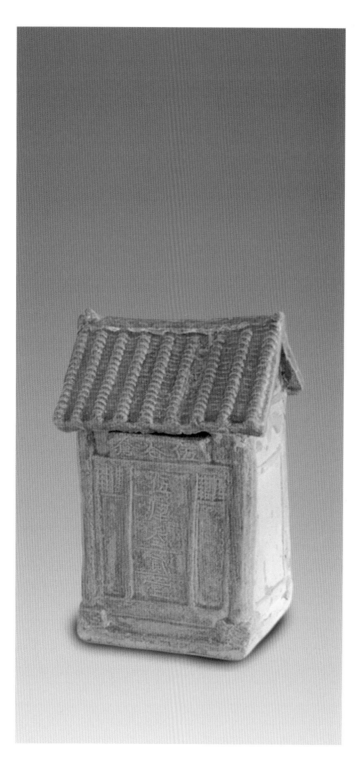

青釉五谷仓

宋

瓷质

面宽 14.1 厘米，进深 12.4 厘米，高 20 厘米

Celadon Granary

Song Dynasty

Porcelain

Facet Width 14.1 cm/ Depth 12.4 cm/

Height 20 cm

通体施青黄釉，山形顶，屋顶正面阴砥九行，阳砥八行，门柜、门槛、窗棂清晰，仓分五层，从上到下印有阳文"伍""肆""叁""贰""壹"字，门楣上部的门额，从右至左印有阳文"伍谷仓"三字。建筑结构节点清晰，比例协调，此类谷仓较少见。

章立平藏

The entire granary is glazed greenish yellow with a gable roof, on the front wall of which are nine rows of convex tiles and eight rows of concave tiles. The door cabinet, the threshold and the window lattice can be clearly identified. This five-storey granary carries incised inscription of five Chinese numerals from the top to bottom floor, "five", "four", "three", "two", "one", respectively. Three characters "Wu Gu Cang" (Five Grains Granary) are cut in relief from right to the left on the forehead of the door lintel. The building has clear structure joints and is arranged in proper proportion, which is rarely found.

Collected by Zhang Liping

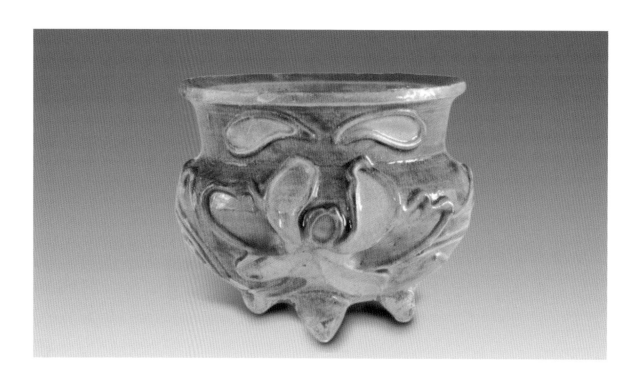

三彩印花三足炉

辽

瓷质

口径 8.5 厘米，高 7 厘米

折沿，短颈，鼓腹，三足稍外折。口沿施酱黄釉，腹间印花分别施酱黄、绿、黄绿彩釉。

罗浩权藏

Three-coloured Tripod Burner with Impressed Floral Design

Liao Dynasty

Porcelain

Mouth Diameter 8.5 cm/ Height 7 cm

The burner is designed with an everted rim, a short neck, a globular body, and three legs turning outwards slightly. The rim is glazed brownish yellow, while the impressed floral motifs on the abdomen are glazed brownish yellow, green, and yellowish green respectively.

Collected by Luo Haoquan

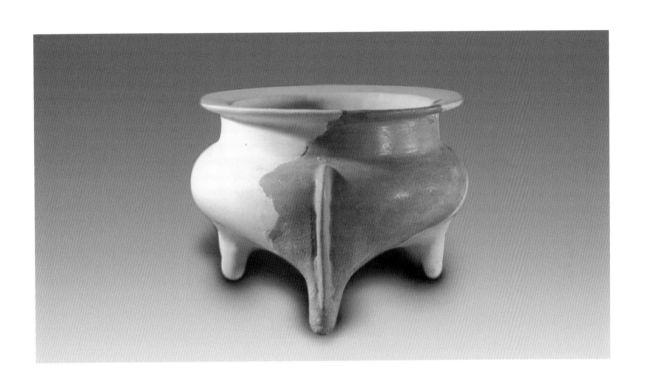

鬲式炉

南宋

瓷质

口径 13.8 厘米，通高 11.6 厘米

米黄夹灰青色釉，底足垫烧。

杭州市园林文物局藏

Cauldron Stove

Southern Song Dynasty

Porcelain

Mouth Diameter 13.8 cm/ Height 11.6 cm

This stove is glazed beige and greyish green, with the fire placed underneath the bottom of the stove. Preserved in the Hangzhou Municipal Bureau of Landscape and Cultural Relics

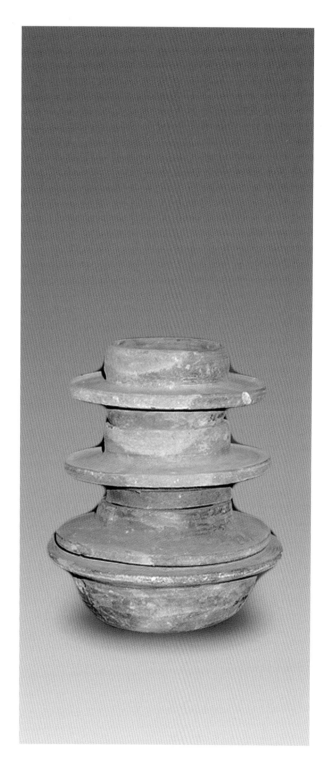

陶锅带笼

元

灰陶质

口径 8.5 厘米，底径 10 厘米，通高 21 厘米，重 1700 克

陶锅一个，蒸笼三层三件，组合成一套炊具。明器，炊具。完整无损。陕西省西安市征集。

陕西医史博物馆藏

Pottery Pot with Steamer

Yuan Dynasty

Grey Pottery

Mouth Diameter 8.5 cm/ Bottom Diameter 10 cm/ Height 21 cm/ Weight 1,700 g

The whole set of cookers are made up of a pottery pot and three tiers of steamers. It is a well-preserved funeral object, and it was collected from Xi'an, Shaanxi Province.

Preserved in Shaanxi Museum of Medical History

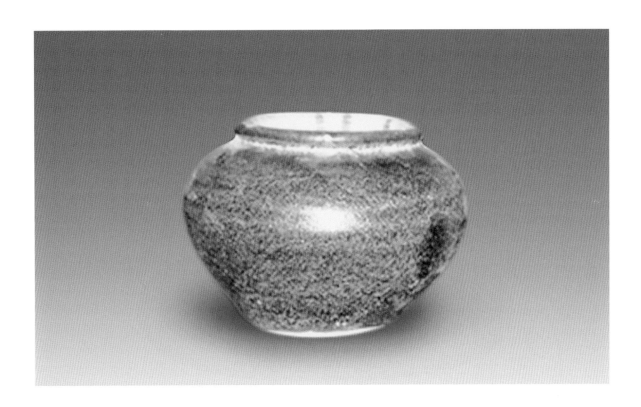

黑釉小瓷罐

宋

瓷质

口径 8 厘米，底径 6 厘米，通高 8.5 厘米，重 350 克

圆唇，鼓腹，圈足，口沿及底无釉。盛贮器。基本完整有裂印。陕西省咸阳市秦都区征集。

陕西医史博物馆藏

Small Black-glazed Porcelain Jar

Song Dynasty

Porcelain

Mouth Diameter 8 cm/ Bottom Diameter 6 cm/ Height 8.5 cm/ Weight 350 g

The jar has a circular rim, a globular abdomen, and a ring foot with the mouth rim and bottom unglazed. It was used as a container, and it is still in good shape except for a few cracks. It was collected from Qindu District of Xianyang, Shaanxi Province. Preserved in Shaanxi Museum of Medical History

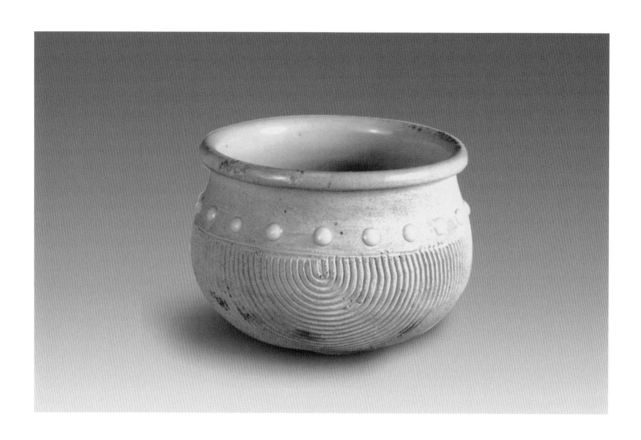

白釉柳斗形罐

北宋

瓷质

口径 10 厘米，底径 2.7 厘米，高 7 厘米

White-glazed Jar with Wicker Patterns

Northern Song Dynasty

Porcelain

Mouth Diameter 10 cm/ Bottom Diameter 2.7 cm/ Height 7 cm

圆唇口，微外卷，束颈，弧腹下收，环底内凹，内壁及唇口满施乳白釉，钵外壁均为素胎，颈部一周饰二十个乳丁纹，并点施白釉，乳丁纹凸起。制作规范，腹部满饰斗纹，柳斗纹雕刻画较深，排列整齐，线条流畅、细腻，立体感强。2000年宝应北宋墓群出土。

宝应博物馆藏

The jar has a slightly everted circular rim, a contracted neck, and a round abdomen narrowing down to an inward concaved bottom. The interior wall and the rim are fully coated with cream glaze, while the exterior wall is unglazed. The neck is decorated with twenty white-glazed nipple patterns in high relief, the production of which is well regulated. The abdomen is fully decorated with whorl patterns which are deeply incised and orderly arranged with smooth fine lines, creating a three-dimensional sense. The jar was excavated from the tombs of the Northern Song Dynasty in Baoying County, Jiangsu Province, in the year 2000.

Preserved in Baoying Museum

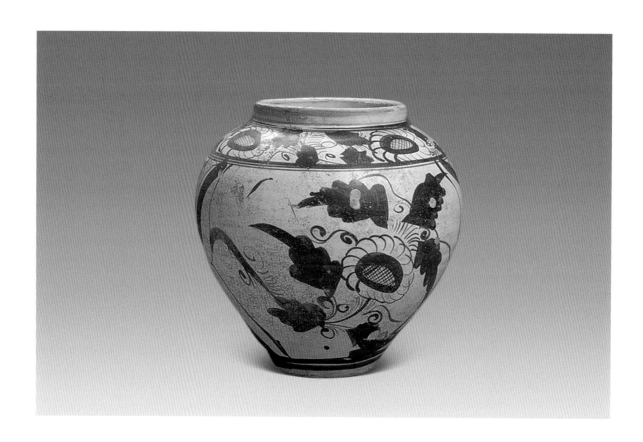

磁州窑菊花纹瓷罐

南宋

瓷质

口径 16.9 厘米，底径 11.2 厘米，高 27.3 厘米

Porcelain Jar with Chrysanthemum Motifs, Cizhou Kiln Ware

Southern Song Dynasty

Porcelain

Mouth Diameter 16.9 cm/ Bottom Diameter 11.2 cm/ Height 27.3 cm

唇口，短直颈，溜肩，鼓腹，圈足。胎呈灰白色，敷化妆土，釉色白中微黄，器身用黑彩满绘；肩部绘缠枝菊，腹部主题纹样为二开光，内绘折枝菊花。此器用毛笔绘画，显得潇洒自如，新颖活泼，具有水墨韵味。白釉下黑彩是磁州窑瓷器的主要装饰方法，其画面装饰具有简练、明快、清新、俊逸的特点，充满了自然美，予人以艺术的享受。江宁陆郎出土。

南京博物院藏

The Jar has a rimmed mouth, a short and straight neck, a sloping shoulder, a swelling belly and a ring foot. The paste of the jar is in pale grey and is covered with engobe. The jar is coated with yellowish white glaze and adorned with black motifs. On the shoulder are interlocking chrysanthemums, while the theme patterns on the belly are chrysanthemum branches in two reserved panels. The brushwork, though casual in style, is elegant, novel and vivid, reflecting the charm of the Chinese ink painting. Black motifs on a white ground are the main technique of decoration of Cizhou kiln ware. Simple and succinct, lucid and lively, neat and exquisite, such decoration is full of natural beauty and brings people artistic enjoyment. The jar was unearthed from Lulang County of Jiangning District of Nanjing, Jiangsu Province.

Preserved in Nanjing Museum

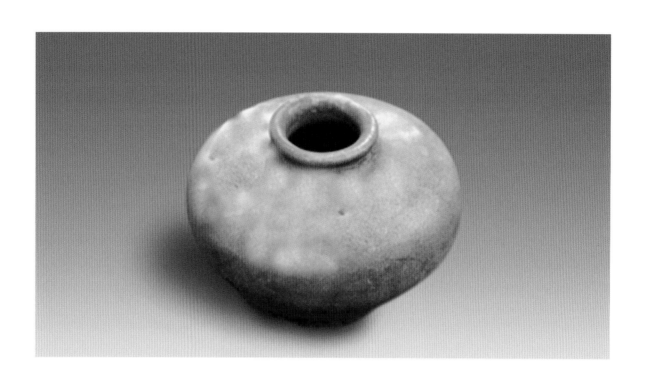

龙泉窑小口罐

宋

瓷质

口外径 4.3 厘米，腹径 11.5 厘米，底径 3.6 厘米，
通高 7.9 厘米，腹深 7.2 厘米

小口，鼓腹，腹上丰下收，平底。盛液体容器。

广东中医药博物馆藏

Small-mouthed Jar, Longquan Kiln Ware

Song Dynasty

Porcelain

Mouth Outer Diameter 4.3 cm/ Belly Diameter
11.5 cm/ Bottom Diameter 3.6 cm/ Height 7.9 cm/
Depth 7.2 cm

The small-mouthed jar has a swelling belly
narrowing down to the flat bottom. It was utilized
as a liquid container.

Preserved in Guangdong Chinese Medicine Museum

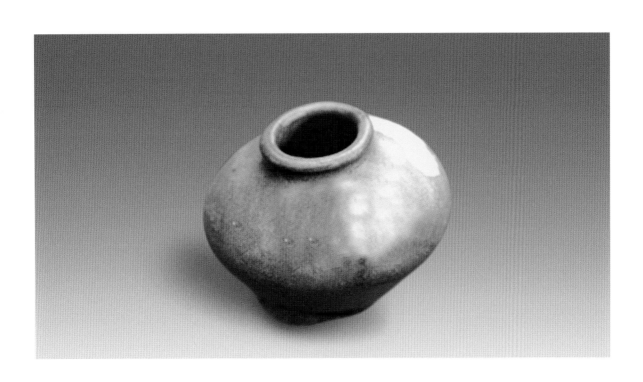

瓷罐

宋

瓷质

口外径 3.4 厘米，腹径 7.5 厘米，底径 3.1 厘米，

通高 5.7 厘米，腹深 4.5 厘米

圆口，鼓腹，平底。盛液体容器。

广东中医药博物馆藏

Porcelain Jar

Song Dynasty

Porcelain

Mouth Outer Diameter 3.4 cm/ Belly Diameter

7.5 cm/ Bottom Diameter 3.1 cm/ Height 5.7 cm/

Depth 4.5 cm

The jar has a circular mouth, a swelling abdomen and

a flat bottom. It was utilized as a liquid container.

Preserved in Guangdong Chinese Medicine Museum

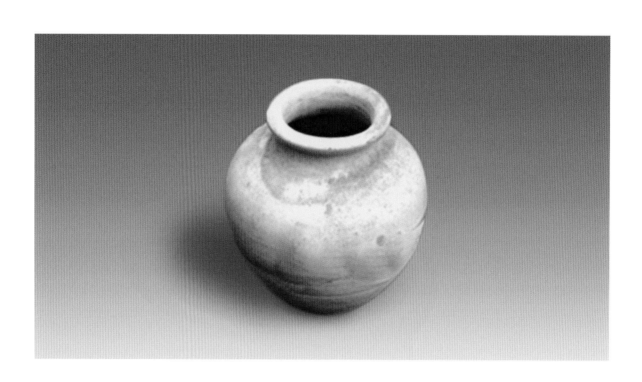

陶罐

宋

陶质

口外径 5.8 厘米，腹径 9.7 厘米，底径 4.3 厘米，

通高 10.4 厘米，腹深 9.2 厘米

圆口，短颈，鼓腹，腹下内收，平底。盛物容器。

广东中医药博物馆藏

Pottery Jar

Song Dynasty

Pottery

Mouth Outer Diameter 5.8 cm/ Belly Diameter 9.7 cm/ Bottom Diameter 4.3 cm/ Height 10.4 cm/ Depth 9.2 cm

The jar has a circular mouth, a short neck, a swelling abdomen narrowing down to the flat bottom. It was utilized as a container.

Preserved in Guangdong Chinese Medicine Museum

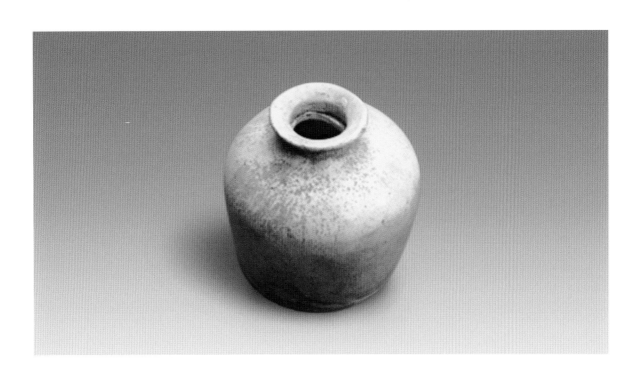

陶罐

宋

陶质

口外径 4.1 厘米，腹径 8.7 厘米，底径 7.8 厘米，
通高 8.6 厘米，腹深 8.2 厘米

敞口，平底。盛液体容器。

广东中医药博物馆藏

Pottery Jar

Song Dynasty

Pottery

Mouth Outer Diameter 4.1 cm/ Belly Diameter
8.7 cm/ Bottom Diameter 7.8 cm/ Height 8.6 cm/
Depth 8.2 cm

The jar with a flared mouth and a flat bottom was
utilized as a liquid container.

Preserved in Guangdong Chinese Medicine Museum

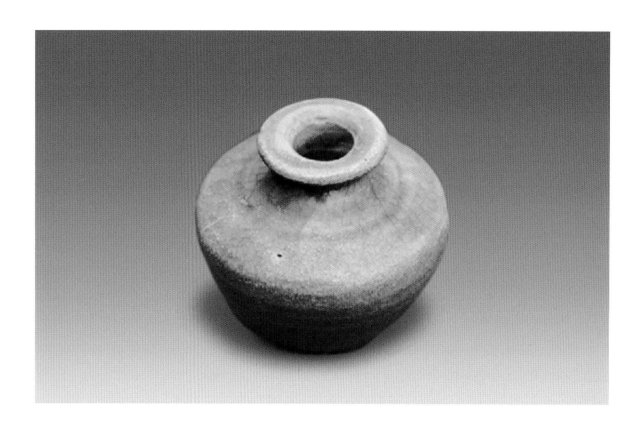

龙泉窑瓷罐

宋

瓷质

口外径 3.75 厘米，腹径 7.6 厘米，底径 4.1 厘米，通高 6.6 厘米，腹深 5.4 厘米，重 169 克

Porcelain Jar, Longquan Kiln Ware

Song Dynasty

Porcelain

Mouth Outer Diameter 3.75 cm/ Belly Diameter 7.6 cm/ Bottom Diameter 4.1 cm/ Height 6.6 cm/ Depth 5.4 cm/ Weight 169 g

盘口，束颈，鼓腹，腹上丰下收，平底。盛细碎物品或液体容器。

广东中医药博物馆藏

The jar has a dish-shaped mouth, a contracted neck, a globular belly narrowing down to a flat bottom. It was used for holding small items or liquid.

Preserved in Guangdong Chinese Medicine Museum

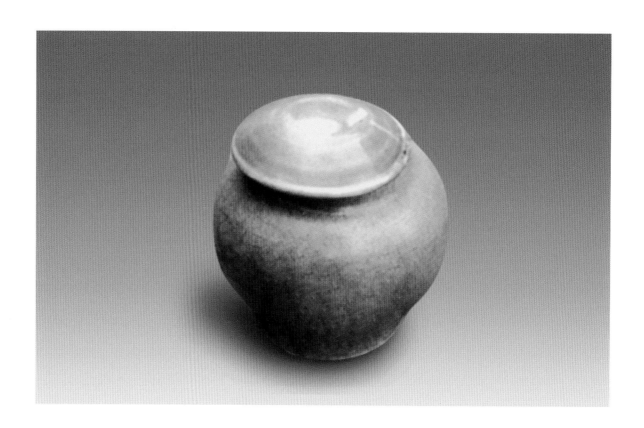

龙泉窑瓷罐

宋

瓷质

口外径 4.7 厘米，腹径 7.2 厘米，底径 4.8 厘米，通高 6.2 厘米，带盖高 7.7 厘米，腹深 4.9 厘米

Porcelain Jar, Longquan Kiln Ware

Song Dynasty

Porcelain

Mouth Outer Diameter 4.7 cm/ Belly Diameter 7.2 cm/ Bottom Diameter 4.8 cm/ Height 6.2 cm/ Height (including the lid) 7.7 cm/ Depth 4.9 cm

直口，鼓腹，腹下部内收，腹面有瓜裂纹路，圈足，带盖。盛物容器。

广东中医药博物馆藏

The porcelain jar has a straight mouth, a lid and a swelling belly narrowing down to the ring foot. On the surface of the abdomen are netted melon patterns. It was used as a container.

Preserved in Guangdong Chinese Medicine Museum

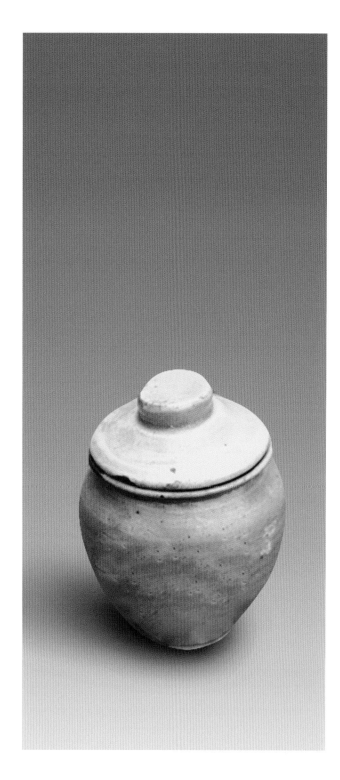

青瓷罐

宋

瓷质

口外径 6.7 厘米，腹径 7.6 厘米，底径 4.1 厘米，

通高 9.7 厘米，腹深 6.4 厘米

Celadon Jar

Song Dynasty

Porcelain

Mouth Outer Diameter 6.7 cm/ Belly Diameter

7.6 cm/ Bottom Diameter 4.1 cm/ Height 9.7 cm/

Depth 6.4 cm

敞口，鼓腹，腹下部内收，平底。盛细碎物
品容器。

广东中医药博物馆藏

The jar has a flared mouth and a swelling belly
narrowing down to the flat bottom. It was used
for holding small items.

Preserved in Guangdong Chinese Medicine
Museum

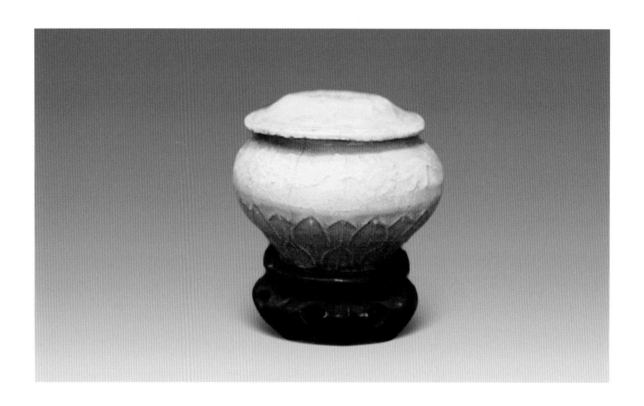

影青窑盖罐

宋

瓷质

口外径 5.8 厘米，腹径 7.7 厘米，底径 4.2 厘米，高 5 厘米，带盖高 6.1 厘米，腹深 4.6 厘米，重 100 克

Misty Blue Lidded Jar

Song Dynasty

Porcelain

Mouth Outer Diameter 5.8 cm/ Belly Diameter 7.7 cm/ Bottom Diameter 4.2 cm/ Height 5 cm/ Height (including the lid) 6.1 cm/ Belly Depth 4.6 cm/ Weight 100 g

罐平口，鼓腹，平底，带底座，带盖，盖似莲叶，

腹上部饰小菊花，下部饰植物叶。用于盛物。

广东中医药博物馆藏

This Misty-blue-glazed jar has a pedestal, a lid
resembling a lotus leaf, a flat mouth, a flat foot
and a drum belly with petty chrysanthemum
decorations on the upper part and leaf motifs on
the lower part. It was used as a container.

Preserved in Guangdong Chinese Medicine
Museum

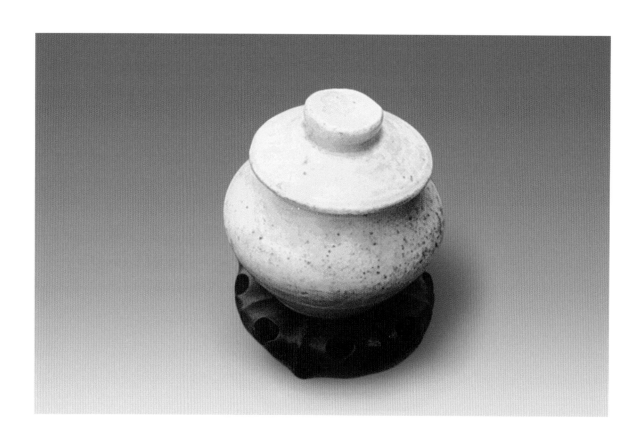

青瓷盖罐

宋

瓷质

口外径 5.6 厘米，腹径 8.2 厘米，底径 4.2 厘米，通高 8 厘米，腹深 4.3 厘米，重 250 克

Lidded Celadon Jar

Song Dynasty

Porcelain

Mouth Outer Diameter 5.6 cm/ Belly Diameter 8.2 cm/ Bottom Diameter 4.2 cm/ Height 8 cm/ Belly Depth 4.3 cm/ Weight 250 g

带盖，盖顶有一圆形平顶纽，鼓腹，平底。用于盛物。

广东中医药博物馆藏

This celadon jar has a lid with a round flat knob on its top, a drum belly and a flat foot. It served as a container.

Preserved in Guangdong Chinese Medicine Museum

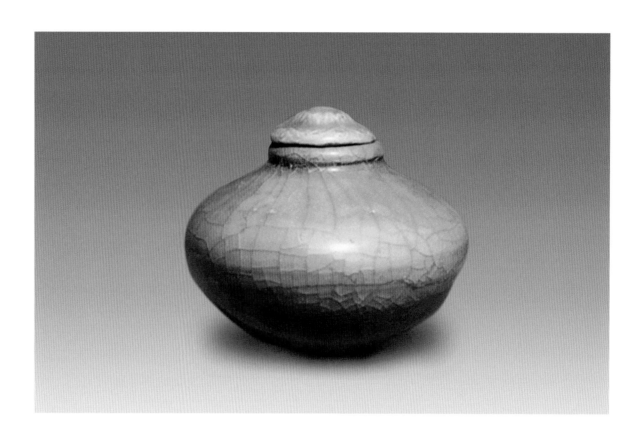

龙泉窑小罐

宋

瓷质

口外径 3.8 厘米，腹径 9.2 厘米，底径 3.2 厘米，带盖高 7.8 厘米，腹深 6 厘米，重 280 克

Small Jar, Longquan Kiln Ware

Song Dynasty

Porcelain

Mouth Outer Diameter 3.8 cm/ Belly Diameter 9.2 cm/ Bottom Diameter 3.2 cm/ Height (including the lid) 7.8 cm/ Belly Depth 6 cm/ Weight 280 g

鼓腹，腹面有瓜裂纹路，平底，带盖，并且
盖边呈莲花状。用于盛物。

广东中医药博物馆藏

This jar has a drum belly with netted melon crackles on the surface, a flat foot and a lid with a lotus-shaped rim. It was used as a container.
Preserved in Guangdong Chinese Medicine Museum

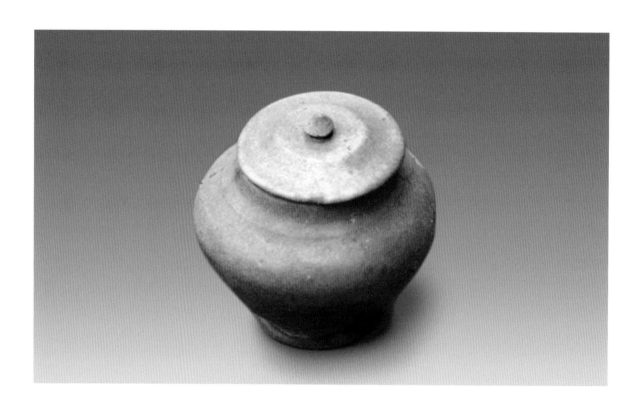

龙泉窑盖罐

宋

瓷质

口外径 6.3 厘米，腹径 10.6 厘米，底径 5.8 厘米，高 9.4 厘米，带盖高 10.9 厘米，腹深 6.6 厘米。重 421 克

Lidded Jar, Longquan Kiln Ware

Song Dynasty

Porcelain

Mouth Outer Diameter 6.3 cm/ Belly Diameter 10.6 cm/ Bottom Diameter 5.8 cm/ Height 9.4 cm/ Height (including the lid) 10.9 cm/ Belly Depth 6.6 cm/ Weight 421 g

鼓腹，腹面有瓜裂纹，平底，底边外延，带盖，盖顶一圆形顶钮。盛物容器。

广东中医药博物馆藏

This jar is made in the design of a drum belly with netted melon crackles on the surface, a flat foot extending outwards, and a lid with a round flat knob on its top. It served as a container.

Preserved in Guangdong Chinese Medicine Museum

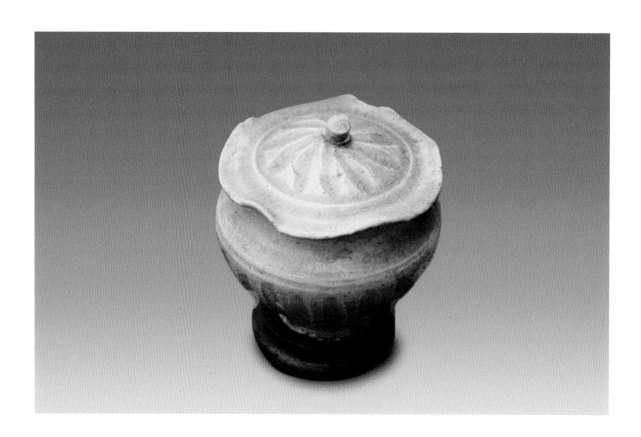

龙泉窑荷叶边盖罐

宋

瓷质

口外径 6.68 厘米，底径 4 厘米，高 6.1 厘米，带盖高 8.2 厘米，腹深 4.6 厘米，重 202 克

Jar with a Lotus-leaf-shaped Lid, Longquan Kiln Ware

Song Dynasty

Porcelain

Mouth Outer Diameter 6.68 cm/ Bottom Diameter 4 cm/ Height 6.1 cm/ Height (including the lid) 8.2 cm/ Belly Depth 4.6 cm/ Weight 202 g

带盖，盖似荷叶，鼓腹，腹面刻有竖向宽条纹，

并有瓜裂纹路，小圈足。用于盛细小物品。

广东中医药博物馆藏

This jar has a lotus leaf-shaped lid, a drum belly incised with broad and vertical stripes and netted melon crackles on the exterior wall, and a small ring foot. It served as a container for holding small items.

Preserved in Guangdong Chinese Medicine Museum

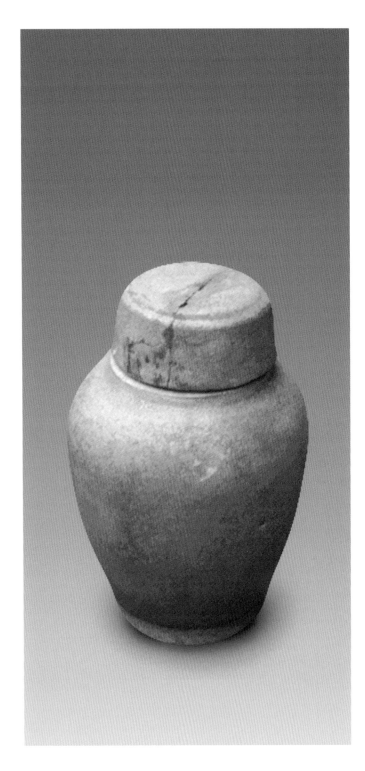

釉陶盖罐

宋

陶质

口外径 5.1 厘米，腹径 11.1 厘米，底径 7.1 厘米，带盖高 16.1 厘米，腹深 13.8 厘米，重 728 克

Glazed Pottery Lidded Jar

Song Dynasty

Pottery

Mouth Outer Diameter 5.1 cm/ Belly Diameter 11.1 cm/ Bottom Diameter 7.1 cm/ Height (including the cover) 16.1 cm/ Belly Depth 13.8 cm/ Weight 728 g

直口，带盖，盖顶平，盖边向下卷，含住罐口，盖与罐口相合，圆肩，肩丰，下收，平底，底边外展。用于盛物。

广东中医药博物馆藏

This jar has a straight mouth, round and plump shoulders, a belly narrowing down to the flat but flared foot. The flat-topped jar lid, with the exterior rim rolling down, exactly fits the mouth of the jar. It served as a container.

Preserved in Guangdong Chinese Medicine Museum

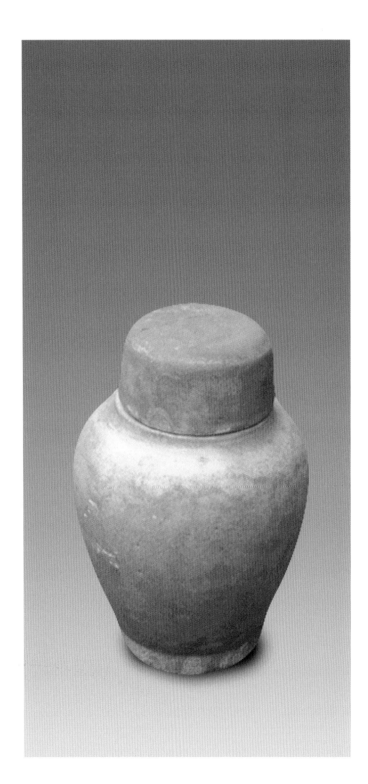

釉陶盖罐

宋

陶质

口外径 5.5 厘米，腹径 11.3 厘米，底径 7.35 厘米，带盖高 16.3 厘米，腹深 13.3 厘米，重 883 克

Glazed Pottery Lidded Jar

Song Dynasty

Pottery

Mouth Outer Diameter 5.5 cm/ Belly Diameter 11.3 cm/ Bottom Diameter 7.35 cm/ Height (including the lid) 16.3 cm/ Belly Depth 13.3 cm/ Weight 883 g

直口，带盖，盖顶平，盖边向下卷，含住罐口，圆肩，肩丰，下收，圈足。用于盛物。

广东中医药博物馆藏

This jar has a straight mouth, round and plump shoulders, a belly narrowing down to the ring foot. It has a flat lid with the edge rolling downward and closing around the mouth of the jar. It was used as a container.

Preserved in Guangdong Chinese Medicine Museum

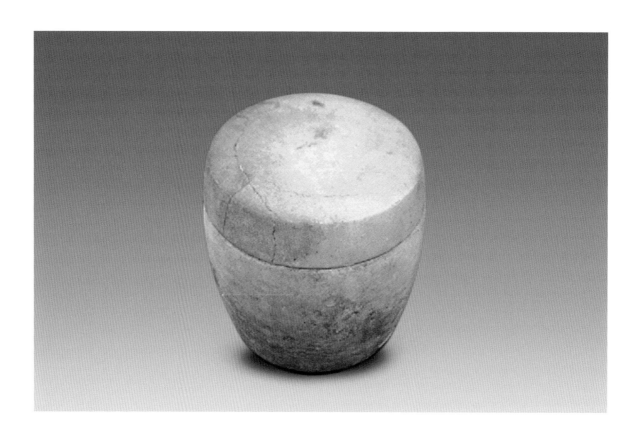

青釉盖罐

宋

陶质

口外径 14.6 厘米，腹径 16.4 厘米，底径 12 厘米，通高 16.5 厘米，腹深 12 厘米，重 1500 克

Celadon Pottery Jar with Lid

Song Dynasty

Pottery

Mouth Outer Diameter 14.6 cm/ Belly Diameter 16.4 cm/ Bottom Diameter 12 cm/ Height 16.5 cm/ Belly Depth 12 cm/ Weight 1,500 g

大口，秃宝字盖，盖与罐相合，罐腹丰，平底。
储物容器。

广东中医药博物馆藏

This jar is designed with a big mouth, a bald lid
fitting on the jar, a swelling belly and a flat foot.
It was used as a storage container.

Preserved in Guangdong Chinese Medicine
Museum

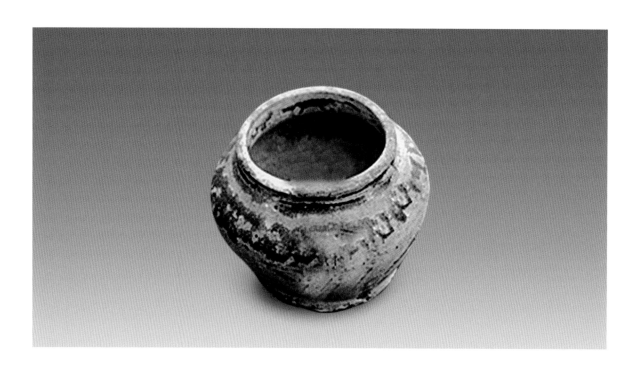

釉陶小罐

宋

陶质

口外径 6.7 厘米，腹径 9.7 厘米，底径 7 厘米，通高 7 厘米，腹深 7.1 厘米

Small Glazed Pottery Jar

Song Dynasty

Pottery

Mouth Outer Diameter 6.7 cm/ Belly Diameter 9.7 cm/ Bottom Diameter 7 cm/ Height 7 cm/ Belly Depth 7.1 cm

大口，口沿圆润，鼓腹，腹上丰下收，平底。
盛物容器。

广东中医药博物馆藏

This jar has a big mouth with rounded and smooth rim, a swelling belly, narrowing down to the flat foot. It was utilized as a storage container.

Preserved in Guangdong Chinese Medicine Museum

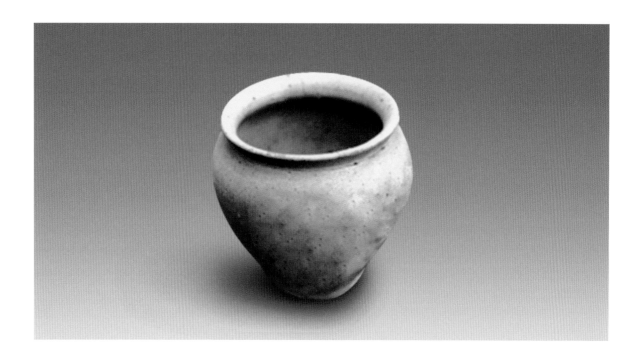

青瓷小罐

宋

瓷质

口外径 7 厘米，腹径 8.1 厘米，底径 4.1 厘米，通高 7.4 厘米，腹深 6.6 厘米

Small Celadon Porcelain Jar

Song Dynasty

Porcelain

Mouth Outer Diameter 7 cm/ Belly Diameter 8.1 cm/ Bottom Diameter 4.1 cm/ Height 7.4 cm/ Belly Depth 6.6 cm

大敞口，鼓腹，腹上丰下收，平底。盛物容器。

广东中医药博物馆藏

This small celadon jar is characterized with a big open mouth and a bulgy belly narrowing down to the flat foot. It was utilized as a storage container.

Preserved in Guangdong Chinese Medicine Museum

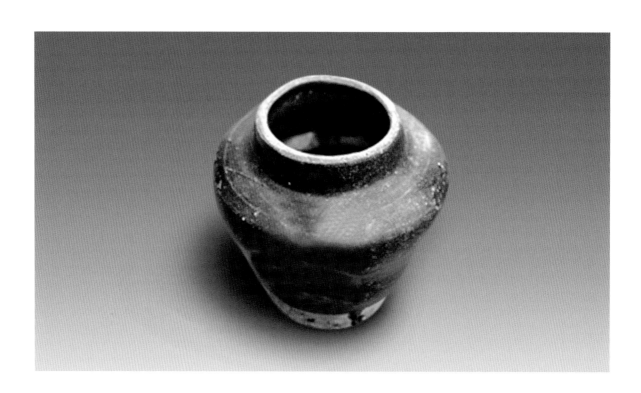

黑釉瓷罐

宋

瓷质

口外径 5.5 厘米，腹径 9.5 厘米，底径 5 厘米，

通高 8.9 厘米，腹深 7 厘米

平口，丰肩，肩下渐收，圈足。盛物容器。

广东中医药博物馆藏

Black-glazed Porcelain Jar

Song Dynasty

Porcelain

Mouth Outer Diameter 5.5 cm/ Belly Diameter 9.5 cm/ Bottom Diameter 5 cm/ Height 8.9 cm/ Belly Depth 7 cm

This jar with a flat mouth, plump shoulders, and a ring foot was used as a storage container.

Preserved in Guangdong Chinese Medicine Museum

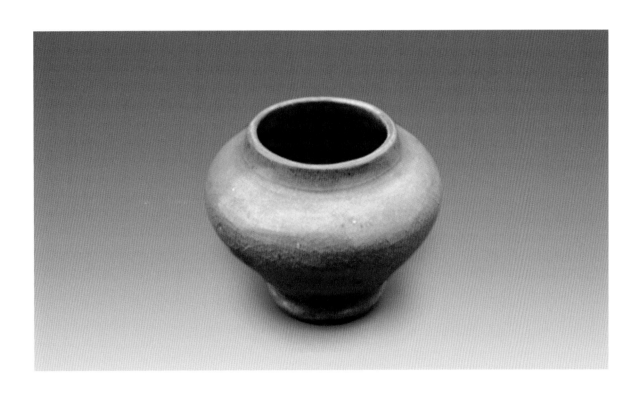

龙泉窑瓷罐

宋

瓷质

口外径 6.1 厘米，腹径 10.2 厘米，底径 5.4 厘米，

通高 7.9 厘米，腹深 6.2 厘米，重 303 克

平口，鼓腹，腹上丰下收，圈足。盛物容器。

广东中医药博物馆藏

Porcelain Jar, Longquan Kiln Ware

Song Dynasty

Porcelain

Mouth Outer Diameter 6.1 cm/ Belly Diameter 10.2 cm/ Bottom Diameter 5.4 cm/ Height 7.9 cm/ Belly Depth 6.2 cm/ Weight 303 g

This jar with a flat mouth and a swelling belly narrowing down to the ring foot was a storage container.

Preserved in Guangdong Chinese Medicine Museum

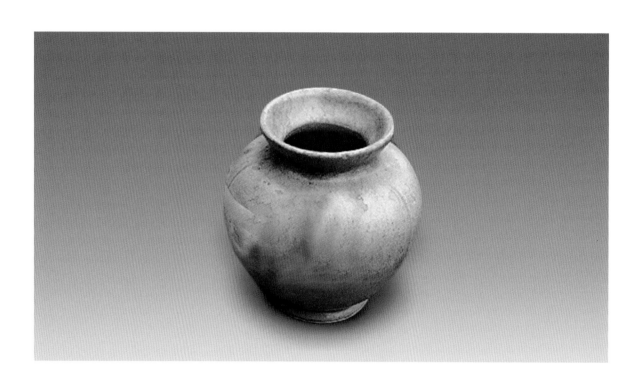

瓜棱陶罐

宋

陶质

口外径 5.7 厘米，腹径 8.9 厘米，底径 4.9 厘米，

通高 8.9 厘米，腹深 8.3 厘米，重 201 克

敞口，鼓腹，腹上丰下收，小圈足。盛细碎物。

广东中医药博物馆藏

Pottery Jar in the Shape of Ribbed Melon

Song Dynasty

Pottery

Mouth Outer Diameter 5.7 cm/ Belly Diameter 8.9 cm/ Bottom Diameter 4.9 cm/ Height 8.9 cm/ Belly Depth 8.3 cm/ Weight 201 g

This jar has an open mouth and a globular belly narrowing down to a small ring foot. It was used as a container for storing small items.

Preserved in Guangdong Chinese Medicine Museum

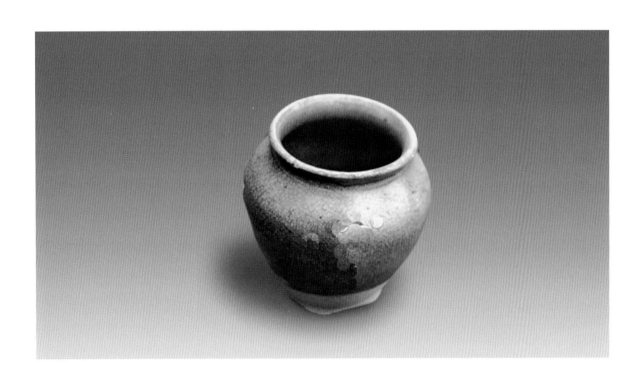

龙泉窑罐

宋

瓷质

口外径 7.1 厘米，腹径 9.6 厘米，底径 6 厘米，

通高 9.6 厘米，腹深 8 厘米

大口，鼓腹，腹下部内收，腹面有瓜裂纹，圈足。

盛物容器。

广东中医药博物馆藏

Jar, Longquan Kiln Ware

Song Dynasty

Porcelain

Mouth Outer Diameter 7.1 cm/ Belly Diameter 9.6 cm/

Bottom Diameter 6 cm/ Height 9.6 cm/ Belly Depth

8 cm

This jar is characterized by a big mouth, a tapered

drum belly with netted melon crackles on the

surface, and a ring foot. It was used as a container.

Preserved in Guangdong Chinese Medicine Museum

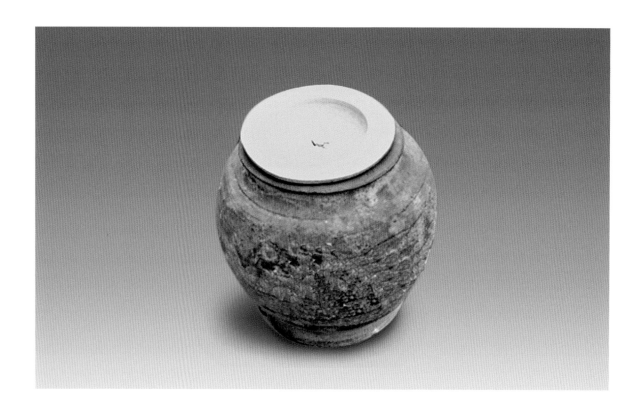

陶罐

宋

陶质

口外径 9.2 厘米，腹径 13.6 厘米，底径 9.3 厘米，通高 11.6 厘米，腹深 10.4 厘米

Pottery Jar

Song Dynasty

Pottery

Mouth Outer Diameter 9.2 cm/ Belly Diameter 13.6 cm/ Bottom Diameter 9.3 cm/ Height 11.6 cm/ Belly Depth 10.4 cm

带盖，盖顶心有裂纹，大口，口沿外侈，鼓腹，腹部有弦棱纹，平底，口沿及底边有破损。盛物容器。

广东中医药博物馆藏

This jar has a cover with a crack at the top centre, a big mouth with a flared rim, a swelling belly decorated with raised bowstring patterns, and a flat foot. Both the mouth rim and the bottom edge are damaged. It was used as a container.

Preserved in Guangdong Chinese Medicine Museum

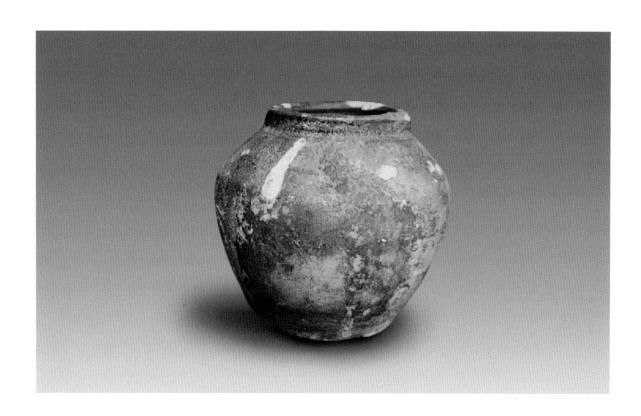

釉陶罐

宋

陶质

口外径 11.2 厘米，腹径 18.5 厘米，底径 11.8 厘米，通高 16.3 厘米，腹深 15.5 厘米，重 1250 克

Glazed Pottery Jar

Song Dynasty

Pottery

Mouth Outer Diameter 11.2 cm/ Belly Diameter 18.5 cm/ Bottom Diameter 11.8 cm/ Height 16.3 cm/ Belly Depth 15.5 cm/ Weight 1,250 g

短颈，口唇外侈，削肩，肩丰下收，平底。

盛物容器。

广东中医药博物馆藏

The jar has a short neck, a wide mouth with a flared rim, a sloping and plump shoulder which narrows down to a flat foot. It was utilized as a container.

Preserved in Guangdong Chinese Medicine Museum

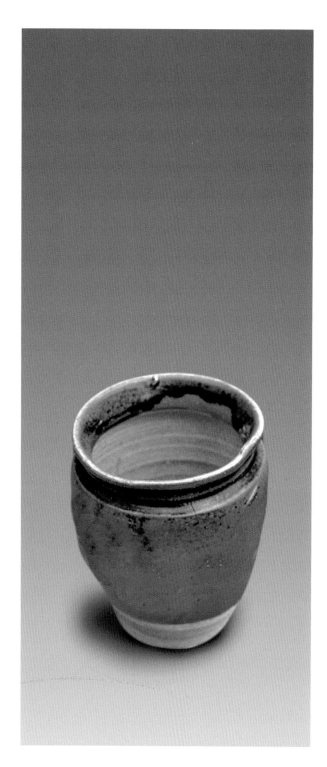

陶罐

宋

陶质

口外径 7.5 厘米，腹径 8.1 厘米，底径 5.1 厘米，
通高 9.9 厘米，腹深 8.6 厘米

Pottery Jar

Song Dynasty

Pottery

Mouth Outer Diameter 7.5 cm/ Belly Diameter
8.1 cm/ Bottom Diameter 5.1 cm/ Height 9.9 cm/
Belly Depth 8.6 cm

大敞口，小圈足，内胎有弦纹。盛物容器。

广东中医药博物馆藏

This jar has a big flared mouth and a small ring foot. The interior wall of the body is decorated with string patterns. It was utilized as a container.

Preserved in Guangdong Chinese Medicine Museum

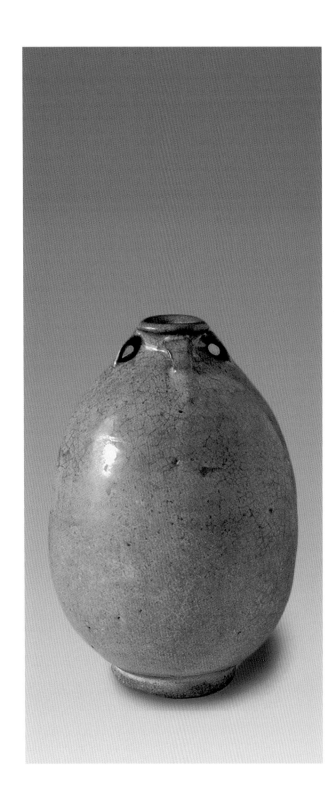

灰白釉四系罐

金

瓷质

口径 5.5 厘米，底径 9.5 厘米，高 25 厘米

Greyish-white-glazed Pot with Four Rings

Jin Dynasty

Porcelain

Mouth Diameter 5.5 cm/ Bottom Diameter

9.5 cm/ Height 25 cm

小口，短颈，丰腹，圈足。口缘至肩部设扁
条状四系。全身施灰白色釉，肥厚莹润，釉
不到足，近脚处和圈足内无釉，露淡淡红色
胎骨，胎质坚细，底足中央呈尖凸状。

周振武藏

The pot has a small mouth, a short neck, a
round belly and a ring foot. Four strip-shaped
rings are attached vertically to the part joining
the mouth-rim and the shoulder. A rich and
creamy greyish-white glaze covers the whole
vessel leaving the foot and the base unglazed,
exposing traces of light red body with hard and
refined texture. The foot is pointed in the centre.
Collected by Zhou Zhenwu

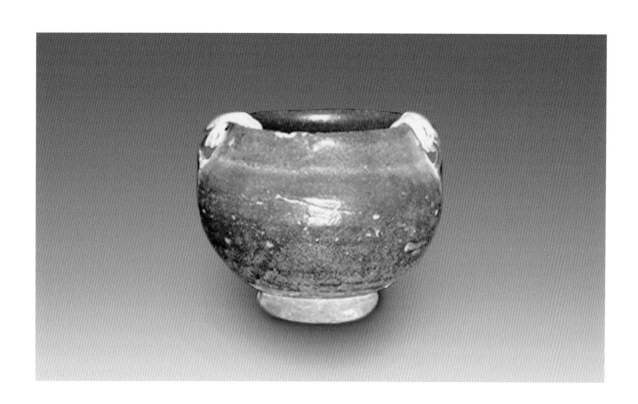

双耳瓷罐

元

瓷质

口径 9 厘米，底径 6 厘米，通高 9.5 厘米，重 400 克

敞口，鼓腹，圈足，肩处有双耳，棕色底无釉。盛贮器。完整无损。

陕西医史博物馆藏

Porcelain Jar with Double Ears

Yuan Dynasty

Porcelain

Mouth Diameter 9 cm/ Bottom Diameter 6 cm/ Height 9.5 cm/ Weight 400 g

This brown-glazed jar is designed with a flared mouth, a swelling belly, a ring foot, and two brown unglazed ears attached to the shoulder. It was used as a storage utensil and is still in good condition.

Preserved in Shaanxi Museum of Medical History

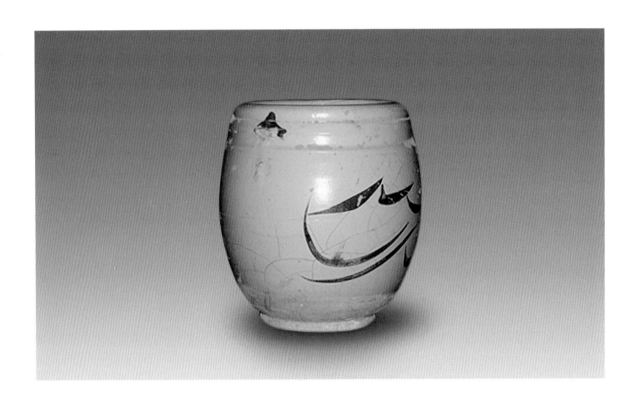

瓷罐

元

瓷质

口径 13 厘米，底径 9 厘米，通高 16.5 厘米，
重 1050 克

圆口，圆腹，双耳白粗瓷，腹上有图案。盛贮器。
一耳残。

陕西医史博物馆藏

Porcelain Jar

Yuan Dynasty

Porcelain

Mouth Diameter 13 cm/ Bottom Diameter 9 cm/
Height 16.5 cm/ Weight 1,050 g

This jar is white coarse porcelain ware with features
of a circular mouth, double ears, and a round belly
decorated with motifs. It was utilized as a storage
utensil with one ear cracked.

Preserved in Shaanxi Museum of Medical History

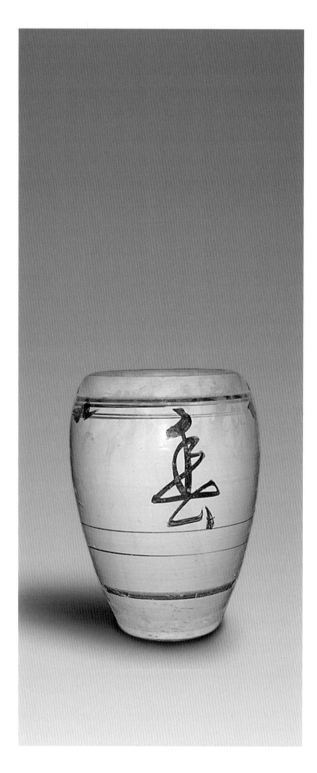

粗瓷罐

元

瓷质

口径 24 厘米，底径 16 厘米，通高 38 厘米，重
4800 克

束口，直腹，圈足，白粗瓷。盛贮器。完整无损。
陕西省西安市征集。

陕西医史博物馆藏

Goarse Porcelain Jar

Yuan Dynasty

Porcelain

Mouth Diameter 24 cm/ Bottom Diameter 16 cm/
Height 38 cm/ Weight 4,800 g

This white coarse porcelain jar has a contracted
mouth, a straight belly and a ring foot. It was used
as a storage utensil and remains intact. It was
collected from the city of Xi'an, Shaanxi Province.

Preserved in Shaanxi Museum of Medical History

粗瓷罐

元

瓷质

口径 24 厘米，底径 16 厘米，通高 38 厘米，重 4800 克

平口，直腹，圈足，白粗瓷。底内有一小孔。盛贮器。陕西省西安市征集。

陕西医史博物馆藏

Goarse Porcelain Jar

Yuan Dynasty

Porcelain

Mouth Diameter 24 cm/ Bottom Diameter 16 cm/ Height 38 cm/ Weight 4,800 g

This white coarse porcelain jar is designed with a flat mouth, a straight abdomen, and a ring foot with a small hole in it. The jar served as a storage utensil. It was collected from the city of Xi'an, Shaanxi Province.

Preserved in Shaanxi Museum of Medical History

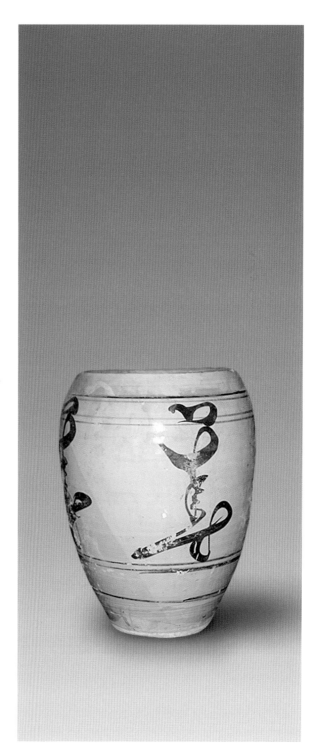

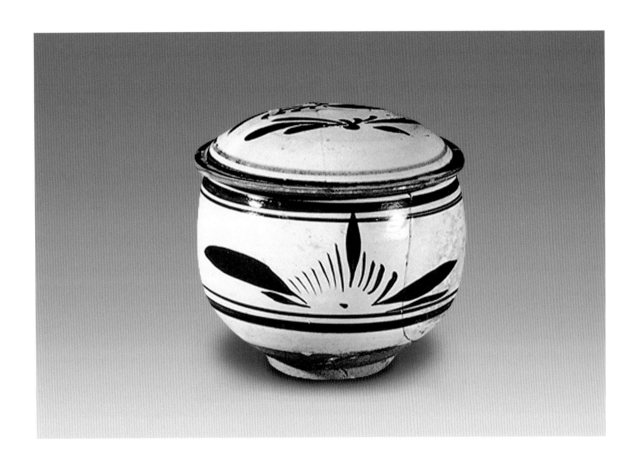

白地黑花瓷罐

元

瓷质

口径 11 厘米，底径 6.4 厘米，通高 11.9 厘米

White Porcelain Jar with Black Floral Designs

Yuan Dynasty

Porcelain

Mouth Diameter 11 cm/ Bottom Diameter 6.4 cm/ Height 11.9 cm

直口微敛，深腹，圈足，白底上绘出两组写
意的蔓草，圆盖上也有同样的构图，色调明快，
笔法流畅。河南省鲁山县段店窑遗址出土。

河南省文物考古研究院藏

This jar has a slightly contracted straight mouth,
a deep belly and a ring foot. Two groups of
freehand creeping weeds are fluently delineated
on a white ground in a bright tone both on
the belly and the surface of the round lid. It
was excavated from Duandian kiln in Lushan
County, Henan Province.

Preserved in Henan Provincial Institute of
Cultural Heritage and Archaeology

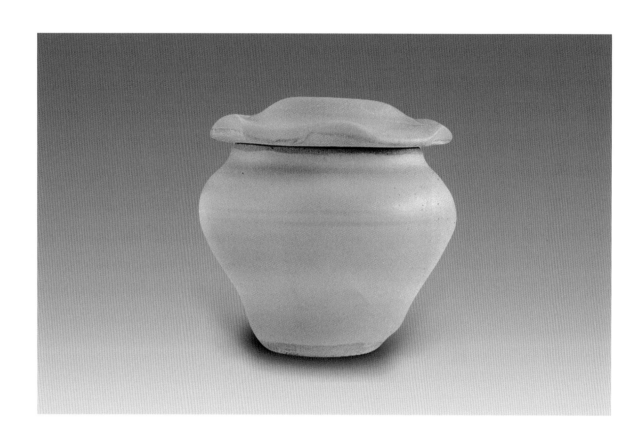

龙泉窑荷叶形盖罐

元

瓷质

口径 5 厘米，高 6.5 厘米

Jar with a Lotus-shaped Lid, Longquan Kiln Ware

Yuan Dynasty

Porcelain

Mouth Diameter 5 cm/ Height 6.5 cm

荷叶形盖，直口，矮颈，丰肩，至足渐收，圈足。
施豆青色釉，甚肥润。

李庆全藏

Glazed pea-green, this jar has a lotus-shaped lid, a straight mouth, a short neck, a plump shoulder which narrows down to the bottom, and a ring foot.

Collected by Li Qingquan

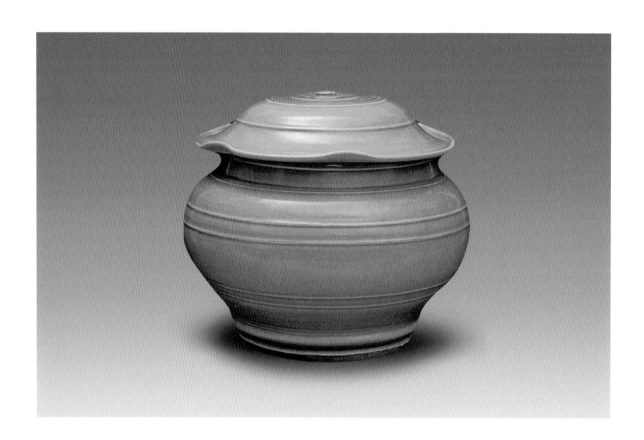

龙泉窑荷叶盖瓷罐

元

瓷质

腹径 30 厘米，通高 24 厘米

Porcelain Jar with a Lotus-shaped Lid, Longquan Kiln Ware

Yuan Dynasty

Porcelain

Belly Diameter 30 cm/ Height 24 cm

直口，鼓腹，圈足。盖呈荷叶形，有钮。器身施青绿色釉，通体饰数道弦纹。釉色晶莹，有玉一般的质感。造型素雅端庄，给人一种恬静的美感。溧水区人民医院建筑工地窖藏出土。

溧水区博物馆藏

This jar is designed with a straight mouth, a drum belly, a ring foot, and a lid in the shape of a lotus leaf with a knob. Covered with a luminous turquoise glaze, the jar is decorated with some string patterns. The colour of the glaze is glittering and translucent like natural jade. The elegant and demure design renders people a sense of beauty and tranquility. It was excavated from the construction site cellar of People's Hospital in Lishui District, Jiangsu Province.

Preserved in Lishui Museum

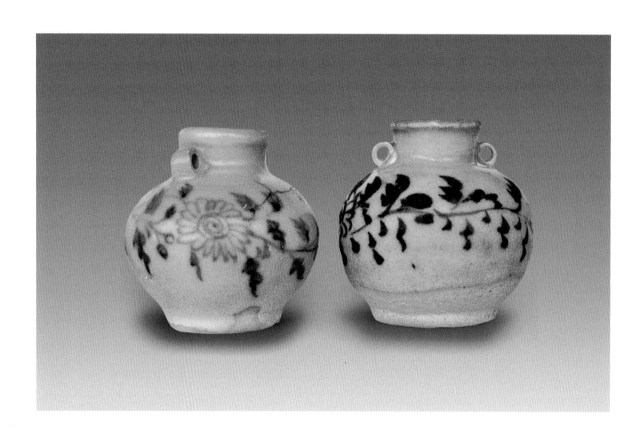

青花缠枝菊纹双耳小罐

元

瓷质

口径 2.7 厘米，底径 3.6 厘米，高 5.5 厘米

Small Double-eared Blue-and-white Jars with Interlocking Chrysanthemum Motifs

Yuan Dynasty

Porcelain

Mouth Diameter 2.7 cm/ Bottom Diameter 3.6 cm/ Height 5.5 cm

唇口，矮颈，鼓腹，圈足，肩至颈部两边置
双环耳。腹间绘缠枝菊花纹一周，青花浓艳。
施白釉不到足，釉色白中泛鸭蛋青色。底无
釉，呈火石红色，杂有褐色斑点，胎质粗糙。
这对元代青花瓷小罐出土于菲律宾。

叶勉均藏

This pair of jars is characterized by a lip-shaped
mouth, a short neck, a swelling belly, a ring
foot, and two ring ears attached symmetrically
to the part between the shoulder and neck.
The abdomen is decorated with a band of
interlocking chrysanthemum motifs in rich
and gaudy blue. The jar, except the foot, is
covered with white glaze with a tinge of duck
egg green. The gritty and unglazed bottom is in
flint red with brown speckles. This pair of small
blue-and-white porcelain jar made in the Yuan
Dynasty was excavated from the Philippines.
Collected by Ye Mianjun

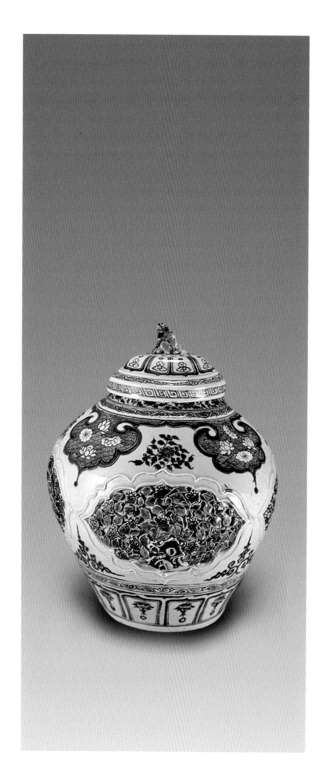

青花开光镂雕红蓝釉花卉大罐

元

瓷质

口径 15.3 厘米，底径 18.7 厘米，高 42.3 厘米

Hollow Engraved Blue-and-white Jug with Reddish Blue-glazed Floral Designs

Yuan Dynasty

Porcelain

Mouth Diameter 15.3 cm/ Bottom Diameter 18.7 cm/

Height 42.3 cm

胎坚硬致密，器表施白釉，釉色细腻润泽。直口，短颈，溜肩，鼓腹下收，平底，覆盆式盖，盖顶堆塑坐狮钮。盖面绘青花莲瓣纹、卷草纹和回纹。颈部绘青花卷草纹和牡丹纹。肩部饰如意形垂云，上有青花绘制的水波纹，用留白手法托出白莲数朵，腹部双勾菱花形串珠开光，内镂雕四季园景，以青花渲染枝叶，釉单红涂绘山石和花朵，色泽浓艳夺目。

河北博物院藏

With a hard and dense texture, this jug is coated with even, transparent, and pure white glaze. It features a straight mouth, a short neck, a sloping shoulder, a drum belly narrowing down to a flat foot and a reversed basin-shaped lid, on which is pasted a knob in the form of a sitting lion. Lotus patterns, floral scrolls and rectangular spirals are painted with cobalt blue on the lid, while floral scrolls and peonies motifs on the neck. The shoulder is decorated with Ruyi-shaped billowing clouds, above which are water ripple patterns in cobalt blue to foil white lotuses through a technique of "blank-leaving". On the abdomen are incised dual sketched strings of beads in water-caltrop flower pattern, within which is hollow engraved a garden view of the four seasons. The branches and leaves are in cobalt blue while rocks and flowers are painted vermeil. The colour of the jug is rich, gaudy and eye-catching.

Preserved in Hebei Museum

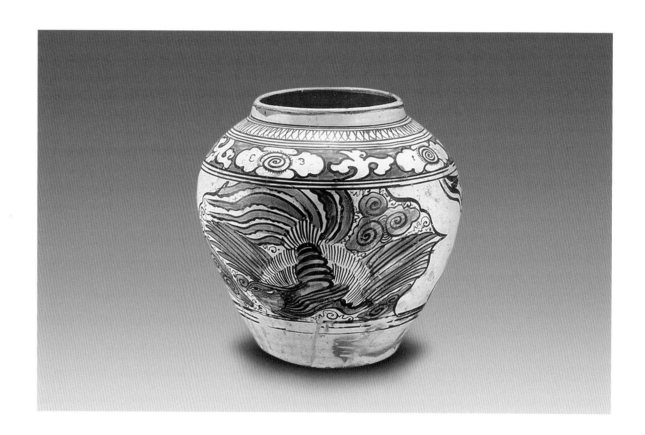

白釉褐彩双凤纹罐

元

瓷质

口径 24 厘米，高 40 厘米

White-glazed Jar with Double Brown Phoenix Designs

Yuan Dynasty

Porcelain

Mouth Diameter 24 cm/ Height 40 cm

直口，溜肩，球形腹，腹下部渐收，玉璧形砂底。器内满施酱釉，器外在白釉上绘褐花。肩部绘凤纹和花叶纹带，腹部两面如意形开光，内绘一展翅飞翔的凤，周围填郑云纹，开光之间饰菊花纹。彩绘用双勾平涂和实笔点画结合起来的笔法，以深褐色渲染。元代磁州窑代表作。1971 年扬州市漕河岸出土。

扬州博物馆藏

This jar has a straight mouth, sloping shoulders, a spheroidal belly narrowing down to a jade disk-shaped buccaro bottom. The interior is fully glazed with caramel, and the exterior is covered with white glaze, on which are painted dark brown flowers. A band of phoenix and leaf patterns is delineated on the shoulders. In both Ruyi-shaped reserved panels on the two opposite sides of the abdomen are painted a flying phoenix surrounded by clouds, and chrysanthemum motifs are painted between the two panels. The motifs are painted with combined techniques of dual sketching and flat colouring, as well as real dots and lines, with dark brown applied to it. This work as a whole exemplifies the craftsmanship of Cizhou Kiln ware in the Yuan dynasty. It was excavated from the bank of Cao River in Yangzhou City, Jiangsu Province, in the year 1971.

Preserved in Yangzhou Museum

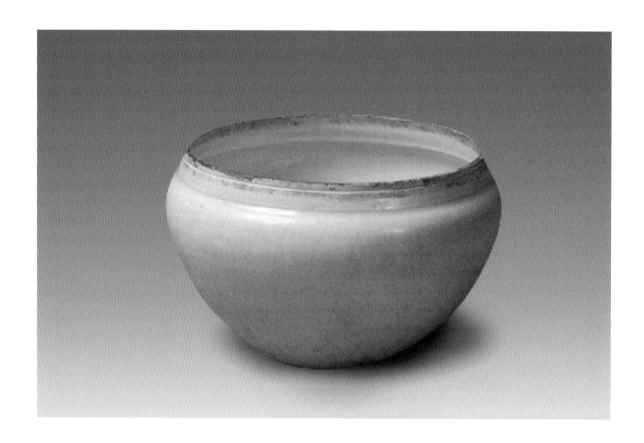

青白瓷汤瓯

北宋

瓷质

口径 11.8 厘米，底径 4.5 厘米，高 8.6 厘米

Greenish-white-glazed Porcelain Soup Bowl

Northern Song Dynasty

Porcelain

Mouth Diameter 11.8 cm/ Bottom Diameter 4.5 cm/ Height 8.6 cm

芒口，内敛。平底及内外壁满施釉，釉面莹润细腻。外壁有交叉竹编纹，近底处饰弦纹三道，口沿饰弦纹一道。器型十分规整，胎薄而透亮，质地坚硬，叩之铿锵有声如钟磬，是宋代青白釉瓷器中之精品。景德镇湖田窑产品。

南京博物院藏

This greenish-white-glazed soup bowl has an inward convergent mouth with an unglazed rim, and a flat foot, which, together with the interior and exterior, is fully coated with even, transparent, and pure glaze. Interlocking bamboo weaving patterns are incised on the exterior wall, while three bands of string patterns on the part close to the bottom, and another band on the mouth rim. This regularly shaped soup bowl with thin and transparent roughcast and solid texture, which can produce a clear ring sound like the clang of chime stones, is an exquisite piece among greenish white porcelain wares in the Song dynasty. It is a product from the Hutian Kiln in Jingdezhen. Preserved in Nanjing Museum

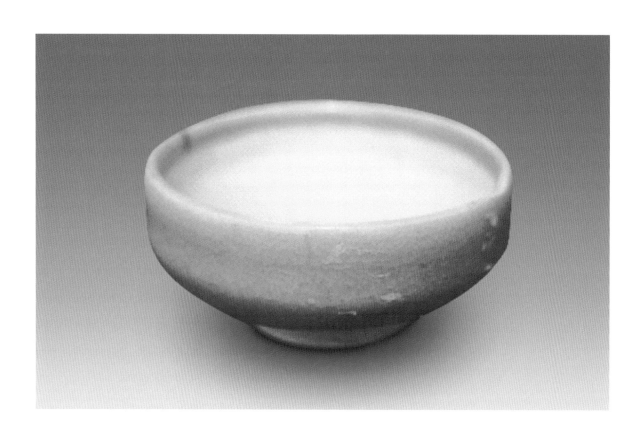

建窑小钵

宋

瓷质

口外径 9.8 厘米，底径 4.65 厘米，通高 4.9 厘米，
腹深 4 厘米，重 160 克

白胎，圈足。食器。

广东中医药博物馆藏

Alms Bowl, Jian Kiln Ware

Song Dynasty

Porcelain

Mouth Outer Diameter 9.8 cm/ Bottom Diameter
4.65 cm/ Height 4.9 cm/ Belly Depth 4 cm/ Weight
160 g

This bowl, featuring a white body and a ring foot,
was utilized as a food container.

Preserved in Guangdong Chinese Medicine Museum

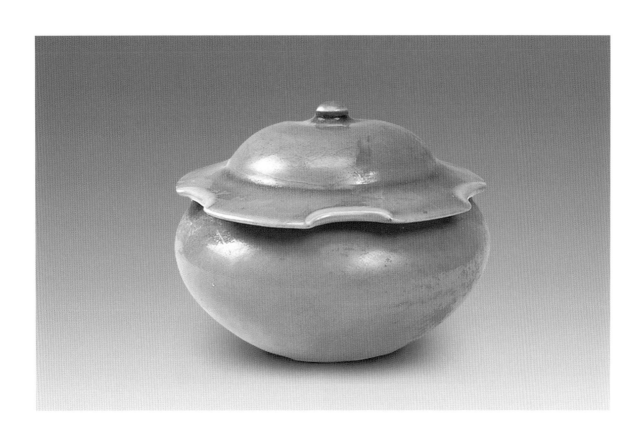

青釉瓷钵

宋

瓷质

口径 10 厘米，底径 4 厘米，通高 12 厘米

青釉，平底，鼓腹，带盖，造型秀丽挺拔。

昭陵博物馆藏

Celadon Bowl

Song Dynasty

Porcelain

Mouth Diameter 10cm/ Bottom Diameter 4cm/ Height 12cm

The bowl, coated with celadon, has a flat bottom, a swelling belly and a cover. It is beautiful, tall and straight.

Preserved in Zhaoling Museum

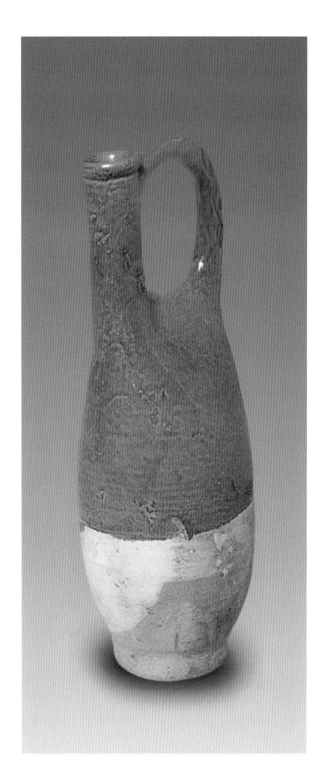

绿釉鸡冠壶

辽

瓷质

口径 3.3 厘米，底径 7.5 厘米，高 36 厘米

Green-glazed Jug with a Comb-shaped Handle

Liao Dynasty

Porcelain

Mouth Diameter 3.3 cm/ Bottom Diameter 7.5 cm/ Height 36 cm

细长直口，秀长腹，口缘与肩间设鸡冠状为把，
圈足。器身上部施绿釉，莹润透亮，身下部无釉，
现淡黄红色细泥胎，还现白色护胎化妆土。

梁剑波藏

This jug has a long, slender and straight mouth,
a long and narrow abdomen, a comb-shaped
handle placed between the mouth edge and the
shoulder, and a ring foot. The upper part of the
body is covered with green glaze which is smooth
and transparent, while the lower part is unglazed,
exposing the bright red and yellow clay body
underneath and the white engobe coating.

Collected by Liang Jianbo

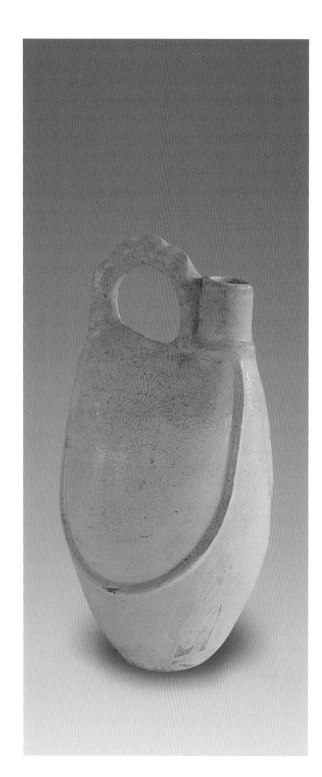

白釉鸡冠壶

辽

瓷质

高 22 厘米

White-glazed Jug with a Comb-shaped Handle

Liao Dynasty

Porcelain

Height 22 cm

秀长扁形腹，身面饰一凸雕条形带，顶部一旁筒状为流，鸡冠状为提梁。浅圈足，全身施白釉，釉莹润。

李明藏

This jug has a slender, oblate and vertical abdomen. The body of the jug is decorated with a strip-shaped belt in high undercut relief. A cannular spout is on one side of the top, beside which is a comb-shaped hoop handle. Bright and smooth white glaze is applied to the whole ware including the shallow ring foot.

Collected by Li Ming

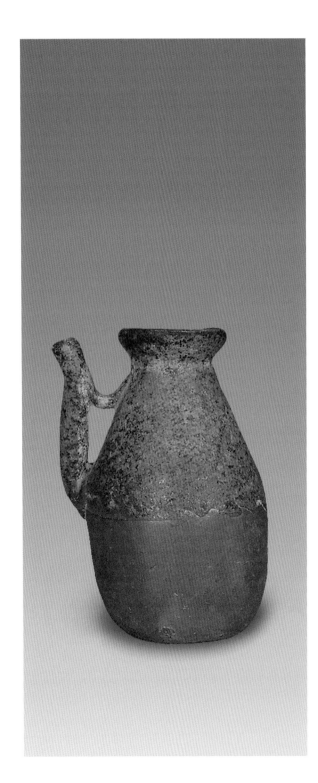

陶酒壶

宋

陶质

口外径 4.5 厘米，腹径 7.3 厘米，宽 8.8 厘米，
高 14.25 厘米

Pottery Wine Pot

Song Dynasty

Pottery

Mouth Outer Diameter 4.5 cm/ Belly Diameter 7.3 cm/

Width 8.8 cm/ Height 14.25 cm

由粗陶烧制，壶形。该壶上半部施土釉，敞口，

平底，长壶嘴，工艺粗糙。盛酒器具。1955

年入藏。保存基本完好。

中华医学会 / 上海中医药大学医史博物馆藏

This ewer-shaped pot is made from crude clay. With the upper part coated with clay glaze, the pot has a flared mouth, a flat foot and a long spout. It is rough in workmanship. This wine vessel was collected in the year 1955 and remains basically intact.

Preserved in Chinese Medical Association/ Museum of Chinese Medicine, Shanghai University of Traditional Chinese Medicine

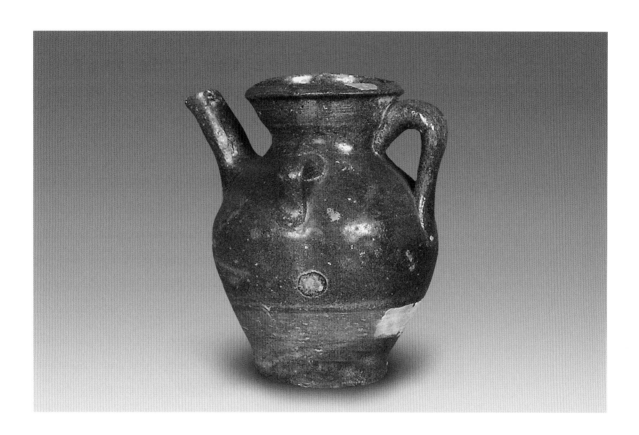

陶酒壶

宋

陶质

口外径 5.7 厘米，口内径 4.3 厘米，腹径 8.6 厘米，宽 10.7 厘米，高 11.6 厘米

Pottery Wine Pot

Song Dynasty

Pottery

Mouth Outer Diameter 5.7 cm/ Mouth Inner Diameter 4.3 cm/ Belly Diameter 8.6 cm/ Width 10.7 cm/ Height 11.6 cm

棕黄陶制，壶形。施墨绿釉，施涂不匀，敞口，平底，斜直形嘴，一端有桥状耳，肩部设两系，工艺粗糙。盛酒器具。1955 年入藏。保存基本完好。

中华医学会 / 上海中医药大学医史博物馆藏

This ewer-shaped wine pot is made of brownish yellow clay and is unevenly glazed black green. It has a flared mouth, a flat foot, an oblique spout, a bridge-shaped ear on one side and two rings on the shoulder. It is rough in workmanship and is well preserved. This wine vessel was collected in the year 1955.

Preserved in Chinese Medical Association/ Museum of Chinese Medicine, Shanghai University of Traditional Chinese Medicine

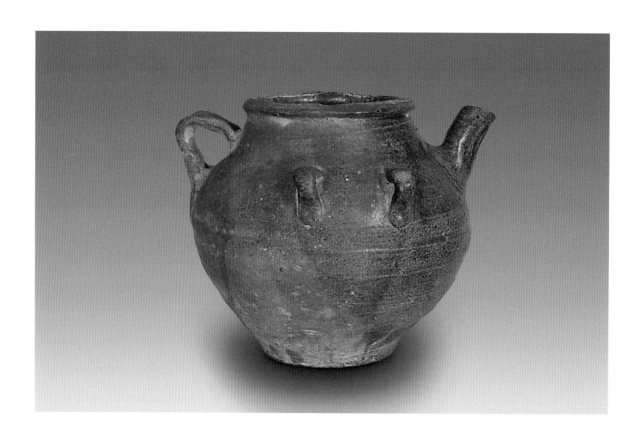

陶壶

宋

陶质

口外径 9.2 厘米，口内径 7.1 厘米，直径 14.1 厘米，通高 15.5 厘米

Pottery Pot

Song Dynasty

Pottery

Mouth Outer Diameter 9.2 cm/ Mouth Inner Diameter 7.1 cm / Diameter 14.1 cm/ Height 15.5 cm

壶形。该藏为夹沙粗陶，壶嘴部分施釉，壶身旋纹清晰，烧制火候较高。壶肩部有壶嘴和壶把及四系。底部无款，无盖。盛药、酒器具。1955 年入藏。基本完好。

中华医学会 / 上海中医药大学医史博物馆藏

This pot is made of gritty sandy clay. The spout is partially glazed and the body is decorated with clear spiral patterns. The pot was fired at a high temperature. There is a spout, a handle and four rings attached to the shoulder. With neither lid on the top nor inscription at the bottom, the pot was used as a medicine or wine container. It was collected in the year 1955 and basically remains intact.

Preserved in Chinese Medical Association/ Museum of Chinese Medicine, Shanghai University of Traditional Chinese Medicine

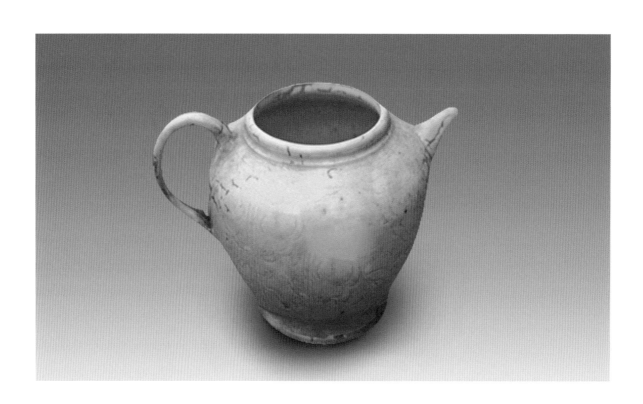

青釉瓷壶

宋

瓷质

口外径 8.15 厘米，腹径 13.25 厘米，底径
8.55 厘米，腹深 11.1 厘米，重 634 克

鼓腹，一半圆形耳，短流，圈足，足边外展。生
活用品。

广东中医药博物馆藏

Celadon Kettle

Song Dynasty

Porcelain

Mouth Outer Diameter 8.15 cm/ Belly Diameter
13.25 cm/ Bottom Diameter 8.55 cm/ Belly Depth
11.1 cm/ Weight 634 g

This celadon porcelain ewer is a household utensil
featuring a swelling belly, a semicircular handle and
a short spout, a ring foot extending outwardly.

Preserved in Guangdong Chinese Medicine Museum

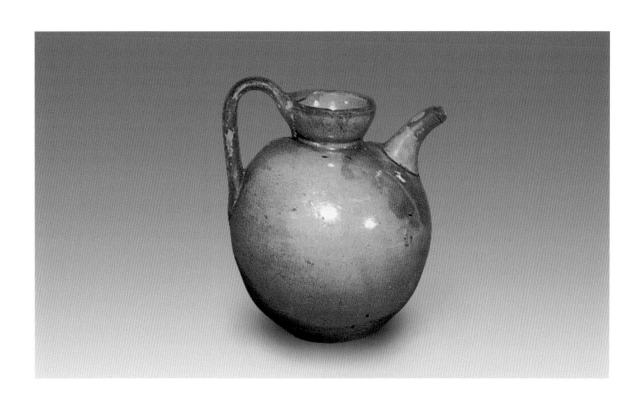

青釉瓷壶

宋

瓷质

腹径 9.8 厘米，高 13.4 厘米

器形较小，窄肩斜溜，圆鼓腹，壶肩部有壶嘴和
壶把。酒具。

广东中医药博物馆藏

Celadon Kettle

Song Dynasty

Porcelain

Belly Diameter 9.8 cm/ Height 13.4 cm

The kettle, small in shape, has a sloping shoulder
and a round swelling belly. On its shoulder is its
spout and handle. It is a wine vessel.

Preserved in Guangdong Chinese Medicine
Museum

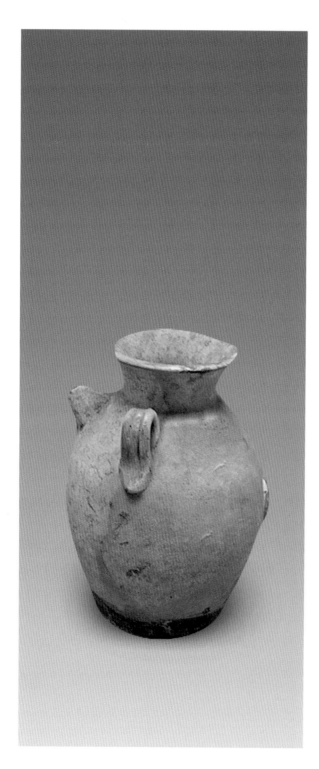

壶

宋

瓷质

高 20 厘米

喇叭形口，腹微鼓，平底，双耳，把已残，六棱形短流，施青釉至腹下半部。由四川省文物考古研究所调拨。

成都中医药大学中医药传统文化博物馆藏

Ewer

Song Dynasty

Porcelain

Height 20 cm

This ewer has a trumpet mouth, a slightly swelling belly, a flat foot, double ears, a handle which is cracked, and a short hexagonal spout. Celadon glaze is applied to the ewer and ends at the lower part of the abdomen. It was allocated from Sichuan Provincial Institute of Cultural Relics and Archeology.

Preserved in Museum of Traditional Chinese Medicine Culture, Chengdu University of Traditional Chinese Medicine

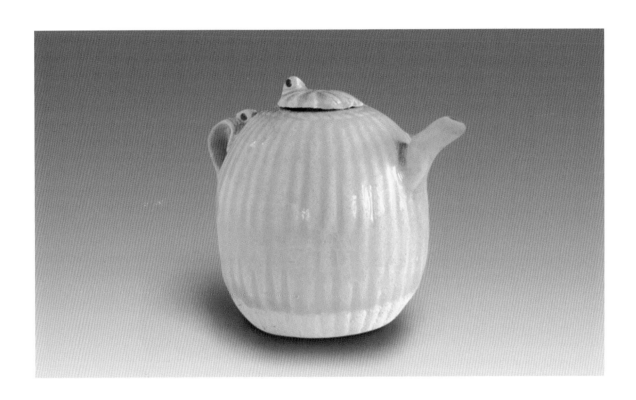

影青印花带盖壶

宋

瓷质

高 8 厘米

敛口，瓜楞腹，曲流，带盖，盖与壶把上各有一带孔纽。饮水用具。

周振武藏

Misty-blue Kettle with Stamped Design and Lid

Song Dynasty

Porcelain

Height 8 cm

The kettle was used as a water vessel, with a contracted mouth, a bent spout, and a lid. Melon-shaped concave lines can be seen on its belly. There is a hole button on the lid and the handle respectively.

Collected by Zhou Zhenwu

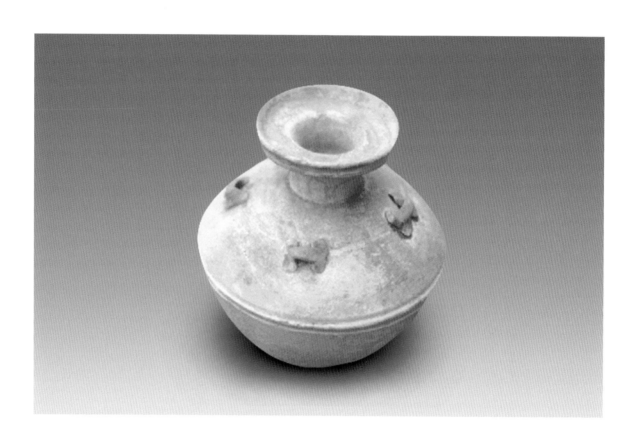

青釉四系陶壶

宋

陶质

口外径 6.5 厘米，腹径 11.7 厘米，底径 6.9 厘米，通高 11.9 厘米，腹深 11 厘米，重 550 克

Celadon Pot with Four Rings

Song Dynasty

Pottery

Mouth Diameter 6.5 cm/ Belly Diameter 11.7 cm/ Bottom Diameter 6.9 cm/ Height 11.9 cm/ Depth 11 cm/
Weight 550 g

陶壶，细直颈，盘口，口唇上卷，鼓腹，上
腹部有四系钮耳，平底。用于盛酒等液体的
容器。

广东中医药博物馆藏

This pot is designed with a thin straight neck, a
dish-shaped mouth with an everted rim angling
upward and a swelling belly. There are four
twisted rings on the upper part of the belly and
the bottom is flat. The pot was utilized as a
container for carrying wine or liquid.

Preserved in Guangdong Chinese Medicine
Museum

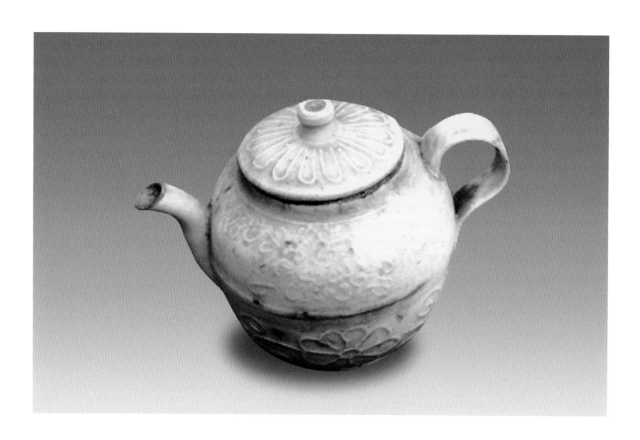

影青窑壶

宋

瓷质

口外径 5 厘米，腹径 8.1 厘米，底径 4.9 厘米，带盖高 9 厘米，腹深 6.5 厘米

Misty-blue-glazed Pot

Song Dynasty

Porcelain

Mouth Outer Diameter 5 cm/ Belly Diameter 8.1 cm/ Bottom Diameter 4.9 cm/ Height(with the lid) 9 cm/

Depth 6.5 cm

带盖，盖顶圆扁钮，盖面有花瓣纹，鼓腹，
腹有花纹，弧形短流，半圆耳。饮水器皿。

广东中医药博物馆藏

This pot has a lid with a flat circular knob on
the top. The lid is decorated with floral petal
designs. The globular body bears floral motifs,
with a curved short spout and an arch-shaped
handle attached to it. It was used as a drinking
vessel.

Preserved in Guangdong Chinese Medicine
Museum

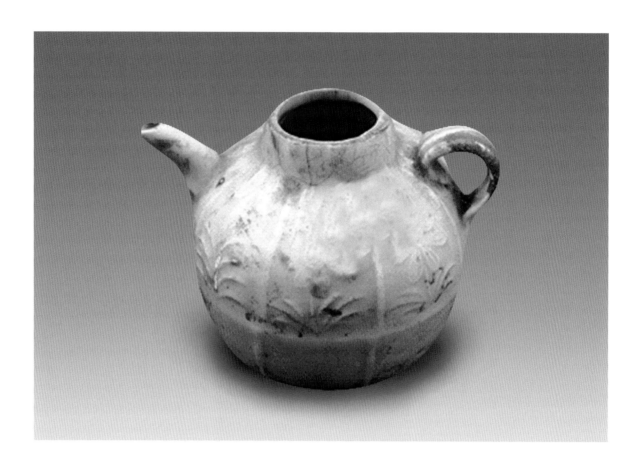

影青瓷壶

宋

瓷质

口外径 4.1 厘米，腹径 9.8 厘米，底径 8.7 厘米，通高 8 厘米，腹深 7.3 厘米，重 242 克

Misty-blue-glazed Porcelain Pot

Song Dynasty

Porcelain

Mouth Outer Diameter 4.1 cm/ Belly Diameter 9.8 cm/ Bottom Diameter 8.7 cm/ Height 8 cm/ Belly Depth 7.3 cm/ Weight 242 g

平口，鼓腹，腹上削下丰，半圆形耳，弧形
长流，腹部瓜棱形，并刻有花纹。饮水用具。

广东中医药博物馆藏

This pot has a flat mouth and a swelling belly,
tapering upward from the rounded belly. A
semicircular handle and a curved long spout
are attached to the belly, which is decorated
with melon ribbed patterns and floral motifs. It
served as a drinking utensil.

Preserved in Guangdong Chinese Medicine
Museum

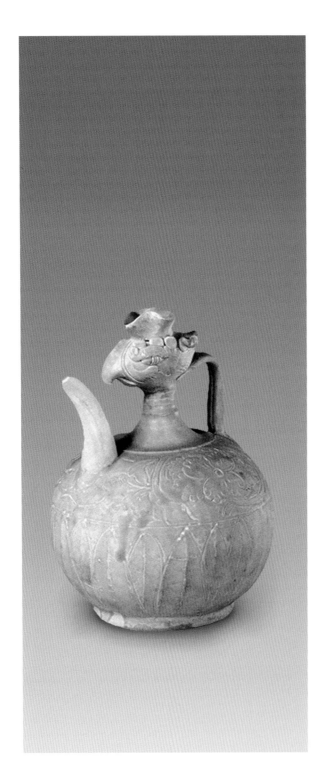

西村窑刻花凤首执壶

宋

瓷质

口径 4.2 厘米，底径 8.3 厘米，高 16.8 厘米

Porcelain Ewer with Carved Phoenix Head Design, Xicun Kiln Ware

Song Dynasty

Porcelain

Mouth Diameter 4.2 cm/ Bottom Diameter 8.3 cm/ Height 16.8 cm

壶口为高冠凤首，大眼曲喙，凤头花冠为注
水口。细颈上凸起弦纹三道。圆腹，上腹部
刻画花卉纹，下腹部刻画仰莲瓣纹。宽圈足。
通体施青白釉。

故宫博物院藏

The mouth of this ewer is in the shape of a
phoenix head with big eyes and decurved beak.
Above the comb of the phoenix head is a water
filling nozzle. There are three bands of string
patterns on the thin neck of the ewer. The ewer
has a broad ring foot and a globular belly, with
incised floral motifs on the upper part, and
upward lotus-petal patterns on the lower part. It
is coated with greenish white glaze.
Preserved in the Palace Museum

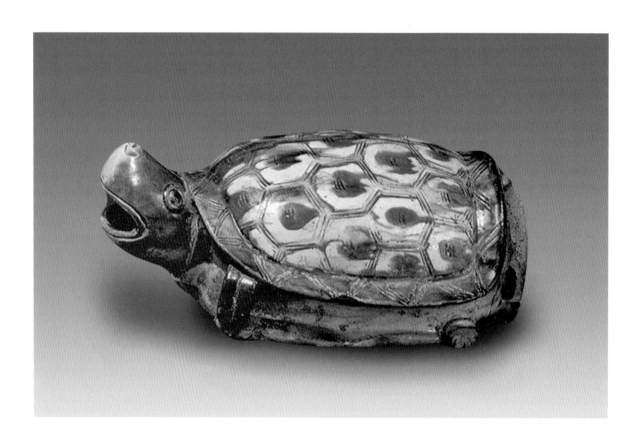

三彩陶龟形壶

金

瓷质

宽 18.1 厘米，厚 11.8 厘米，高 28.5 厘米

Three-colour-glazed Turtle-shaped Water Dropper

Jin Dynasty

Porcelain

Width 18.1 cm/ Thickness 11.8 cm/ Height 28.5 cm

胎体厚重，壶体做成龟形。龟头为壶口，龟体为壶身，一面圆鼓，用绿色彩釉绘甲纹，另一面扁平，用黄褐色彩釉绘龟腹，两侧附龟足形穿系，尾部做成圈足式。龟形壶竖立，可穿绳提携。济宁市东门出土。

济宁市博物馆藏

The body of this turtle-shaped water vessel is heavy and thick with a turtle-head spout and a belly in the shape of a turtle body. The round and bulging side of the belly is glazed green and yellow in tortoiseshell patterns, while the other side is coated with yellowish brown glaze. Two turtle-foot rings are attached to both sides of the body, with the turtle bottom as the ring foot. When in upright position, this turtle-shaped water dropper can be carried with strings. It was excavated from the East Gate of Jining City, Henan Province.

Preserved in Jining Museum

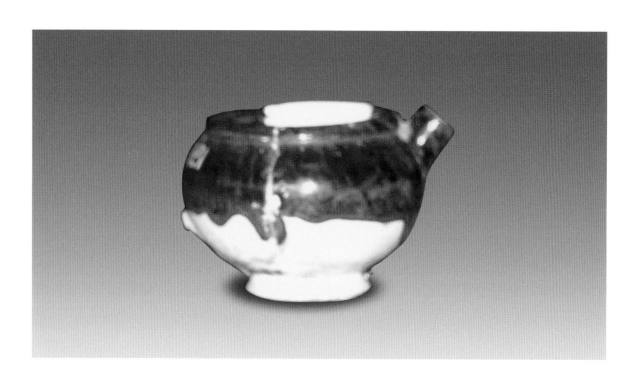

小黑瓷壶

元

瓷质

口径 5 厘米，底径 3.2 厘米，通高 4.5 厘米，重 50 克

弇口，圆唇，鼓腹，平底，肩部有一水流，下部无釉。生活用器。有修补。陕西省西安市大雁塔出土。

陕西医史博物馆收藏

Small Black-glazed Porcelain Pot

Yuan Dynasty

Porcelain

Mouth Diameter 5 cm/ Bottom Diameter 3.2 cm/ Height 4.5 cm/ Weight 50 g

This black-glazed pot has a small circular mouth, a swelling belly and a flat bottom with a spout attached to the shoulder. Its lower part is unglazed. On the pot can be seen marks of restoration. The pot, a household utensil, was excavated from the Wild Goose Pagoda of Xi'an, Shaanxi Province.

Preserved in Shaanxi Museum of Medical History

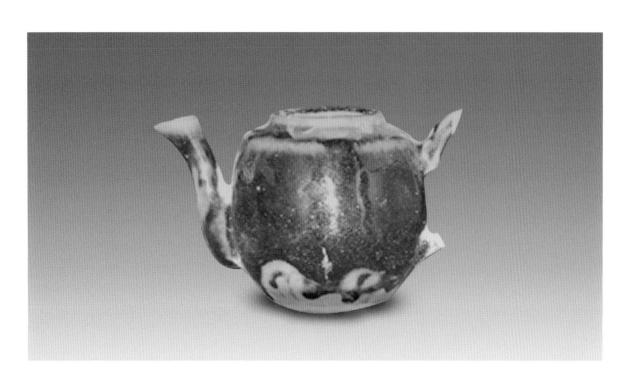

黑釉小瓷壶

元

瓷质

口径 5 厘米，底径 5 厘米，通高 8.2 厘米，重
250 克

弇口，小折肩，略直腹，浅圈足，中腹有一壶把
及流。水器。壶把有残。陕西省澄城县征集。

陕西医史博物馆藏

Small Black-glazed Porcelain Pot

Yuan Dynasty

Porcelain

Mouth Diameter 5 cm/ Bottom Diameter 5 cm/
Height 8.2 cm/ Weight 250 g

This pot has a small mouth, a slightly angular
shoulder, a straight belly and a shallow ring foot.
Attached to the middle part of the pot are a handle
and a spout. The handle is cracked. This water
vessel was collected from Chengcheng County in
Shaanxi Province.

Preserved in Shaanxi Museum of Medical History

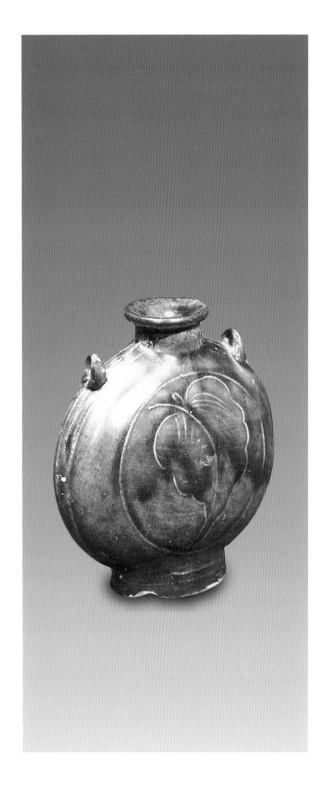

游牧用釉陶水壶

元

陶质

黄釉。壶体为扁鼓形，上刻有叶片饰图。壶体上方两侧有穿孔壶耳。

中国医史博物馆藏

Glazed Pottery Flask for Nomads

Yuan Dynasty

Pottery

This oblate drum-shaped flask is glazed yellow with leaf-shaped motifs incised on the belly. There are two hoop handles on both sides of the upper part of the body.

Preserved in Chinese Medical History Museum

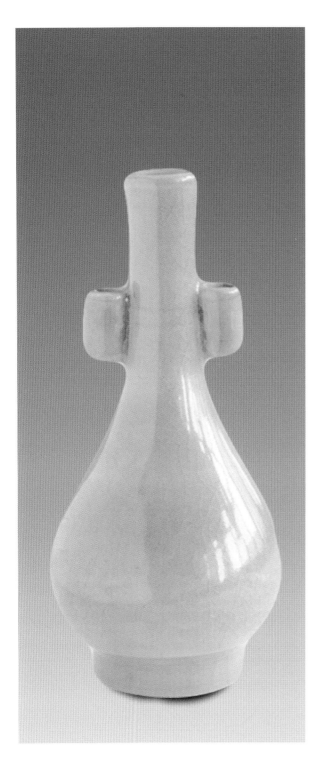

龙泉窑黄釉双贯耳瓶

南宋

瓷质

高 23 厘米

直口，长颈，胆形腹，圈足，颈部饰双弦纹，装双贯耳，里外施青黄色釉，开冰裂纹片，釉色晶莹明亮。

邓其根藏

Yellow-glazed Vase with Two Tubular Ears, Longquan Kiln Ware

Southern Song Dynasty

Porcelain

Height 23 cm

This pot has a straight mouth and an elongated bottleneck, a gall bladder-shaped belly and a ring foot. There are two incised string bands on the bottleneck where two tubular ears are set. The interior and exterior are coated with lustering yellow celadon glaze with broken-ice crackles.

Collected by Deng Qigen

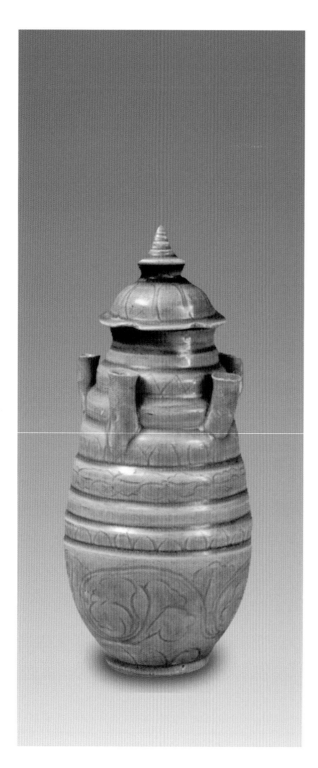

青釉六管瓶

北宋

瓷质

口径 8.3 厘米，底径 9 厘米，通高 34.7 厘米

Celadon-glazed Vase with Six Tubes

Northern Song Dynasty

Porcelain

Mouth Diameter 8.3cm/ Bottom Diameter 9 cm/

Height 34.7 cm

胎体较厚重，呈灰色。通体施釉，青中闪黄色。器体细高似塔形，直口，高颈作节状，并出六管（与颈末通），鼓腹，平底。盖作子口，宽沿，钮作塔刹状。通体刻画纹饰，腹部饰缠枝花卉纹，叶内辅以篦划纹。龙泉窑（今浙江省龙泉市）产品。

山东博物馆藏

The grey-coloured body is thick and heavy. The whole vase is coated with yellow celadon glaze. The vase is tall and thin in the shape of a tower with features of a straight mouth, an elongated bottleneck with multiple layers, six tubes connected to the neck, a swelling belly and a flat bottom. There is a booby hatch lid with a broad edge and a knob in the shape of a stupa top. The whole vase is decorated with incised motifs, and on the belly are found motifs of interlocking branches and flowers with comb patterns carved in the flower leaves.This vase was produced in Longquan Kiln (Longquan City, Zhejiang Province).

Preserved in Shandong Museum

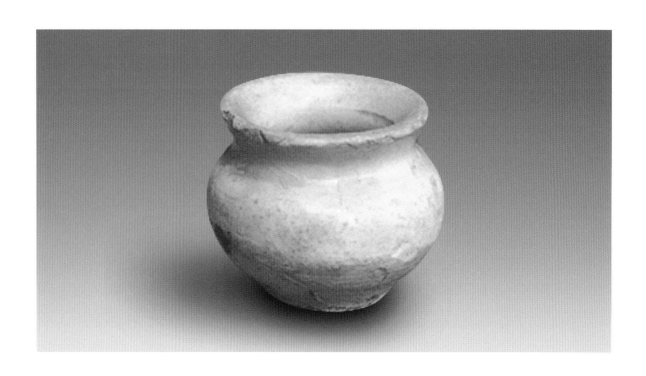

磁州小瓶

宋

瓷质

口外径 3.2 厘米，腹径 3.7 厘米，底径 1.9 厘米，
通高 2.9 厘米，重 20 克

盘口，鼓腹，平底。盛物容器。

广东中医药博物馆藏

Small Vase, Cizhou Kiln Ware

Song Dynasty

Porcelain

Mouth Outer Diameter 3.2 cm/ Belly Diameter
3.7 cm/ Bottom Diameter 1.9 cm/ Height 2.9 cm/
Weight 20 g

This small vase is designed with a dish-shaped
mouth, a swelling belly and a flat bottom. It was
utilized as a storage container.

Preserved in Guangdong Chinese Medicine Museum

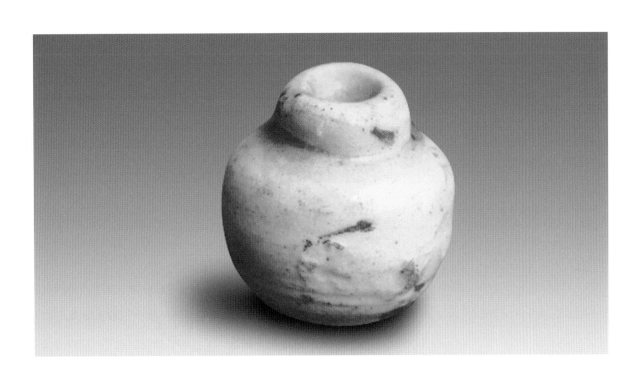

磁州小瓶

宋

瓷质

腹径 1.9 厘米，通高 1.9 厘米，重 5.1 克

直口，平肩，鼓腹，平底。盛物容器。

广东中医药博物馆藏

Small Vase, Cizhou Kiln Ware

Song Dynasty

Porcelain

Belly Diameter 1.9 cm/ Height 1.9 cm/ Weight 5.1 g

This small vase has a straight mouth, a flat shoulder, a swelling belly and a flat bottom. It was utilized as a container.

Preserved in Guangdong Chinese Medicine Museum

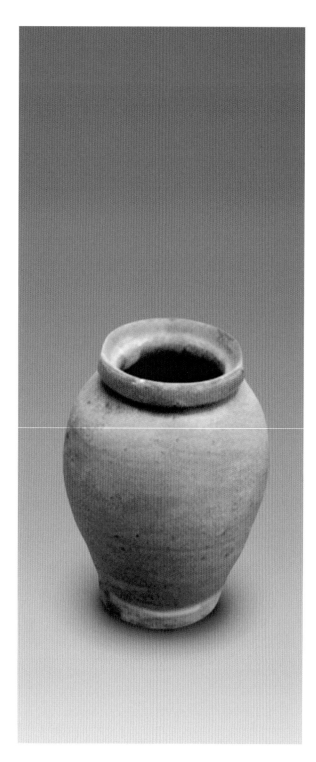

黄釉瓶

宋

陶质

口外径 5.5 厘米，腹径 8.3 厘米，底径 5.4 厘米，

通高 10.8 厘米，腹深 9.7 厘米，重 273 克

小敞口，鼓腹，腹上丰下敛，小圈足。盛物容器。

广东中医药博物馆藏

Yellow-glazed Vase

Song Dynasty

Pottery

Mouth Outer Diameter 5.5 cm/ Belly Diameter
8.3 cm/ Bottom Diameter 5.4 cm/ Height 10.8 cm/
Depth 9.7 cm/ Weight 273 g

This vase has a small flared mouth and a swelling
belly which narrows down to a ring foot. It served
as a container.

Preserved in Guangdong Chinese Medicine Museum

青瓷瓶

宋

瓷质

口外径 4.9 厘米，腹径 7 厘米，底径 4.4 厘米，

通高 9.7 厘米，腹深 8 厘米

圆口，平肩，肩丰，肩以下渐内敛，瓜裂纹路。

广东中医药博物馆藏

Celadon Vase

Song Dynasty

Porcelain

Mouth Outer Diameter 4.9 cm/ Belly Diameter

7 cm/ Bottom Diameter 4.4 cm/ Height 9.7 cm/

Depth 8 cm

This vase is designed with a rounded mouth, a flat

but plump shoulder which narrows down slightly.

The vase bears netted melon pattern on the outside

surface.

Preserved in Guangdong Chinese Medicine Museum

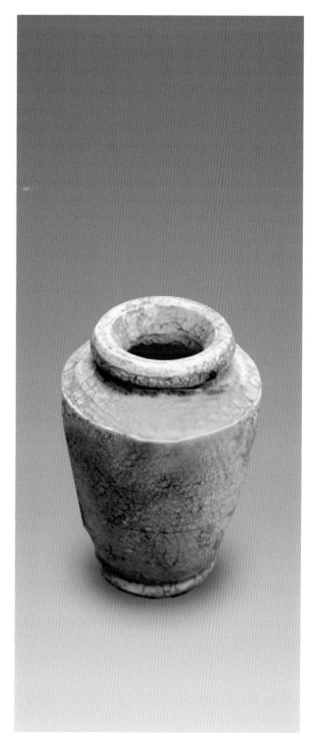

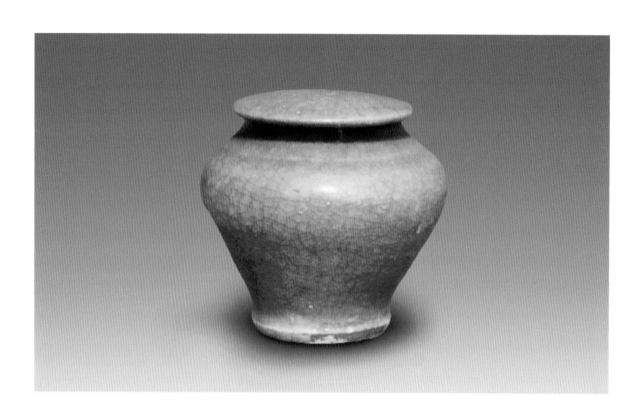

梅青龙泉盖瓶

宋

瓷质

口径 5 厘米，腹径 8.05 厘米，底径 4.4 厘米，通高 6.8 厘米，腹深 4.7 厘米，重 755 克

Plum-green-glazed Vase with a Lid, Longquan Kiln Ware

Song Dynasty

Porcelain

Mouth Diameter 5 cm/ Belly Diameter 8.05 cm/ Bottom Diameter 4.4 cm/ Height 6.8 cm/ Depth 4.7 cm/ Weight 755 g

平口，削肩，鼓腹，下收敛，圈足，带圆扁盖。

盛物容器。

广东中医药博物馆藏

This vase is designed with a flat mouth, a sloping shoulder, a swelling belly narrowing down to a ring foot, and a round flattened lid. It served as a container.

Preserved in Guangdong Chinese Medicine Museum

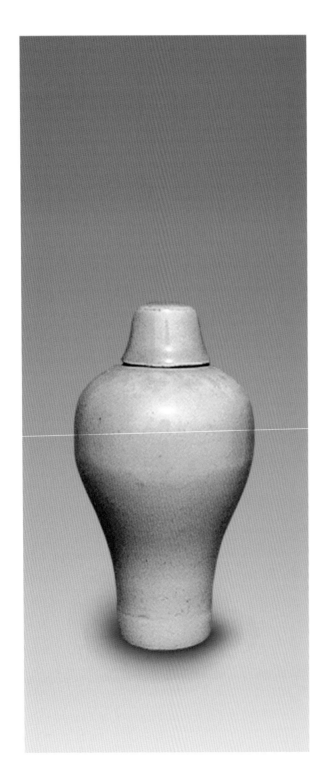

龙泉窑酒瓶

宋

瓷质

口外径 2.8 厘米，腹径 9.6 厘米，底径 5.5 厘米，

通高 17.7 厘米，腹深 14.8 厘米，重 447 克

Wine Vase, Longquan Kiln Ware

Song Dynasty

Porcelain

Mouth Outer Diameter 2.8 cm/ Belly Diameter

9.6 cm/ Bottom Diameter 5.5 cm/ Height 17.7 cm/

Depth 14.8 cm/ Weight 447 g

直口，圆肩，腹部上直下束，带盖，宝字盖，
盖与肩合，平底。用于盛酒。

广东中医药博物馆藏

This wine vessel has a straight mouth a circular
shoulder, a flat bottom,. The upper part of the
belly is straight but tightly contracted at the
lower part. The lid is trapezoid-shaped, fitting
closely with the shoulder. It was used as a wine
container.

Preserved in Guangdong Chinese Medicine
Museum

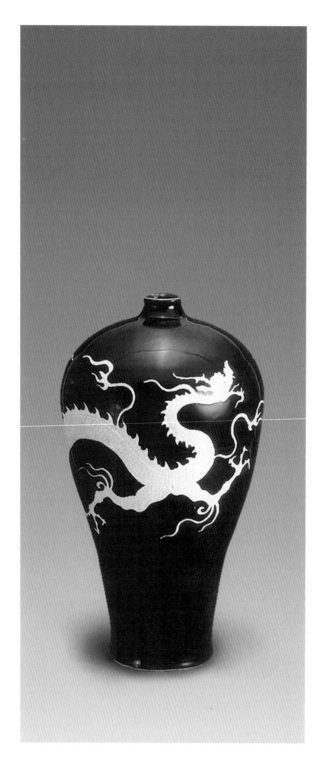

霁蓝釉白龙纹梅瓶

元

瓷质

口径 5.5 厘米，底径 14 厘米，高 43.5 厘米

Sapphire-glazed Prunus Vase with White Dragon Pattern

Yuan Dynasty

Porcelain

Mouth Diameter 5.5 cm/ Bottom 14 cm/ Height 43.5 cm

口小，颈短，肩丰。肩以下逐渐收敛，至近底部微微外撇。浅底内凹。通体施霁青白釉，两种釉色对比鲜明、强烈。在国内外收藏的三件元霁蓝釉白龙纹梅瓶中，此瓶器型最大，造型秀挺，釉色净润，纹饰精美且又生动活泼，气势磅礴，是梅瓶中的极品。1984 年从扬州市文物商店收购。

扬州博物馆藏

This prunus vase is small-mouthed, short-necked, and broad-shouldered. The belly narrows from the shoulder down and is slightly flared at the shallow concave bottom. The vase is coated with glazes of two colours in strong contrast-sapphire and white. This vase is the biggest among the three similar works of the Yuan Dynasty collected both at home and abroad, and enjoys pretty shape with clear and smooth glaze. Decorated with exquisite and vivid dragon design, full of power and grandeur, this object is regarded as a masterpiece of prunus vases. It was purchased from an antique shop in Yangzhou City, Jiangsu Province. Preserved in Yangzhou Museum

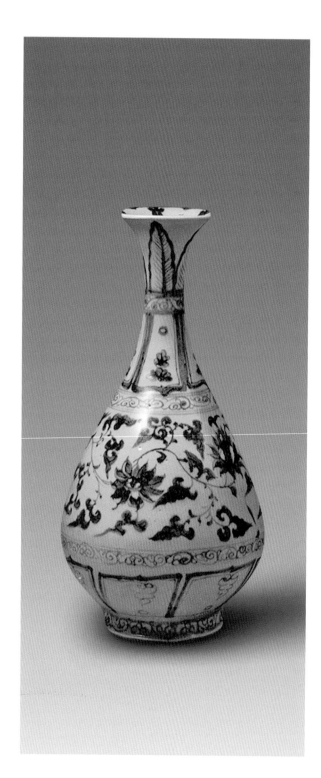

青花玉壶春瓶

元

瓷质

口径 8.3 厘米，底径 9.1 厘米，高 29.4 厘米

Blue and White Pear-shaped Vase with Flared Lip

Yuan Dynasty

Porcelain

Mouth Diameter 8.3 cm/ Bottom Diameter 9.1 cm/ Height 29.4 cm

通体施青白釉。喇叭形口，细颈，流肩，鼓腹，圈足。绘青花蕉叶纹、缠枝莲纹及莲瓣纹。纹饰匀称丰满，线条自然流畅，青花色调深沉。景德镇窑烧制。1972 年于莱州市东安乡出土。

烟台市博物馆藏

This green-white glazed vase has a trumpet-shaped mouth, a narrow neck, a sloping shoulder, a swelling belly and a ring foot. Adorned with patterns of blue and white plantain leaves, interlocking lotus branches and petals, the vase is prominent in well-proportioned motif design, smooth lines and the dark tones of blue and white glaze. It was fired and made in the Jingde zhen kiln and excavated from Dong'an Township of Laizhou City, Shandong Province, in 1972.

Preserved in Yantai Museum

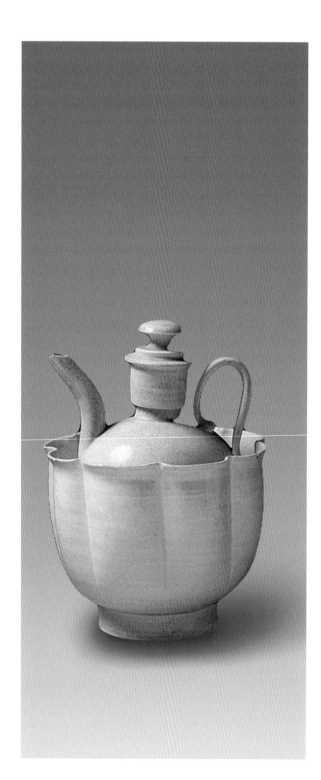

青白釉带温碗注子

北宋早期

瓷质

通高 17.5 厘米

Green-white-glazed Wine Pot with Warming Bowl

Early Northern Song Dynasty

Porcelain

Height 17.5 cm

直口，球形腹，浅圈足。流上翘而弯曲，双带式扁平
柄。在注子表面用泥条堆塑了一支卷草，从壶嘴分两
支向柄部伸展而去，布满全器。套盖，盖钮作蘑菇形，
盖壁上有两小孔用以穿绳系盖。圈足上留有红色的垫
烧痕。有十个莲瓣组成的莲花形口，如一朵仰莲绽开。
碗内底有七个支钉痕，外底有垫圈痕迹，胎骨细白坚致，
釉色青润淡雅，是北宋初期景德镇湖田窑的产品。

溧水区博物馆藏

This wine pot has a straight mouth, a globular belly, a
shallow ring foot, an upward bending spout and a twin-
belt flat handle. The pot is adorned with two clay-strip
floral scrolls in relief extending from the spout to the
handle respectively, covering the entire pot. The mouth
is entangled by the lid with a mushroom-shaped knob.
There are two holes on the lid for ease of tying a tether.
There are red firing marks on the ring foot. The bowl is in
the shape of a blooming lotus with ten petals. The bottom
of the bowl bears marks of a gasket and seven positioning
pins. The fine and solid body is covered with elegant and
lustrous greenish white glaze. It was made in Hutian Kiln
of Jingdezhen in the early Northern Song Dynasty.
Preserved in Lishui Museum

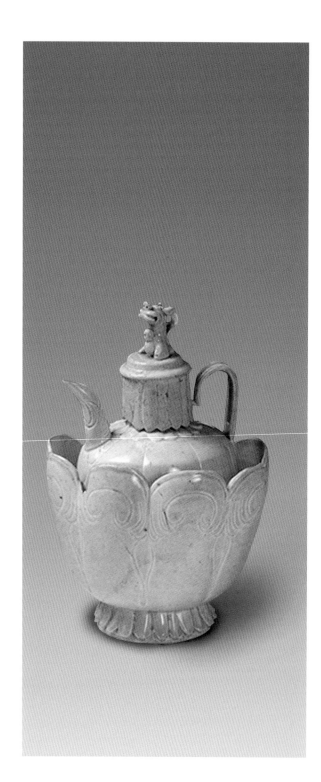

青白瓷注子

宋

瓷质

注高 21.6 厘米，托高 17.5 厘米

Green-white Porcelain Wine Pot

Song Dynasty

Porcelain

Pot: Height 21.6 cm/ Warming Bowl: Height

17.5 cm

圆腹，直流微曲，流口略高于注口，釉色白而闪黄，下腹内收。扁平的带形把上饰二道细弦纹，流与器把的根部均置叶状图案。注表面成八瓣瓜棱形。盖钮状如蹲狮，阔嘴，昂首，翘尾，胸抱一圆球。莲瓣形圈足，底部留有四个支烧痕迹。高淳区沧溪夹埂村出土。

高淳博物馆藏

The wine pot is designed with a rounded belly which narrows down in the lower part and a slightly curved spout whose end is taller than the mouth. The whole body of the pot is coated with yellowish-white glaze. The belt-shaped handle is adorned with two thin bowstring patterns. Both the spout and the handle end are incised with leaf-shaped motifs. The surface of the wine pot is divided into eight melon rib pieces. The lid knob is in the shape of a squat lion whose mouth opens wide, with the head perked, tail raised, and a ball in its breast. Spur (kiln support) marks are found on the lotus-petal-shaped ring foot. It was excavated from Jiageng Village in Cangxi District of Gaochun County, Jiangsu Province.

Preserved in Gaochun Museum

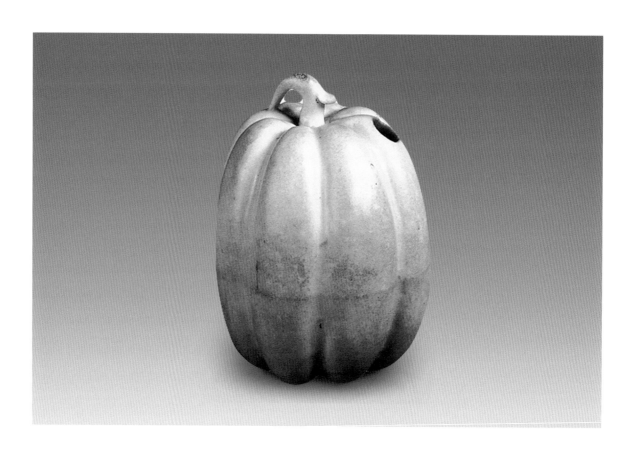

青白釉瓜形水注

北宋

瓷质

底径 6.9 厘米，高 8.8 厘米

Green-white-glazed Water Dropper in the Shape of Melon

Northern Song Dynasty

Porcelain

Bottom Diameter 6.9 cm/ Height 8.8 cm

全器成八瓣瓜楞形，顶部为一弯曲的瓜蒂，肩部有一注孔，腹部有接痕，系分段制作粘接成器，底心内收，胎细白，满施青白色薄釉，莹亮。此水注设计独特，造型优美。1995 年宝应宋墓出土。

宝应博物馆藏

This water dropper is in the shape of a ribbed melon with eight ridges and a curved stalk-shaped knob on the top. There is a hole on the shoulder for water injection. A welding defect on the belly indicates that the subsections of the vessel were made separately and then bonded together. The bottom is inwardly concaved. The fine white body is covered with a thin layer of bright green-white glaze. The water dropper has an appealing design and elegant shape. It was excavated from a tomb of the Song Dynasty in Baoying County, Jiangsu Province, in 1995.

Preserved in Baoying Museum

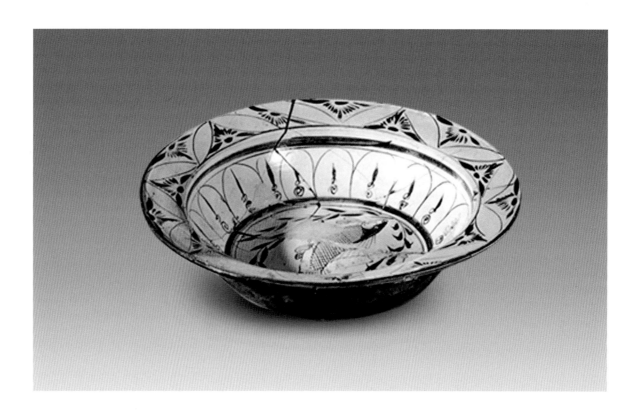

白地黑花瓷盆

元

瓷质

口径 41.6 厘米，底径 23.7 厘米，高 10.2 厘米

White Porcelain Basin with Black Floral Designs

Yuan Dynasty

Porcelain

Mouth Diameter 41.6 cm/ Bottom Diameter 23.7 cm/ Height 10.2 cm

宽平沿，浅腹，大平底，盆内施釉绘画。中
心画面是一尾嬉戏于蔓草间的游鱼，环绕着
的是盆壁一周的莲瓣，莲与鱼相配，颇具匠
心。盆沿上则是布局工整的草叶纹。整个图
幅虽满布盆壁，但疏密有序，主次得当，是
民间绘画艺术的上乘之作。河南省鲁山县段
店遗址出土。

河南省文物考古研究院藏

This basin is designed with a broad flat edge,
a shallow belly and a big flat bottom. The
interior is first glazed and then painted with
fish playing among water weeds, surrounded
by a band of lotus petals on the sidewall of the
basin. The lotus flowers with the matching fish
are designed with great ingenuity. The edge of
the basin is covered with leaf patterns in a neat
layout. The motifs are painted on the basin in
an orderly and structured manner, making the
bowl a masterpiece of the folk art paintings. It
was excavated from the relics of Duandian Kin
in Lushan County, Henan Province.
Preserved in Henan Provincial Institute of
Cultural Heritage and Archaeology

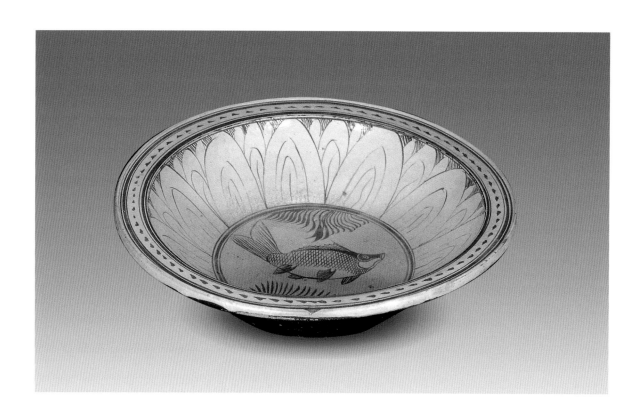

白地黑花鱼藻纹折沿盆

元

瓷质

口径 46.7 厘米，高 11.5 厘米

White Everted-rimed Basin with Black Fish and Water Weed Decoration

Yuan Dynasty

Porcelain

Mouth Diameter 46.7 cm/ Height 11.5 cm

胎粗松厚重。盆外壁施褐色釉，色泽浓厚。内壁施白釉，呈乳白色。宽折沿，浅腹，平底微内凹。口沿饰弦纹和点纹，内壁为宽莲瓣纹，内底绘鱼藻纹。

河北博物院藏

The body of this basin is gritty, loose and heavy, with the exterior covered with dense and thick brown glaze and the interior wall coated with opalized white glaze. The basin has a broad everted angular rim, a shallow belly and an inwardly concaved bottom. The mouth rim is adorned with bowstring and dot patterns while the interior wall is decorated with a wide band of lotus-petal motifs. The internal bottom is painted with fish and water weed as decorations. Preserved in Hebei Museum

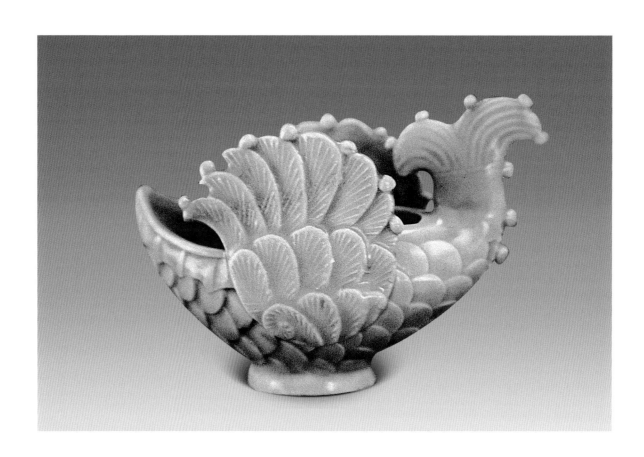

耀州窑飞鱼形水盂

北宋

瓷质

长 14 厘米，宽 7.4 厘米，高 9.3 厘米

Flying-fish-shaped Water Pot, Yaozhou Ware

Northern Song Dynasty

Porcelain

Length 14 cm/ Width 7.4 cm/ Height 9.3 cm

龙鱼形，上颚向上翻卷，双翅高振呈飞翔状，鱼尾商桥，呈 "U" 字形，器内隔成前后两室，底置小圈足。足根无釉。 1971 年于辽宁北票辽墓出土。

辽宁省博物馆藏

The pot is in the shape of a dragonfish, its palate rolling upward, its wings vibrating highly and ready to flying away. The fishtail is U-shaped. Sitting on a small ring foot, its body is divided into two rooms. The bottom of the foot is unglazed. It was unearthed from the tomb of Liao in Beipiao City, Liaoning Province. Preserved in Liaoning Provincial Museum

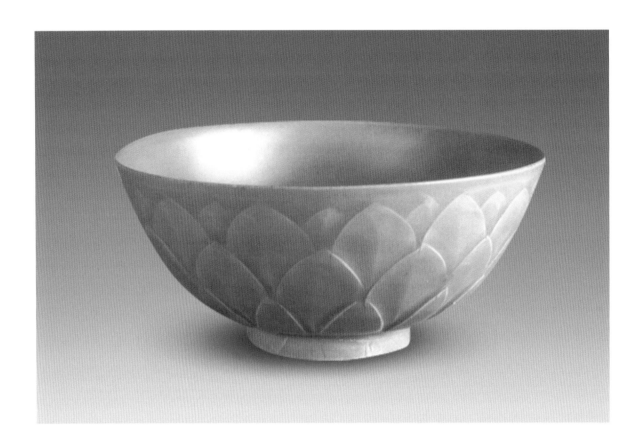

青釉仰莲碗

北宋

瓷质

口径 14.8 厘米，底径 5.8 厘米，高 6.7 厘米

Celadon Bowl with Upward Lotus Design

Northern Song Dynasty

Porcelain

Mouth Diameter 14.8 cm/ Bottom Diameter 5.8 cm/ Height 6.7 cm

敞口，弧腹，矮圈足，腹外壁刻饰四层浮雕莲瓣状，中间两层瓣叶较大，上下两层略小，莲瓣错落有致，雕刻规整，线条流畅，竖刀、偏刀技法运用娴熟，莲瓣纹有线浮雕效果，内外均施青色釉，微黄，釉质莹润，胎致密，灰白。1995 年宝应宋墓出土，为北宋时期临汝窑产品。

宝应博物馆藏

This bowl is designed with an open mouth, a round belly and a short ring foot. The exterior wall is decorated with four bands of overlapping lotus petals in relief, among which petals in the middle are bigger than that of the upper and lower bands. The lotus petals are well-spaced and incised in a neat and tidy way with smooth lines. The low relief carving techniques, such as shallow cut and stop cut, are used skilfully. Covered inside and out with a glaze of yellowish celadon, the bowl has a glossy and smooth appearance. The greyish white body of the pottery is very dense and fine-grained. It was excavated in the tomb of the Song Dynasty in Baoying County, Jiangsu Province, in 1995.

Preserved in Baoying Museum

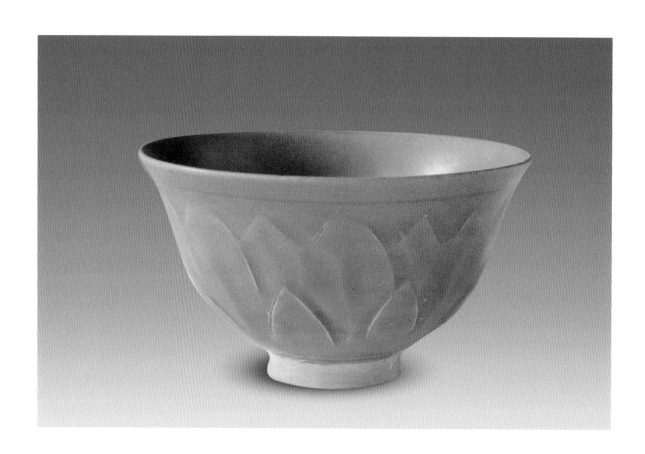

耀州窑青釉莲花瓣纹碗

北宋

瓷质

口径 13 厘米，高 7.3 厘米

Celadon Bowl with Lotus Petal Motifs, Yaozhou Kiln Ware

Northern Song Dynasty

Porcelain

Mouth Diameter 13 cm/ Height 7.3 cm

敞口，口沿稍外撇，由沿至足渐收，圈足规
整稍高。腹部刻多重莲花瓣纹，立体感甚强，
施青绿色釉，晶莹润泽。灰白胎甚坚实。
此碗为陕西省铜川市黄堡镇耀州窑产品。

谢志峰藏

The bowl has an open mouth with a flared rim
and a tall, neat ring foot. The external wall
tapers down slightly from the mouth rim to the
foot. The belly is incised with overlapping lotus
petals, giving out a strong three-dimensional
sense. The bowl is coated with glossy and
smooth blue-and-green glaze, and the body
of the pottery is solid in greyish white. It was
made in Yaozhou Kiln, Huangbao County,
Tongchuan City, Shaanxi Province.
Collected by Xie Zhifeng

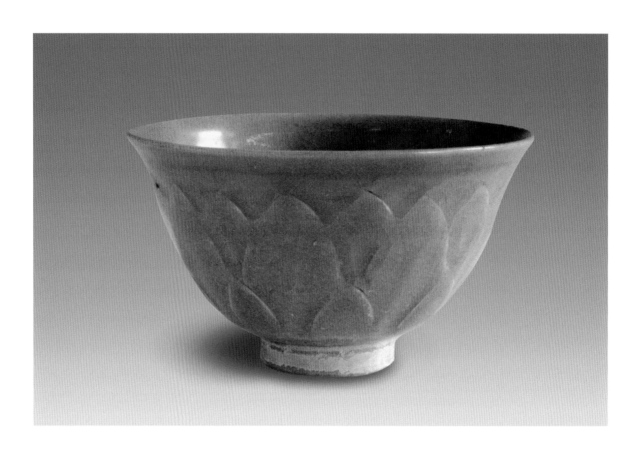

耀州窑青釉莲花瓣碗

北宋

瓷质

口径 13 厘米，底径 4.5 厘米，高 7.5 厘米

Celadon Bowl with Lotus Petal Motifs, Yaozhou Kiln Ware

Northern Song Dynasty

Porcelain

Mouth Diameter 13 cm/ Bottom Diameter 4.5 cm/ Height 7.5 cm

敞口，口沿至足渐收，圈足稍高甚规整。腹部刻多重莲瓣纹。碗内外满施青色釉至足，足内亦有釉。胎灰白。此碗为陕西铜川市黄堡镇耀州窑的产品。

李鸿基藏

This bowl is designed with an open mouth and a neat, tall ring foot. The external wall tapers slightly from the mouth rim to the foot. The belly is incised with overlapping lotus petals. Celadon glaze is applied to both the interior and the exterior with even the inside of the bottom glazed. The body of the pottery is greyish white. It was made in Yaozhou Kiln, Huangbao County, Tongchuan City, Shaanxi Province.

Collected by Li Hongji

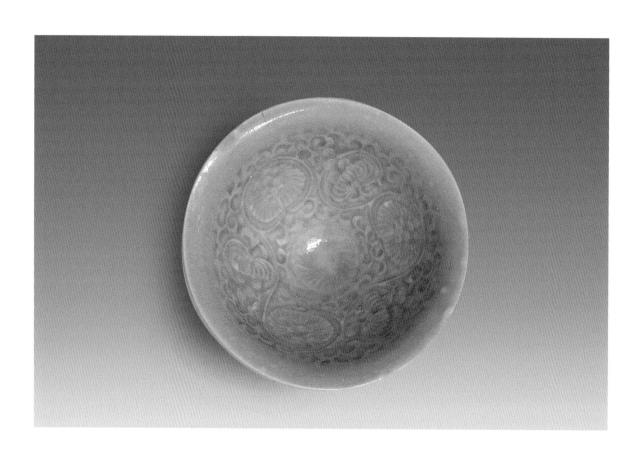

耀州窑青釉印花碗

北宋

瓷质

口径 13.8 厘米，高 5.8 厘米

Celadon Bowl with Impressed Floral Designs, Yaozhou Kiln Ware

Northern Song Dynasty

Porcelain

Mouth Diameter 13.8 cm/ Height 5.8 cm

敞口，沿稍外折，弧形腹，小圈足较规整，
内壁印缠枝菊花，装饰清晰，满施青绿色釉，
甚莹亮。此碗为耀州窑产品。

林存义藏

This bowl is designed with an open mouth with
a slightly everted rim, an arch-shaped belly and
a small and neat ring foot. The interior wall
is impressed with clear motifs of interlocking
branches of chrysanthemum. The bowl is fully
coated with glossy and bright green glaze. It
was made in Yaozhou Kiln.

Collected by Lin Cunyi

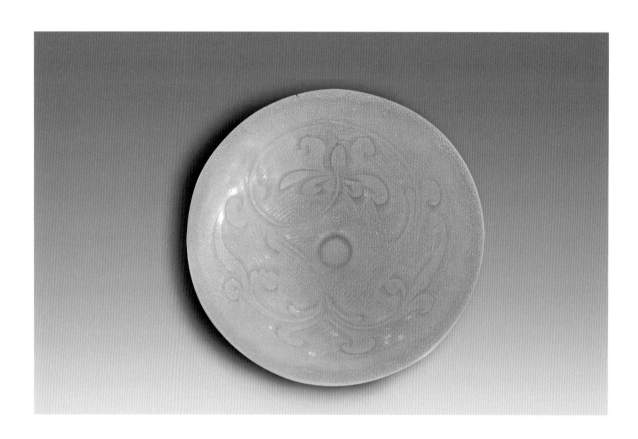

青釉刻花碗

北宋

瓷质

口径 14.5 厘米，高 4.4 厘米

Celadon Bowl with Incised Floral Design

Northern Song Dynasty

Porcelain

Mouth Diameter 14.5 cm/ Height 4.4 cm

撇口，斜腹至足渐收，小圈足。内壁刻有花卉，

底心一凹弦纹。里外施满青釉，稍泛黄色，

足底无釉。灰白胎。

梁茂年藏

This bowl with a flared mouth has an oblique belly which narrows down to a small ring foot. The interior wall is incised with floral designs and right in the centre is a concaved bowstring pattern. The inside and the outside are covered with celadon glaze tinged with yellow except the unglazed foot. The body of the pottery is in greyish-white.

Collected by Liang Maonian

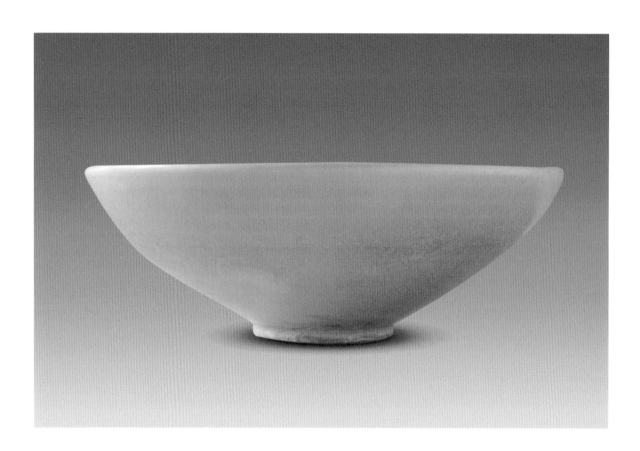

临汝窑刻花碗

北宋

瓷质

口径 20.5 厘米，底径 6.3 厘米，高 7 厘米

Bowl with Incised Floral Design, Linru Kiln Ware

Northern Song Dynasty

Porcelain

Mouth Diameter 20.5 cm/ Bottom Diameter 6.3 cm/ Height 7 cm

敞口，弧形腹，圈足。里外满施青釉，釉至
底足，足内有釉，浅处闪黄色。口沿釉薄处
稍泛黄色，青釉莹润，有棕眼。碗内刻海浪纹，
外壁可见拉坯痕迹。圈足较规整。造型为北
宋典型的临汝窑碗。

林荫璋藏

This bowl has an open mouth, an arch-shaped
belly and a ring foot. The inside and the outside
are fully glazed celadon including the foot, of
which the thinly glazed part sheds yellowish
tinge. The thinly glazed areas on the rim also
has a tint of yellow. The celadon glaze is glossy
and smooth with some pinholes. Incised with
wave motifs on the inside wall, this bowl bears
marks of wheel-throwing on the outside surface.
This kind of design is the most common type of
Linru Kiln ware in the Northern Song Dynasty.
Collected by Lin Yinzhang

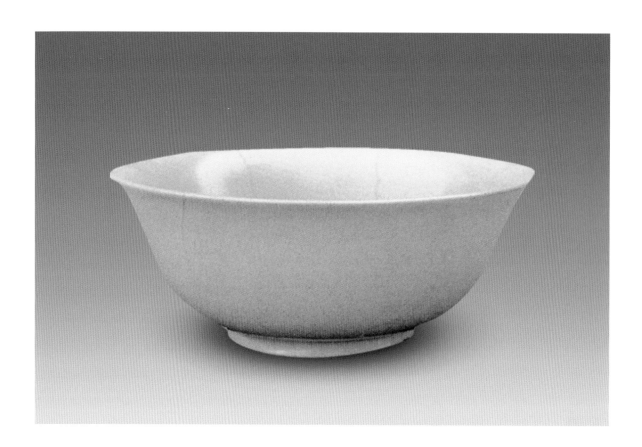

天青釉汝瓷碗

北宋

瓷质

口径 17.1 厘米，高 6.7 厘米

Celeste-glazed Porcelain Bowl, Ru Kiln Ware

Northern Song Dynasty

Porcelain

Mouth Diameter 17.1 cm/ Height 6.7 cm

口唇外敞，腹线饱满，底足外撇，造型端庄雅致。其胎体轻而薄，内外满饰天青色釉，釉色晶莹纯净，釉面有细碎的开片。底足有五个细如芝麻粒大小的支钉，即汝官瓷标准的"芝麻钉"。规整的造型、精良的工艺与典雅的色调，使之成为传世的宋宫廷御用汝瓷的代表作。足部保存有清代乾隆皇帝的御题诗。

故宫博物院藏

This bowl, with a flare-rimmed open mouth, a round belly and a ring foot with flaring sides, shows elegant and dignified style. The thin and light body is covered with glossy and pure celeste glaze with some small crackles. On the bottom are five fine and tiny spurs like sesame seeds, namely the typical "sesame seed-shaped spurs" of the mandarin porcelain from Ru Kiln. This very bowl became known as a masterpiece handed down from the royal court of the Song Dynasty for its neat shape, sophisticated workmanship and elegant hue. In addition, there is an inscription of a poem written by Emperor Qianlong of the Qing Dynasty on the bottom.

Preserved in the Palace Museum

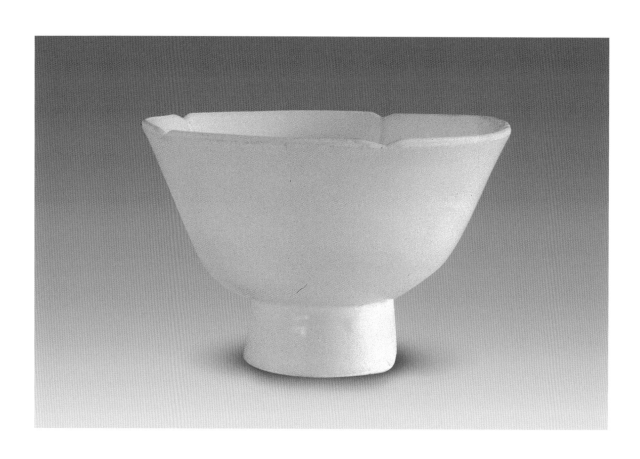

影青花瓣口高足碗

北宋

瓷质

口径 9 厘米，底径 3.8 厘米，高 6 厘米

Misty Blue High Stem Bowl with Five-lobed Rim

Northern Song Dynasty

Porcelain

Mouth Diameter 9 cm/ Bottom Diameter 3.8 cm/ Height 6 cm

敞口，斜腹，圈足稍高，碗沿为五瓣花口，
内壁有凸起的五条线与瓣口及内底弦纹相接，
把内壁分成五等份。里外施隐隐发青的影青
釉，莹洁明亮，足内无釉呈浅黄色，胎质坚细。

黄卓文藏

This bowl is designed with an open mouth,
an oblique belly and a high ring foot. The rim
of this bowl is in the shape of a five-petalled
flower. The interior wall is divided into five
equal parts by five raised lines connecting the
petal mouth to the bowstring pattern on the
inside middle bottom. The inside and the outside
are coated with lustrous misty blue glaze,while
the millet-coloured bottom unglazed. The bowl
has a fine-grained solid clay body.

Collected by Huang Zhuowen

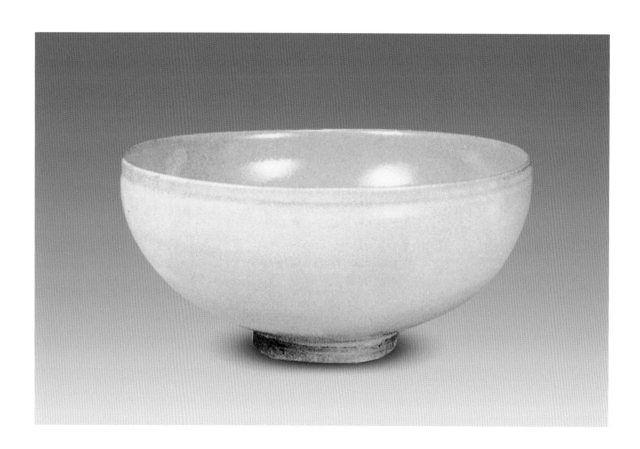

钧瓷碗

北宋

瓷质

口径 25.4 厘米，底径 9.2 厘米，高 11.8 厘米

Bowl, Jun Ware

Northern Song Dynasty

Porcelain

Mouth Diameter 25.4 cm/ Bottom Diameter 9.2 cm/ Height 11.8 cm

大口，深腹，形体厚重。盘的釉色天蓝，碗的釉色则为天青，釉层均匀，色调晶莹，虽是单一色调，却极富韵致。此碗为钧瓷青釉器中的代表作。河南省长葛市石固遗址出土。

河南省文物考古研究院藏

This bowl has a heavy and thick body with a big mouth and a deep belly. The plate is coated with sky blue glaze while the bowl is covered with a thin uniform layer of celeste glaze. With the glaze glittering and translucent, the simple yet charming bowl is representative of celadon Jun ware. It was excavated from Shigu Relic Site in Changge, Henan Province.

Preserved in Henan Provincial Institute of Cultural Heritage and Archaeology

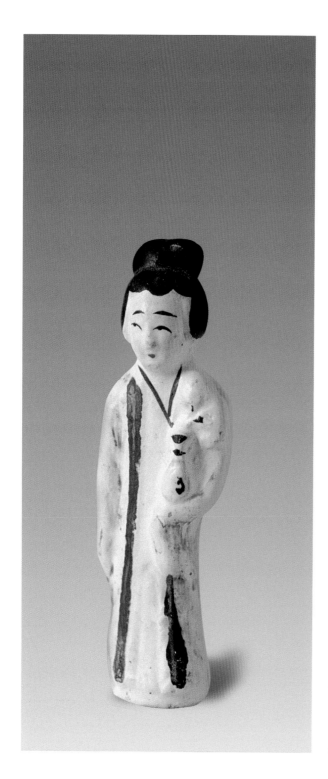

磁州窑加彩小立人

北宋

瓷质

高 13 厘米

Colored Figurine of a Standing Person
Made in Cizhou Kiln

Northern Song Dynasty

Porcelain

Height 13cm

立俑，头梳黑色发髻。衣纹、眉、眼均画黑彩，口点红彩，服饰再加红绿彩绘。施白釉稍泛黄色，灰黄胎。女立俑造型简练生动，黑彩用笔潇洒豪放。磁州窑红绿彩绘是釉上彩绘较早的彩绘工艺，对后来景德镇窑釉上彩有较大的影响。

杨广祥

The standing lady wears a black chignon with her eyes, eyebrows and the lines of her clothes painted black. Her lips are painted red. Her clothes are painted red and green. The glaze is yellowish white and the green ware is grayish yellow. The image is molded concisely and vividly. The color of black has been used in a natural and unrestrained way. The colored glazed painting on ceramics produced at Cizhou Kiln is an earlier technique of color painting on china. It has had a great impact on the colored glazed ceramics produced at Jingdezhen kilns.

Preserved by Yang Guangxiang

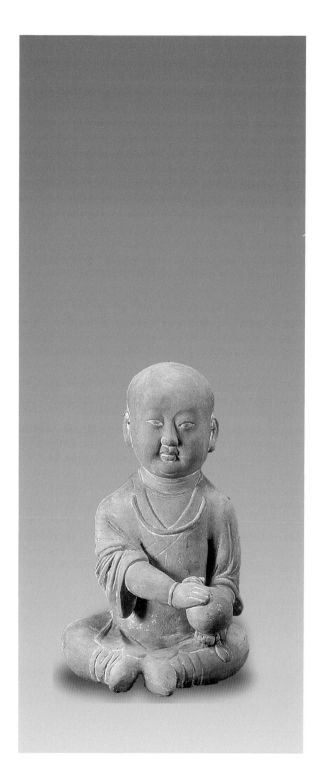

红陶坐童

宋

陶质

高 29 厘米

Red Pottery Figurine of a Sitting Boy

Song Dynasty

Pottery

Height 29 cm

坐童颐满目秀，颈佩项链，臂腕饰镯，双手
持球，天真可爱。

旬邑县博物馆藏

The chubby sitting boy wears a necklace and a
bracelet. His hands hold a ball. He is naive and cute.
Preserved in Xunyi Museum

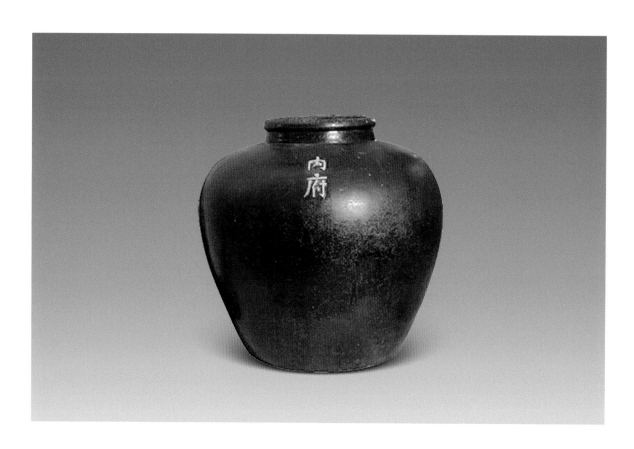

"内府" 黑釉大药酒坛

宋

瓷质

直径 60 厘米，高 60 厘米

Black-glazed Big Medical Wine Pot of "Nei Fu"

Song Dynasty

Porcelain

Diameter 60cm/ Height 60cm

直口，平唇，短直颈，溜肩，鼓腹，平底，圈足。胎体为黑色，外壁肩部有"内府"二字并涂以白釉。"内府"是皇宫内负责监管制造器具的部门，即"内务府"。盛器，为宫廷中贮存药酒的容器。

北京御生堂中医药博物馆藏

The pot has a flat mouth, a short and straight neck, a narrow and inclined shoulder, a bulged belly, a flat bottom and a ring foot. The body is covered with black glaze and the shoulder is painted with white glaze with the inscriptions of "Nei Fu". "Nei Fu" was the department of regulating the tool-made, known as "Imperial Household Department". It was used for storing wine for the royalty.
Preserved in Chinese Medicine Museum of Beijing Yu Sheng Tang Drugstore

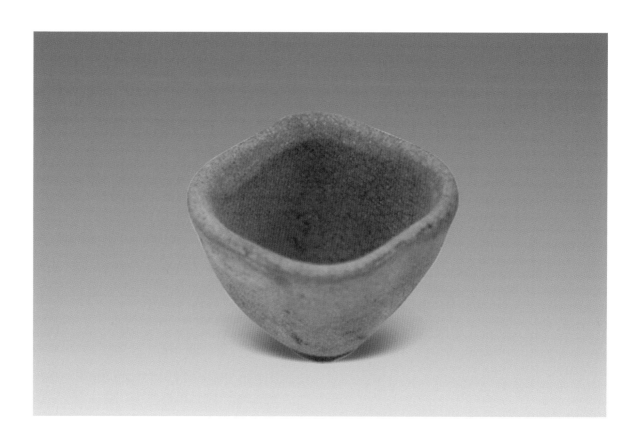

洗眼杯

宋

瓷质

长 5 厘米，宽 3 厘米，高 6 厘米，

Eye-cleaning Cup

Song Dynasty

Porcelain

Length 5cm/ Width 3cm/ Height 6cm

近方形杯口，用于治疗眼疾用，杯口形状恰
和眉骨相吻合，做工巧妙。

北京御生堂中医药博物馆藏

The relatively square cup was used for the
treatment of eye disease and the shape of cup
mouth matches to the brow perfectly, which is
exquisite and delicate.

Preserved in Chinese Medicine Museum of
Beijing Yu Sheng Tang Drugstore

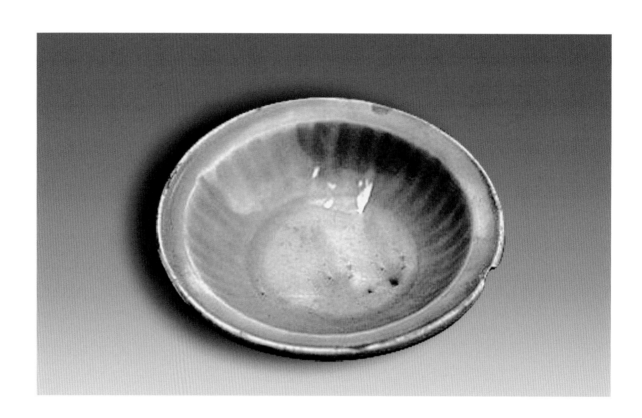

龙泉窑小碗

宋

瓷质

口外径 12.6 厘米，底径 5.6 厘米，通高 4.4 厘米，

腹深 2.4 厘米

盘口，圈足。饮食用具。

广东中医药博物馆藏

Small Bowl, Longquan Kiln Ware

Song Dynasty

Porcelain

Mouth Outer Diameter 12.6 cm/ Bottom Diameter

5.6 cm/ Height 4.4 cm/ Depth 2.4 cm

This small bowl has a dish-shaped mouth and a ring

foot. It served as a food vessel.

Preserved in Guangdong Chinese Medicine Museum

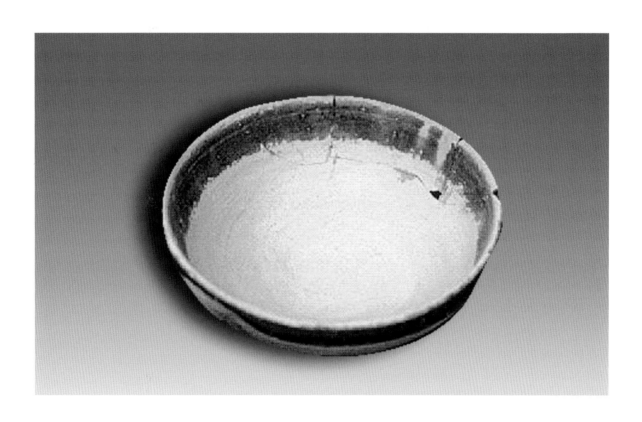

黄釉瓷碗

宋

瓷质

口外径 17.2 厘米，底径 5.5 厘米，通高 6.3 厘米，

腹深 5.3 厘米，重 594 克

黄釉瓷碗，带底座。食具。

广东中医药博物馆藏

Yellow-glazed Porcelain Bowl

Song Dynasty

Porcelain

Mouth Outer Diameter 17.2 cm/ Bottom Diameter

5.5 cm/ Height 6.3 cm/ Depth 5.3 cm/ Weight 594 g

This yellow-glazed bowl sits on a pedestal. It

served as a food vessel.

Preserved in Guangdong Chinese Medicine Museum

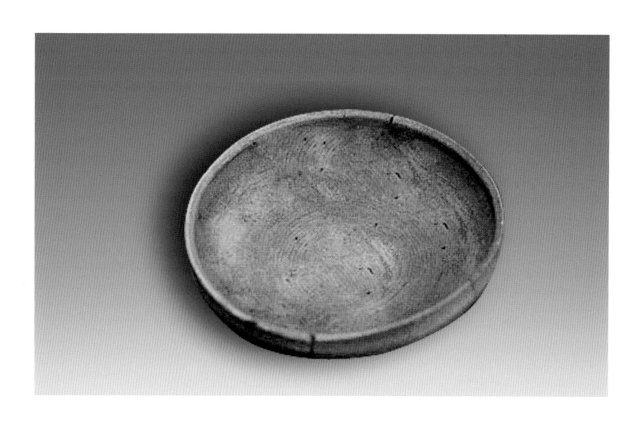

瓷碗

宋

瓷质

口外径 13.9 厘米，底径 6.8 厘米，通高 4.2 厘米，

腹深 3.7 厘米，重 377 克

盘形，碗边沿上卷，平底。饮食用具。

广东中医药博物馆藏

Porcelain Bowl

Song Dynasty

Porcelain

Mouth Outer Diameter 13.9 cm/ Bottom Diameter

6.8 cm/ Height 4.2 cm/ Depth 3.7 cm/ Weight 377 g

This dish-shaped bowl has an everted rim and a flat

bottom. It was used as a food vessel.

Preserved in Guangdong Chinese Medicine Museum

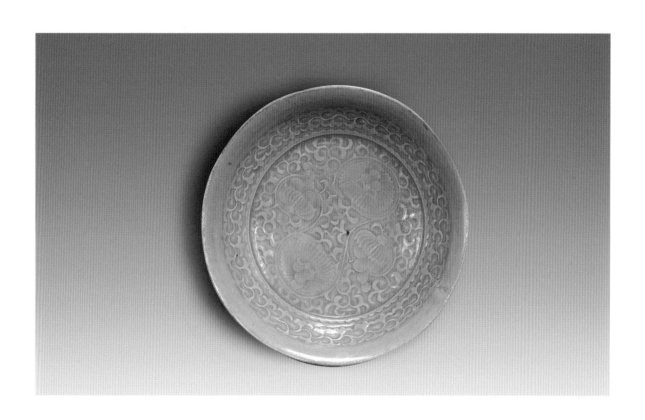

青釉印花瓷碗

宋

瓷质

口径 13 厘米，底径 4 厘米，高 3.6 厘米

敞口，浅腹，小圈足。内壁印缠枝花纹。胎质细腻，釉面均匀，图案布局严谨，线条流畅。

旬邑县博物馆藏

Celadon Bowl with Stamped Design

Song Dynasty

Porcelain

Mouth Diameter 13 cm/ Bottom Diameter 4 cm/ Height 3.6 cm

The bowl has a flared mouth, a shallow body and a small ring foot. It is stamped with interlocking floral patterns. Its body is fine and smooth, with even coating. The patterns are arranged carefully and have smooth lines.

Preserved in Xunyi Museum

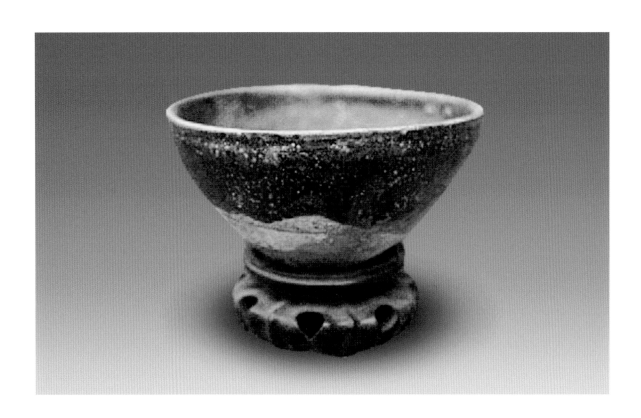

钧窑碗

宋

瓷质

口外径 12 厘米，底径 3.65 厘米，通高 6.3 厘米，

腹深 4.5 厘米，重 218 克

带底座，平口。食具。

广东中医药博物馆藏

Bowl, Jun Kiln Ware

Song Dynasty

Porcelain

Mouth Outer Diameter 12 cm/ Bottom Diameter 3.65

cm/ Height 6.3 cm/ Depth 4.5 cm/ Weight 218 g

This pedestal bowl with a flat mouth was used as a

food vessel.

Preserved in Guangdong Chinese Medicine Museum

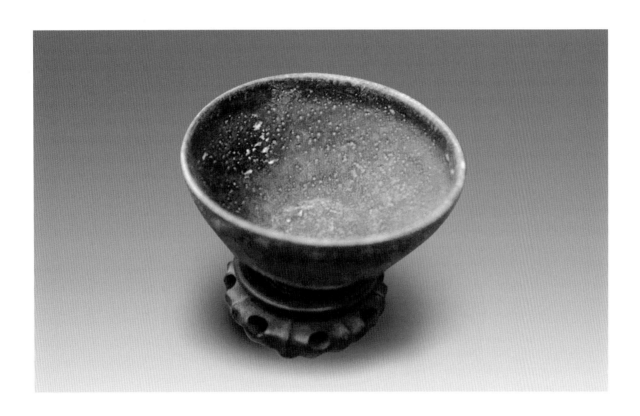

钧窑碗

宋

瓷质

口外径 5 厘米，底径 3.65 厘米，通高 9 厘米，

腹深 3.4 厘米，重 105 克

釉色红中带蓝，小圈足。食器。

广东中医药博物馆藏

Bowl, Jun Kiln Ware

Song Dynasty

Porcelain

Mouth Outer Diameter 5 cm/ Bottom Diameter 3.65 cm/

Height 9 cm/ Depth 3.4 cm/ Weight 105 g

This bowl is red-glazed with a dash of blue and has

a small ring foot. It served as a food vessel.

Preserved in Guangdong Chinese Medicine Museum

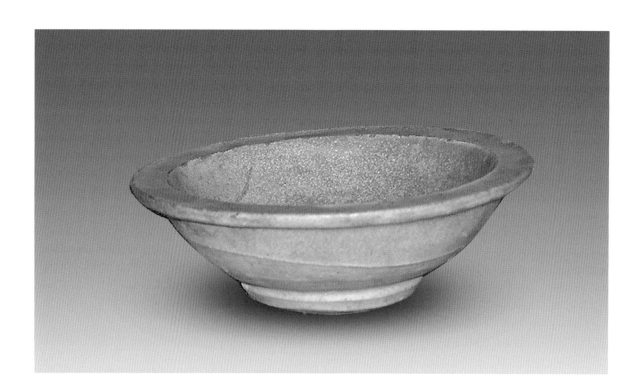

豆青瓷碗

宋

瓷质

口径 12 厘米，底径 5 厘米，高 3.7 厘米，重 200 克

Pea-green-glazed Porcelain Bowl

Song Dynasty

Porcelain

Mouth Diameter 12 cm/ Bottom Diameter 5 cm/ Height 3.7 cm/ Weight 200 g

平口沿，敞口，斜腹，浅足圈，碗外施釉不
到底，豆青釉。食器。口沿略残。陕西省西
安市古玩市场征集。

陕西医史博物馆藏

This bowl has a flat and open mouth, an oblique
belly and a shallow ring foot. The pea-green
glaze is applied to the outside surface close to
the bottom. It was used as a food vessel and its
mouth rim is slightly cracked. It was collected
from the Antique Market of Xi'an, Shaanxi
Province.

Preserved in Shaanxi Museum of Medical History

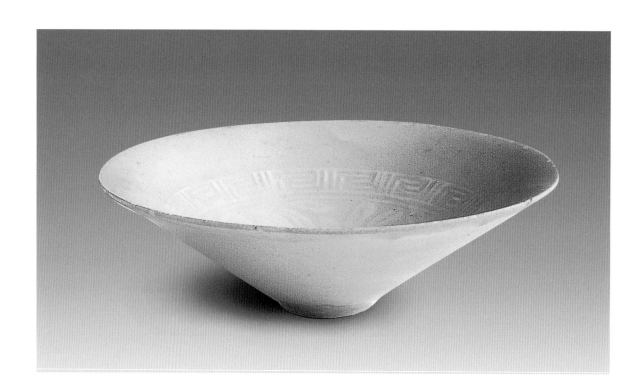

影青印花卉纹碗

宋

瓷质

口径 9.7 厘米，底径 3.2 厘米，高 6.4 厘米

Misty-blue-glazed Bowl with Stamped Floral Design

Song Dynasty

Porcelain

Mouth Diameter 9.7 cm/ Bottom Diameter 3.2 cm/ Height 6.4 cm

大敞口，小圈足。碗内腰部印回纹一周，中
央印菊花纹，纹饰清楚，施釉厚润，色略闪青。
瓷化程度高，叩之声音清脆。

梁茂年藏

The bowl has a wide flared mouth and a small
ring foot. One circular of rectangular spiral
patterns is clearly stamped in the middle of its
interior wall and a chrysanthemums pattern in
the centre of its interior bottom. Coated with
thick glaze, the bowl sheds a slightly cyan tint.
With a high degree of vitrification, it produces a
clear ring sound.

Collected by Liang Maonian

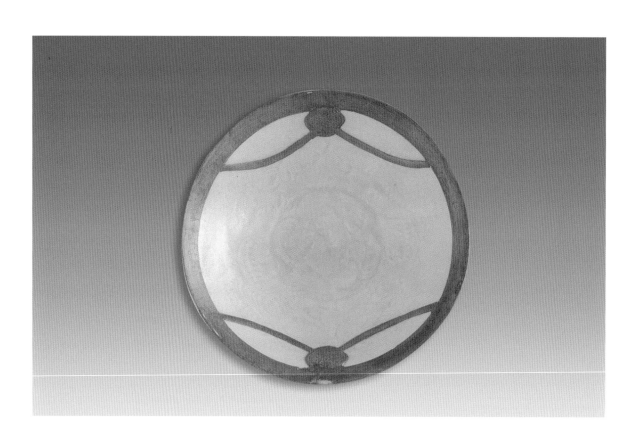

影青刻花碗

宋

瓷质

口径 21 厘米

Misty-blue-glazed Bowl with Carved Design

Song Dynasty

Porcelain

Mouth Diameter 21 cm

撇口，口沿镶银，深腹，圈足。内刻娃娃海
浪纹，刀法有力，形象生动，釉莹澈闪青色。

周振武藏

The bowl has a flared mouth with a silver-bound
mouth rim, a deep belly and a ring foot. The
interior of the bowl is skillfully incised with
vivid and lively designs of babies and waves.
The jade-like glaze looks transparent and sheds
a tint of cyan.

Collected by Zhou Zhenwu

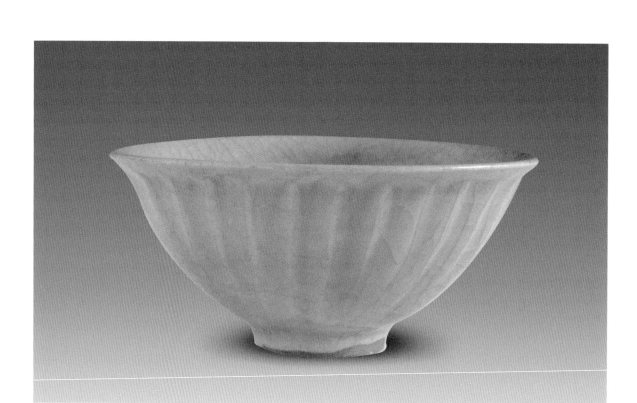

龙泉窑粉青釉菊瓣纹碗

南宋

瓷质

口径 14.8 厘米，高 7 厘米

Lavender-grey-glazed Bowl with Chrysanthemum-petal Pattern, Longquan Ware

Southern Song Dynasty

Porcelain

Mouth Diameter 14.8 cm/ Height 7 cm

敞口，弧形腹，露足，外壁刻印菊花瓣纹，
里外施粉青釉，青翠莹润，莹亮而不刺眼。
圈足内亦施釉，中心有一凸起。足沿露胎处
呈火石红，为典型的龙泉窑胎质呈色。该碗
外沿处有黄土痕，是经过长期土浸之故，当
为出土之物。

梁戊年藏

The bowl has a flared mouth, an arc-shaped
belly and an unglazed bottom. Its exterior wall
is decorated with a pattern of chrysanthemum-
petal. Lavender-grey glaze is applied to both
its inside and outside. The jade-like glaze looks
bright and transparent yet not dazzling to the
eye. A glaze is also enameled inside the ring
foot whcrc a bulge emerges at the centre. The
unglazed foot rim reveals its flint red body
which is the typical body colour of Longquan
Ware. Earth marks, resulting from long-term
burial, can be found on the outer rim of the
bowl, indicating that the bowl should be an
unearthed item.

Collected by Liang Wunian

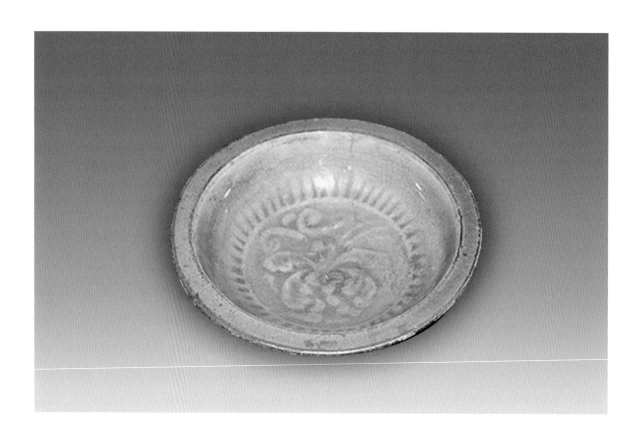

耀瓷碗

宋

瓷质

口径 11.6 厘米，底径 5.5 厘米，通高 3 厘米，重 100 克

Porcelain Bowl, Yao Ware

Song Dynasty

Porcelain

Mouth Diameter 11.6 cm/ Bottom Diameter 5.5 cm/ Height 3 cm/ Weight 100 g

平口沿，斜腹，浅圈足，黄釉碗内有菊花图，足部无釉。食器。有裂印。陕西省咸阳市秦都区征集。

陕西医史博物馆藏

The bowl has a flat mouth rim, a sloping belly and a short ring foot. A chrysanthemum pattern can be seen inside the yellow-glazed bowl. Its foot is unglazed and on the body can be seen some cracks. It served as a food container and was collected from Qindu District, Xianyang, Shaanxi Province.

Preserved in Shaanxi Museum of Medical History

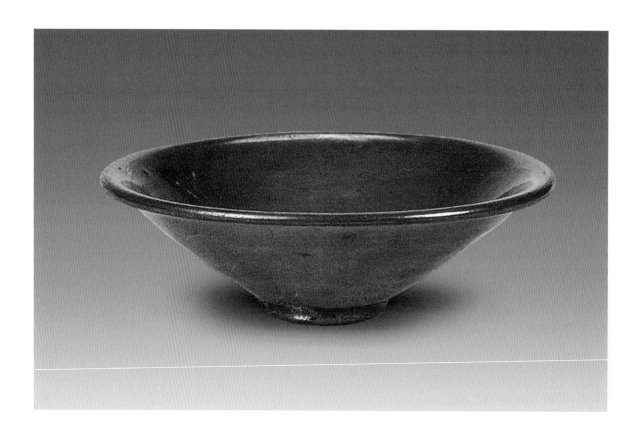

酱釉碗

宋

瓷质

口径 14.6 厘米，高 4.6 厘米

Brown-glazed Bowl

Song Dynasty

Porcelain

Mouth Diameter 14.6 cm/ Height 4.6 cm

白瓷胎，酱釉。侈口，直壁，圈足。陕西省
澄城县出土。

陕西医史博物馆藏

This bowl has a white body and is coated
with a brown glaze. It has a flared mouth, a
straight wall and a ring foot. It was unearthed in
Chengcheng County, Shaanxi Province.
Preserved in Shaanxi Museum of Medical History

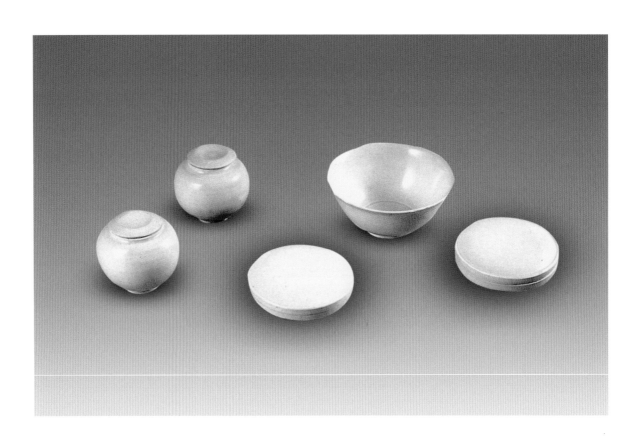

白瓷食具

金前期

瓷质

碗：口径 10.5 厘米，高 4 厘米

盒：口径 8.8 厘米，高 3 厘米

罐：口径 3.4 厘米，高 6.5 厘米

White Porcelain Food Utensils

Early Jin Dynasty

Porcelain

Bowl: Mouth Diameter 10.5 cm/ Height 4 cm

Box: Mouth Diameter 8.8 cm/ Height 3 cm

Jar: Mouth Diameter 3.4 cm/ Height 6.5 cm

薄白胎，釉层光洁而有泪痕，釉色温润而白中闪黄。其中碗的口部做成六曲花瓣口，口沿露胎无釉，小圈足；盒素而无饰，为子母口相扣；罐腹部圆鼓，口上有下凹的小盖。这些特征，都是宋金时期的定窑产品所特有。北京市海淀区南辛庄二号墓出土。

北京大学赛克勒考古与艺术博物馆藏

The white thin bodies of the utensils are coated with bright and clean glaze, on which can be seen glaze drips like "tear stains". The white glazes, soft and smooth, shed a tint of yellow. Among all the utensils, the bowl has a small ring foot and a flower-petal-shaped six-lobed mouth rim, which is unglazed. With no decorations, the buckle-lidded boxes look plain. And the jars have round bellies and concave covers on the top. All the above features belong specifically to the products made in Ding kiln of the Song Dynasty and the Jin Dynasty. The food utensils were unearthed from No.2 Tomb in Nanxin zhuang, Haidian District, Beijing. Preserved in Arthur M.Sackler Museum of Art and Archaeology at Peking University

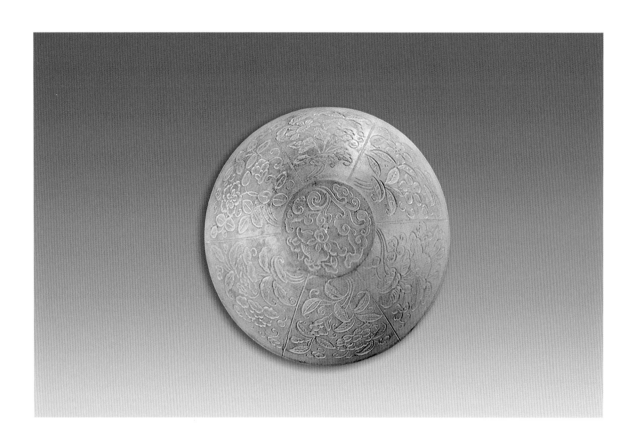

定窑四季花卉印花碗模

金

瓷质

口径 18.6 厘米，底径 6.1 厘米，高 7.3 厘米

Bowl Mould with Stamped Floral Designs, Ding Ware

Jin Dynasty

Porcelain

Mouth Diameter 18.6 cm/ Bottom Diameter 6.1 cm/ Height 7.3 cm

胎色白，质坚，胎体厚重。口内敛，深腹，平底。
外壁刻牡丹、荷花、菊花、月季花等六组不
同的花卉纹饰，底刻石榴花，纹饰繁而不乱。
内壁刻"泰和丙寅岁辛丑月二十四日画，张
记"，为金章宗泰和六年 (1206) 所制。

河北博物院藏

The body of the bowl is white, hard and heavy.
It has a contracted mouth, a deep belly and a flat
bottom. Floral patterns of six different groups,
such as peony, lotus, chrysanthemum, Chinese
rose etc, are stamped on its exterior wall and
patterns of pomegranate flowers at its bottom.
Though complicated, these patterns are well-
ordered. On its interior wall are incised "Made
by Zhang's" and made in the year 1206 under
the reign of Emperor Wanyan Jing of the Jin
Dynasty".
Preserved in Hebei Museum

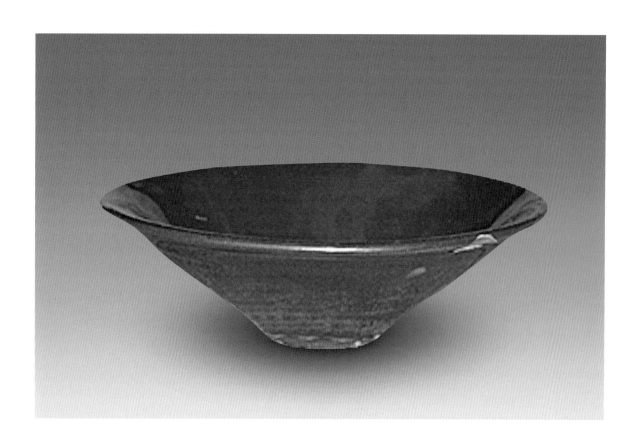

耀瓷碗

金

瓷质

口径 14.5 厘米，底径 4 厘米，通高 5 厘米，重 150 克

Porcelain Bowl, Yao Ware

Jin Dynasty

Porcelain

Mouth Diameter 14.5 cm/ Bottom Diameter 4 cm/ Height 5 cm/ Weight 150 g

敞口，圆唇，斜腹，小圈足，碗呈棕色无纹
饰。食具，生活用具。三级文物，口沿小残。
1986年入藏。陕西省澄城县盖化乡马村征集。

陕西医史博物馆藏

This bowl has a flared mouth with a round
rim, a sloping belly and a small ring foot. It is
brown-glazed with no decorations. It served
as a food utensil for daily use. It is a piece of
the third-class cultural relic and the rim of its
mouth was slightly damaged. The bowl was
collected from Ma Village, Gaihua Township,
Chengcheng County, Shaanxi Province, in
1986.

Preserved in Shaanxi Museum of Medical History

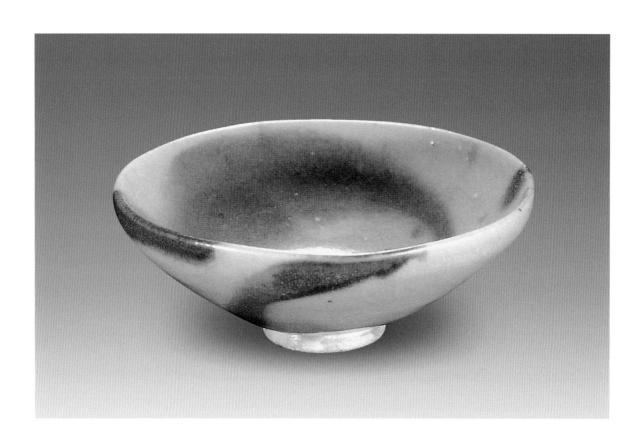

钧窑天蓝釉红斑碗

金

瓷质

口径 13.4 厘米，底径 3.9 厘米，高 4.9 厘米

Sky-blue-glazed Bowl with Red Specks, Jun Ware

Jin Dynasty

Porcelain

Mouth Diameter 13.4 cm/ Bottom Diameter 3.9 cm/ Height 4.9 cm

敛口，深腹斜壁，小圈足。胎质细腻坚硬，
色浅灰。碗施天蓝色釉，足露胎，器表有不
规则的深红色彩斑，色泽绚丽夺目。

河北博物院藏

The bowl has a contracted mouth, a deep belly,
a sloping wall and a small ring foot. The pale
grey body of the bowl is exquisite and hard.
The bowl is sky-blue-glazed with its bottom left
unglazed. Irregular dark red speckles, brilliant
and dazzling in colour, can be seen on the
surface of it.

Preserved in Hebei Museum

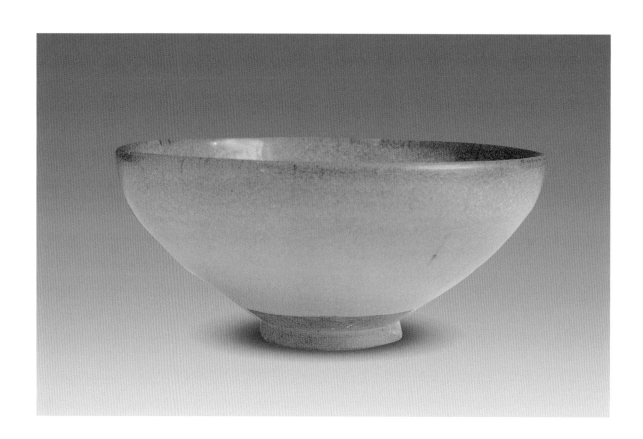

钧窑天蓝釉碗

元

瓷质

口径 16 厘米

Sky-blue-glazed Bowl, Jun Ware

Yuan Dynasty

Porcelain

Mouth Diameter 16 cm

敛口，弧形腹，圈足。里外施天蓝色乳浊釉，釉面布满小气泡，有棕眼。口沿釉薄处为浅黄褐色并杂有黑褐点，釉有流淌，近足处釉甚厚，莹亮如玉，圈足和外底无釉，胎呈灰黄色底，内心有一尖凸起，是元代碗盘器物中常见的一个特点。

伍玉琪藏

This bowl has a contracted mouth, an arc-shaped belly and a ring foot. Sky-blue opacified glaze is applied to both its inside and outside. Minute bubbles are scattered all over the glaze and pinholes can be seen on it. The glaze on the mouth rim is thin and in light yellowish-brown where it is mingled with blackish-brown dots. Due to the flowing of the glaze, the bottom is covered with thicker glaze. The ring foot and the exterior bottom are unglazed. The body of the bowl is in greyish yellow. The interior centre has a convex bulge, which is a feature commonly seen in bowls and plates of the Yuan Dynasty.

Collected by Wu Yuqi

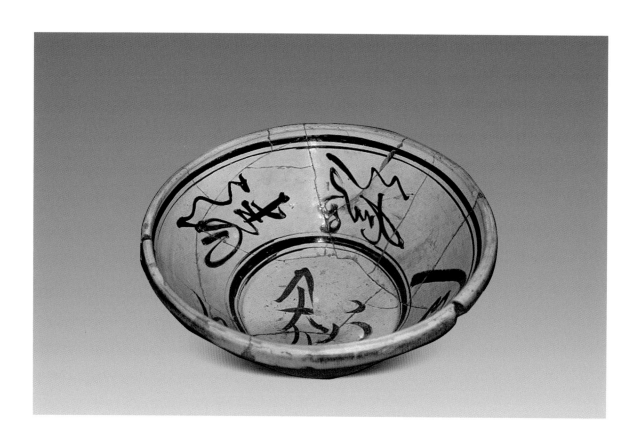

洗三盆

元

瓷质

底径 50 厘米，深 26 厘米

Xi San Pen

Yuan Dynasty

Porcelain

Bottom Diameter 50cm/ Depth 26cm

敞口，白釉褐彩，磁州窑生产。内侧绘"道德清静"
四字，盆底书"忍"字。新生儿出生第三天举办的
洗礼仪式的用具，称"洗三盆"，有点儿受洗的意思。
元代是蒙古族统治，对于汉族人来说，尽管是异族
统治，但汉人尊崇的仍旧是儒家思想，盆内侧周边
的四个字"道德清静"，盆底还有一个大大的"忍"
字，用这个盆给孩子洗礼，是要在孩子小的时候，
就要把儒家思想传递给他，同时还有让孩子从小就
有忍耐，不要惹来杀身之祸的意思。

北京御生堂中医药博物馆藏

The white-glazed basin with brown patterns has a
flared mouth and was produced in Cizhou Kiln. The
interior is carved with inscriptions of "Dao De Qing
Jing" and the bottom is carved with "Ren" (endure).
It was a tool used for infant baptism after a child was
born for three days, named "Xi San Pen". People in
Yuan Dynasty were ruled by Mongolian. However,
Han people respected the Confucianism. The basin
and the baptism meant to pass down the value of the
Confucianism since the birth of an infant and having
the virtue of endurance could prevent them from
getting into troubles as they grow up.
Preserved in Chinese Medicine Museum of Beijing Yu
Sheng Tang Drugstore

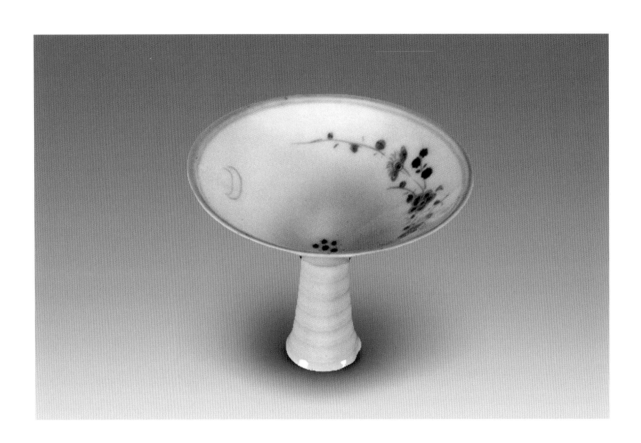

青花新月折枝梅纹高足碗

元

瓷质

口径 11.8 厘米，底径 4.5 厘米，高 9.5 厘米

Blue-and-white Stem Bowl with Crescent and Plum Blossom Designs

Yuan Dynasty

Porcelain

Mouth Diameter 11.8 cm/ Bottom Diameter 4.5 cm/ Height 9.5 cm

胎薄而坚致，洁白细腻，釉色白中闪青，晶
莹润泽，敞口，斜直壁，竹节状高足，足端
露胎，造型小巧秀丽。内壁绘青花月影梅纹，
画面明朗清幽，发色淡雅明快。

河北博物院藏

The body of the bowl is thin and hard, white
and smooth. It is glazed white with a tint of
blue, looking bright, crystal-clear, and mellow.
With a flared mouth, a sloping and straight wall,
a bamboo-like tall foot and an unglazed foot
rim, the bowl is beautiful and exquisite. Blue-
and-white crescent and plum blossom patterns
are painted on its interior wall, creating a bright
and quiet picture, in a simple, elegant and lively
colour.

Preserved in Hebei Museum

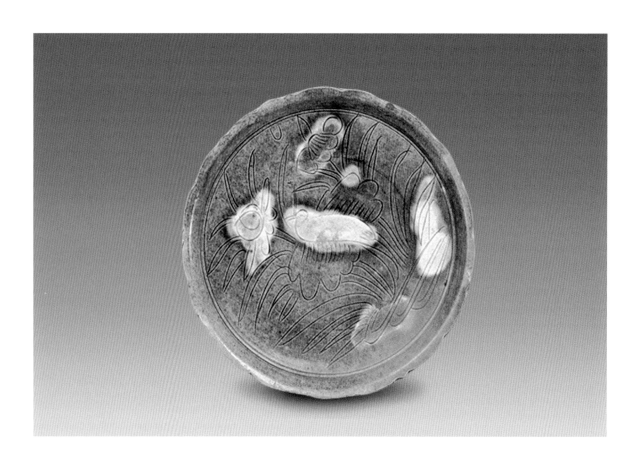

陶三彩刻花鹭莲纹盘

辽

瓷质

口径 18.2 厘米，足径 10.7 厘米，高 2.2 厘米

Tricolour Pottery Plate Incised with Design of Egret and Lotus

Liao Dynasty

Porcelain

Mouth Diameter 18.2 cm/ Foot Diameter 10.7 cm/ Height 2.2 cm

陶盘浅式，九瓣菱花口，盘心平坦，圈足。内底以细线划出荷塘景色，水中一只鹭鸶穿游荷莲中，鹭鸶与莲花涂黄色，荷叶涂葡萄紫色，其余地方施绿釉。

故宫博物院藏

This plate is shallow, wide and flat with a ring foot. Its mouth rim is in the shape of a nine-petal water-chestnut flower. Scenery of lotus pond is carved in fine lines on its interior bottom. And an egret is swimming in the pond among lotus flowers. Both the egret and lotus flowers are painted yellow and the lotus leaf grape-purple. The rest of the interior is green-glazed.

Preserved in the Palace Museum

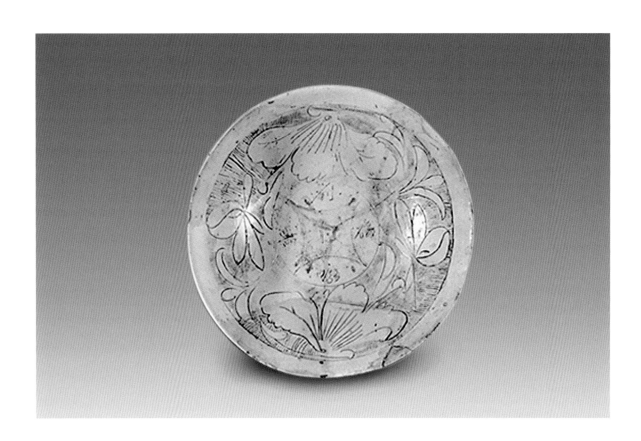

白釉划花"刘家磁器"盘

北宋

瓷质

口径 28.5 厘米，底径 8.7 厘米，高 9 厘米

White-glazed Plate with Incised Inscriptions of "Porcelain Ware of the Liu Family"

Northern Song Dynasty

Porcelain

Mouth Diameter 28.5 cm/ Bottom Diameter 8.7 cm/ Height 9 cm

盘底划出一枚铜钱，钱文为"刘家磁器"。

钱文之外的周壁上，是两两相对的四朵莲花，

以篦刷纹为地。花纹内部是化妆土的白色，

花纹的轮廓线则是胎体的深灰色，对比鲜明

而有层次。民用食具。河南省鹤壁市鹤壁集

窑出土。

河南省文物考古研究院藏

On the interior bottom of the plate is incised a
coin with the inscription of "Porcelain ware by
the Liu family". Two pairs of symmetrical lotus
flowers are carved on the plate's interior wall
with a background of comb patterns. The pale
white flower patterns are in sharp contrasts to
their dark grey contour lines. The plate served
as a food utensil and was unearthed from Hebi
Ji Kiln in Hebi, Henan Province.
Preserved in Henan Provincial Institute of
Cultural Heritage and Archaeology

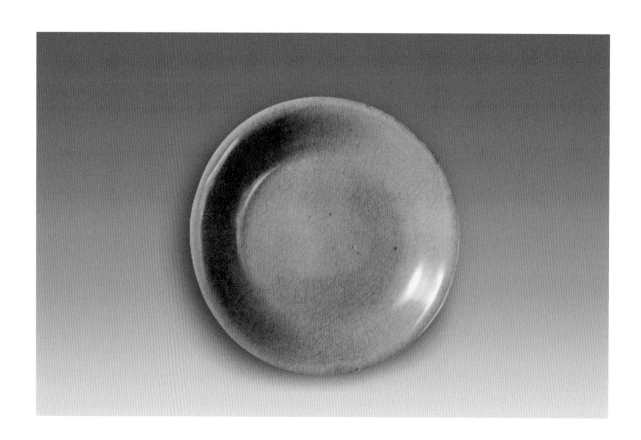

天青釉汝瓷盘

北宋

瓷质

口径 17.1 厘米，高 2.9 厘米

Greyish-celadon-glazed Porcelain Plate, Ru Ware

Northern Song Dynasty

Porcelain

Mouth Diameter 17.1 cm/ Height 2.9 cm

敞口，浅腹，坦底圈足，此外便无其他的线条。盘内外满饰淡青色乳浊釉，满身细碎开片，色调温润深邃。品味大雅之极。北宋汝瓷的雅致与唐三彩的富丽实为中国传统瓷业的并峙双峰。

上海博物馆藏

With a flared mouth, a shallow belly, a wide and flat bottom and a ring foot, the plate has no decoration. Both the interior and exterior of this plate are coated with opaque celadon glaze with small crackles. The mild and mellow colour of the glaze reflects an elegant taste. Refined porcelain Ru ware of the Northern Song Dynasty and gorgeous tricolour porcelain of the Tang Dynasty represent the two peaks in the traditional Chinese ceramics industry. Preserved in Shanghai Museum

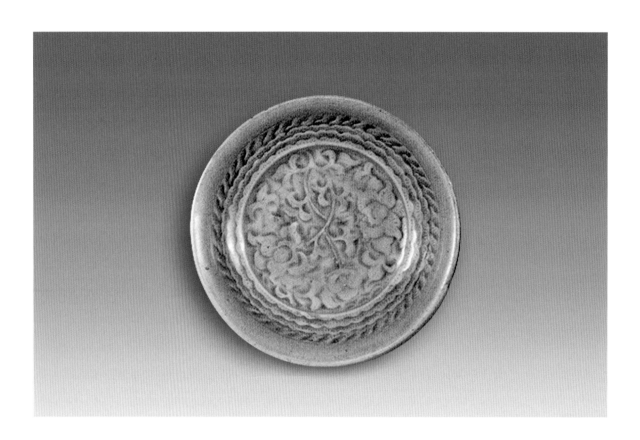

豆青釉印花盘

北宋

瓷质

口径 14.6 厘米，底径 5.3 厘米，高 2.8 厘米

Pea-green-glazed Plate with Stamped Floral Design

Northern Song Dynasty

Porcelain

Mouth Diameter 14.6 cm/ Bottom Diameter 5.3 cm/ Height 2.8 cm

敞口，弧壁，平底，圈足，盘心模印出折枝花卉，周围环绕着水波纹，内外满施豆青色釉，但底足处露出稍泛黄色的胎体，足部也粘有砂粒而略显粗糙，但具有浓郁的生活气息，是民间汝瓷的典型器皿。

广东省博物馆藏

The plate has a flared mouth, a curved wall, a flat bottom, and a ring foot. A pattern of flower branches surrounded by ripple patterns is stamped on the plate's interior bottom. Both the interior and exterior of this plate are coated with pea green glaze, while its bottom is unglazed revealing a slight yellowish body. Grains of sand can also be seen on its foot which shows a bit of roughness of the vessel. Nevertheless, the plate is brimmed with strong flavour of life and is typical of Ru folk ware.

Preserved in Guangdong Museum

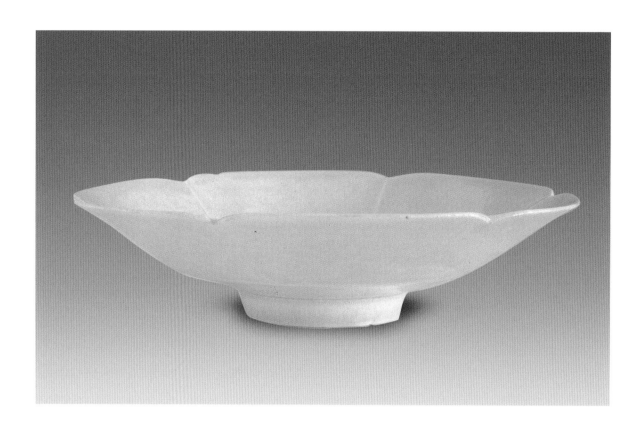

影青釉刻花瓣口盘

北宋

瓷质

口径 12.3 厘米，高 5.5 厘米

Misty-blue-glazed Plate with a Flower-petal-shaped Mouth

Northern Song Dynasty

Porcelain

Mouth Diameter 12.3 cm/ Height 5.5 cm

撇口，六瓣形口沿，斜腹，矮圈足。内壁六直道纹与花口和内底相连，盘中刻花卉，花瓣上划以篦纹，此种刻画法盛于北宋中晚期。盘里外施影青釉，白中显青，十分莹亮，有如青白玉般的质感。底无釉，切削工整，胎质细洁，应是江西湖田窑的产品。影青装饰除江西湖田窑生产外，还有江西南羊窑、吉州窑，安徽繁昌窑，广东潮州窑，福建、湖南、湖北、广西、河南等地都有生产，而以江西湖田窑最负盛名。

李庆全藏

The plate has a flared mouth with a six-lobed rim, a sloping belly and a short ring foot. There are six straight lines on the interior wall linking the mouth rim and the interior bottom. Inside the plate are carved floral patterns, with comb patterns on the petals. This kind of carving style prevailed during the middle and late Northern Song Dynasty. Both the interior and the exterior of the plate are misty-blue-glazed shedding a tint of cyan. The plate looks lustrous and bright resembling a light greenish-white jade. Its bottom is unglazed and neatly cut. With an exquisite and clean body, the plate should be made in Hutian kiln of Jiangxi Province. Besides Hutian kiln, there were many other kilns that could produce misty-blue-glazed porcelain ware, such as Nanyang kiln and Jizhou kiln of Jiangxi Province, Fanchang kiln of Anhui Province, Chaozhou kiln of Guangdong Province and other regions in Fujian Province, Hunan Province, Hubei Province, Guangxi Province and Henan Province. However, of all these kilns, Hutian kiln is the most famous.

Collected by Li Qingquan

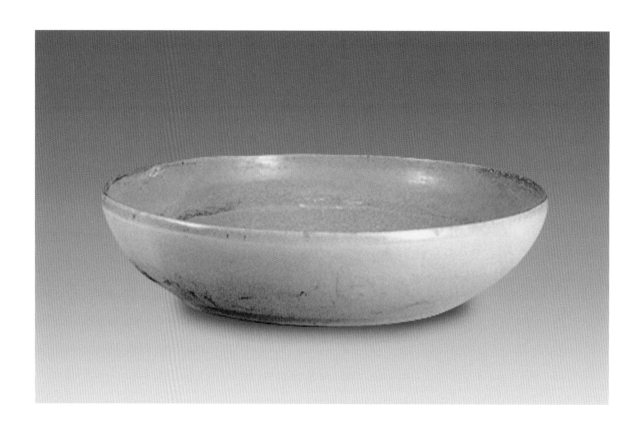

钧瓷盘

北宋

瓷质

口径 27.4 厘米，底径 18.5 厘米，高 6.8 厘米

Porcelain Plate, Jun Ware

Northern Song Dynasty

Porcelain

Mouth Diameter 27.4 cm/ Bottom Diameter 18.5 cm/ Height 6.8 cm

厚厚的质料与乳浊状的天蓝釉，既有沉重的历史感，又富有神秘的气息。底足露出的赭色胎骨和五个乳突状支烧痕更透出沧桑与古朴。其胎釉、造型，都是钧瓷的典型风格。同时出土的还有 2 个烙饼子的铁鏊、4 个盛饭的瓷碗、2 个盛菜的瓷盘。1978 年裴李岗文化石固遗址出土。

河南省文物考古研究院藏

The thick body together with the sky-blue opaque glaze not only carries a strong sense of history but is also full of mystery. The ochre body revealed from the unglazed bottom and the five papilla-shaped firing marks caused by the holder during the kilning process further show its vicissitudes and primitive simplicity. Its glaze colour and shape are typical of Jun ware. Besides, two frying pans used for baking pancakes, four porcelain bowls for containing rice and two porcelain plates for containing dishes were unearthed together with this plate. They were all excavated from the historical site of Peiligang Culture in 1978.

Preserved in Henan Provincial Institute of Cultural Heritage and Archaeology

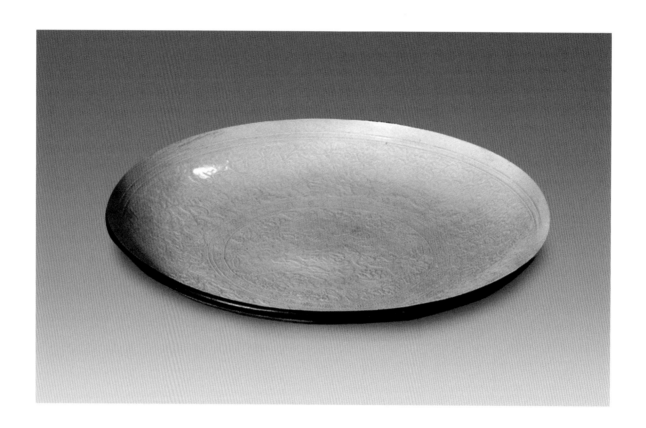

定窑印花缠枝莲大盘

北宋

瓷质

口径 30.1 厘米，底径 13.5 厘米，高 5.6 厘米

Large Plate Stamped with Interlocking Lotus Design, Ding Ware

Northern Song Dynasty

Porcelain

Mouth Diameter 30.1 cm/ Bottom Diameter 13.5 cm/ Height 5.6 cm

胎洁白细腻而致密，釉色白中微闪黄，积釉处有"泪痕"。敞口，斜弧腹，圈足。口部镶铜沿，内壁印缠枝花，底心印折枝莲纹，两组纹饰间以回纹相隔，纹饰层次清晰，线条流畅，是宋代定窑印花工艺的典型作品。

河北博物院藏

The white body of the plate is of exquisite and compact texture. Its white glaze shines a tint of yellow and glaze drips like "tear stains" are formed where the glaze coagulated. The plate has a flared mouth with copper-bound mouth rim, a sloping and curved belly and a ring foot. Interlocking floral patterns are stamped on its interior wall and a pattern of lotus branches at its bottom centre. Between the above two groups of patterns is found a ring of rectangular spiral pattern. All the decorations are clearly layered and smoothly lined, which is typical of stamped Ding ware of the Song Dynasty.

Preserved in Hebei Museum

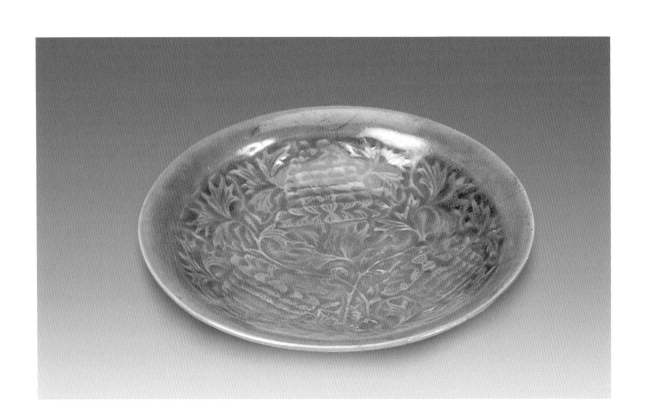

青釉牡丹纹瓷盘

宋

瓷质

口径 19.5 厘米，底径 5.8 厘米，高 4.8 厘米

宽大厚重，腹部平浅，平底，圈足，绘牡丹纹。

昭陵博物馆藏

Celadon Plate with Peony Patterns

Song Dynasty

Porcelain

Mouth Diameter 19.5 cm/ Bottom Diameter 5.8 cm/ Height 4.8 cm

The plate, wide, thick, and heavy, has a flat and shallow belly, a flat bottom, and a ring foot. It is painted with peony patterns.

Preserved in Zhaoling Museum

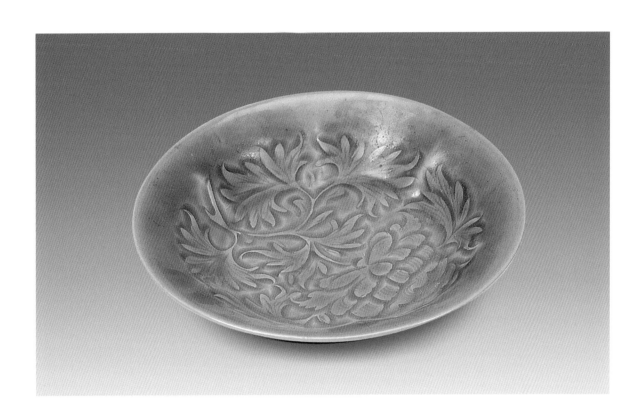

青釉缠枝牡丹纹瓷盘

宋

瓷质

口径 18 厘米，底径 5.5 厘米，高 3.5 厘米

敞口，浅腹，平底，圈足，绘缠枝牡丹纹。

昭陵博物馆藏

Celadon plate with interlocking peony patterns

Song Dynasty

Porcelain

Mouth Diameter 18 cm/ Bottom Diameter 5.5 cm/ Height 3.5 cm

The plate has a flared mouth, a shallow body, a flat bottom and a ring foot. It is stamped with interlocking peony patterns.

Preserved in Zhaoling Museum

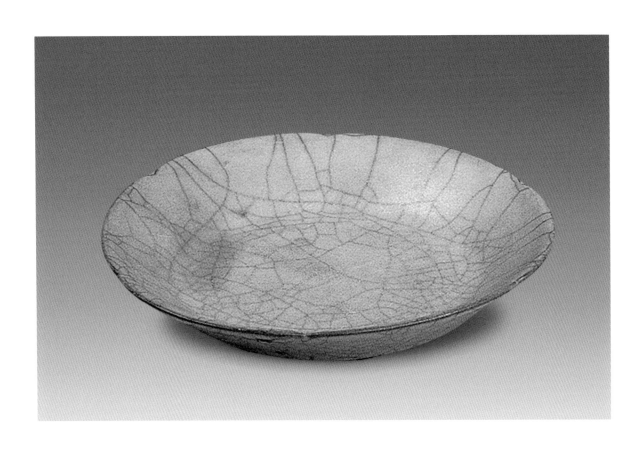

官窑青釉冰裂纹瓷盘

宋

瓷质

口径 13.9 厘米，底径 7.1 厘米，高 2.5 厘米

Celadon-glazed Porcelain Plate with Ice Cracks, Guan Ware

Song Dynasty

Porcelain

Mouth Diameter 13.9 cm/ Bottom Diameter 7.1 cm/ Height 2.5 cm

灰色胎，青灰色釉。釉面平滑，釉质光滑如玉，六股葵瓣口。口稍外撇，浅壁，折腰，矮圈足，圈足内有六支烧钉痕迹。盘内外施釉，自然开裂的纹片横竖交织如网。整个盘的造型极规整，制作精细，为南宋时期官窑之佳作。南京中央门外汪兴祖墓出土。

南京博物院藏

This plate has a grey body, coated with greyish celadon glaze, which is as smooth as jade. The plate has a slightly flared mouth with a six-lobed rim in the shape of mallow petals, a shallow wall, an angular waist and a short ring foot. Six firing nail marks can be seen in the ring foot. Both the interior and exterior of the plate are glazed with crackles intertwining like a net. Neatly shaped and exquisitely designed, the plate is a masterpiece made in the Guan kiln of the Southern Song Dynasty. It was unearthed in the ancestral tomb of Wang Xing, outside the central gate of Nanjing, Jiangsu Province.

Preserved in Nanjing Museum

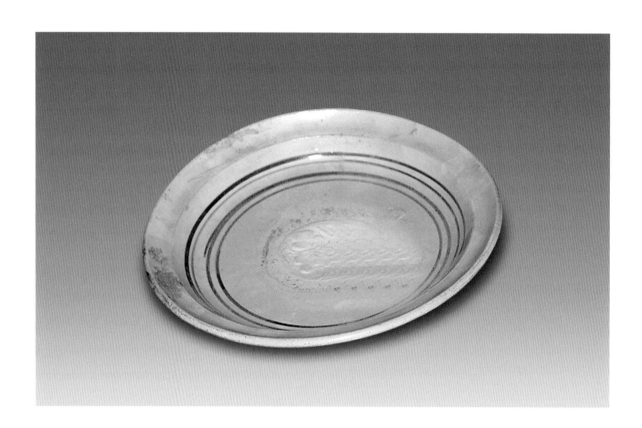

粗瓷大盘

元

瓷质

口径 21 厘米，底径 8 厘米，通高 4 厘米，重 500 克

Large Coarse Porcelain Plate

Yuan Dynasty

Porcelain

Mouth Diameter 21 cm/ Bottom Diameter 8 cm/ Height 4 cm/ Height 500 g

内粗白瓷，外黑釉，盘内为四周弦纹，圈足。

食器。完整无损。

陕西医史博物馆藏

The interior of the plate is coated with a white coarse glaze and the exterior with a black glaze. The plate has a ring foot and a pattern of four circles of strings are found inside the plate. It served as a food container and is well-preserved.

Preserved in Shaanxi Museum of Medical History

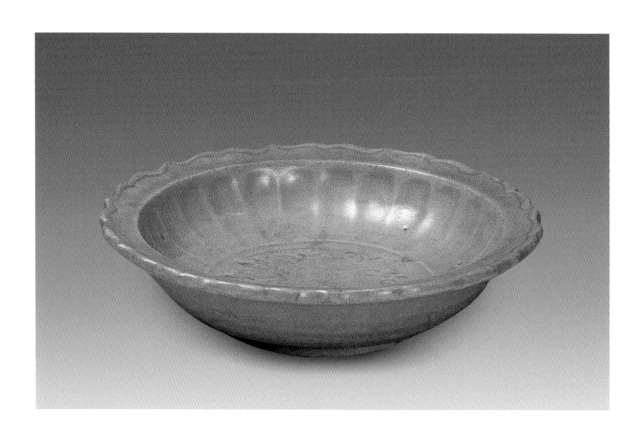

龙泉窑瓷盘

元

瓷质

口径 24.3 厘米，高 4.7 厘米

Porcelain Plate, Longquan Ware

Yuan Dynasty

Porcelain

Mouth Diameter 24.3 cm/ Height 4.7 cm

盘口为十瓣菱花口，盘心平坦，中心微凸，圈足。
盘心正中模印十字形小花，外为一圈模印卷草纹
带。整个大盘施青绿色釉，釉色较为晶莹。圈足
内无釉，呈火石红色。该盘造型规整，胎厚骨重，
全器显得浑厚、古朴。溧水区人民银行大楼王地
窖藏出土。

溧水区博物馆藏

This plate has a ten-lobed mouth rim in the shape of
a water-chestnut flower, and a ring foot. Its bottom
is wide and flat, with the centre raised slightly.
Small cross-shaped flowers are stamped right in
the centre of the plate surrounded by one circle
of scrolled grass pattern. The plate is coated with
bright and lustrous celadon glaze with the flint red
inside of the ring foot unglazed. Neatly shaped with
a thick and heavy body, the plate looks dignified and
simple. It was unearthed from the cellar under the
building of People's Bank of China, Lishui District,
Jiangsu Province.

Preserved in Lishui Museum

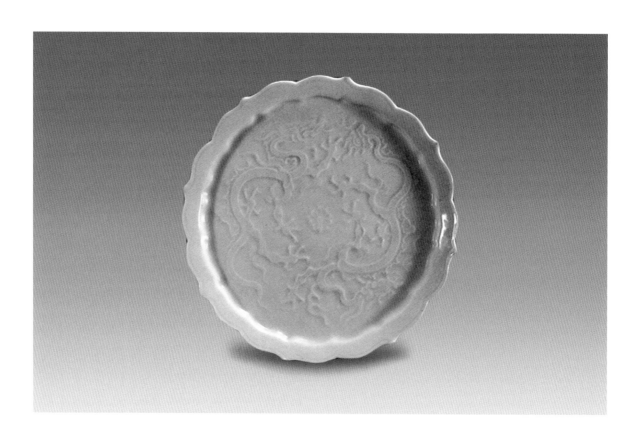

青白釉印龙纹菱花形盘

元

瓷质

口径 16.2 厘米，底径 13.5 厘米，高 1.9 厘米

Bluish-white-glazed Plate with Stamped Dragon and Water-chestnut Flower Designs

Yuan Dynasty

Porcelain

Mouth Diameter 16.2 cm/ Bottom Diameter 13.5 cm/ Height 1.9 cm

胎体轻薄，胎质洁白坚硬而致密，青白釉，
釉面莹润光亮。盘为八瓣菱花形，浅腹，平底，
内模印二龙戏珠。

河北博物院藏

The white thin body of the plate is of solid and
compact texture and covered with bright and
smooth bluish-white glaze. The plate is in the
shape of a water-chestnut flower with eight
petals. It has a shallow belly and a flat bottom.
A pattern of two dragons playing with a pearl is
stamped on its interior bottom.

Preserved in Hebei Museum

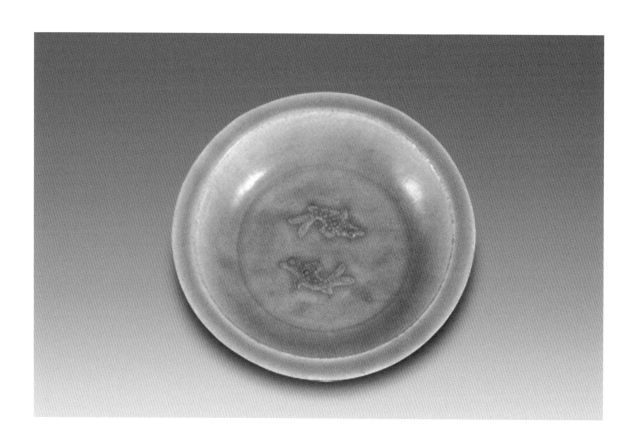

青釉双鱼盘

元

瓷质

口径 22.2 厘米，高 4.9 厘米

Celadon-glazed Plate with Twin-fish Design

Yuan Dynasty

Porcelain

Mouth Diameter 22.2 cm/ Height 4.9 cm

盘为传世品。盘宽折沿，浅弧腹，平底，盘
内底贴首尾相对的模印双鱼。胎青灰细腻，
满施青绿色釉，厚润晶莹，有细开片，游
鱼刻画精美自然，为元代龙泉窑特色产品。

扬州博物馆藏

This plate is handed down from the ancient
times. It has a wide angular mouth rim, a
shallow and curved belly and a flat bottom. A
head-to-tail twin-fish motif is stamped on its
interior bottom. The greenish grey body of the
plate is exquisite, and coated with celadon glaze
with small crackles. The glaze looks smooth
and bright and the stamped fish looks subtle and
natural. The plate is a featured product made in
Longquan Kiln of the Yuan Dynasty.
Preserved in Yangzhou Museum

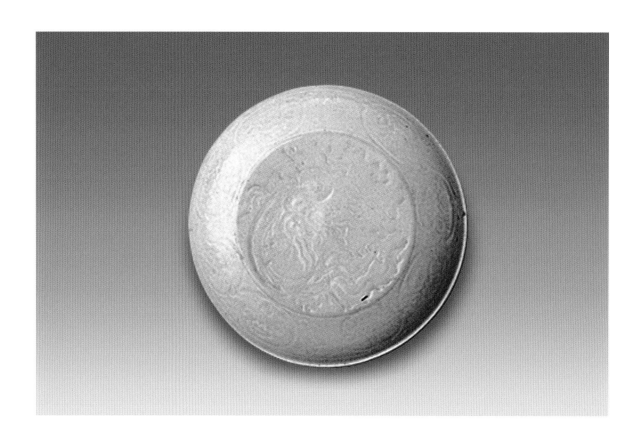

卵白釉印花瓷盘

元

瓷质

口径 17.8 厘米，底径 11.4 厘米

Egg-white-glazed Porcelain Plate with Stamped Flower Design

Yuan Dynasty

Porcelain

Mouth Diameter 17.8 cm/ Bottom Diameter 11.4 cm

浅腹，矮足，胎质细腻。内外施卵白色釉，釉层较厚而局部泛青，釉面光润，盘底内模印独龙戏珠纹样，周壁上印出变体缠枝莲花纹，莲纹上托"八宝"，纹间印有"太禧"2字。盘外壁刻有一周"八大码"纹。传世有"太禧"字样的枢府瓷，目前所知仅有两件（另一件存故宫博物院），此为其中之一。其底内所印龙纹为五爪二角，应是御用之器。

北京大学赛克勒考古与艺术博物馆藏

The plate has a shallow belly, a short foot and an exquisite body. Both its interior and exterior are coated with thick and smooth egg-white glaze with a cyan shine at some parts. A pattern of a dragon playing with a pearl is stamped on the interior bottom of the plate and variant interlocking lotus patterns on the interior wall. "Babao" (Eight Buddhist Emblems) emerge on the lotus patterns, among which are stamped two Chinese characters "Tai Xi" (An Executive Branch of the Royal Court). The exterior wall of the plate is incised with one circle of lotus petal design. This plate is one of the only two porcelain vessels with the Chinese characters of "Taixi" made for the Privy Council of the Yuan Dynasty (the other one is Preserved in the Palace Museum). The dragon pattern stamped on the interior bottom of the plate has five claws and two horns, indicating that the plate was used by the imperial family.

Preserved in Arthur M.Sackler Museum of Art and Archaeology at Peking University

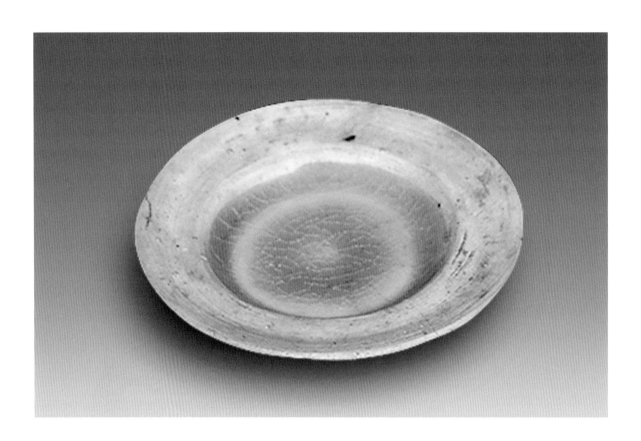

小瓷碟

宋

瓷质

口径 8 厘米，底径 4 厘米，高 1 厘米，重 500 克

Small Porcelain Dish

Song Dynasty

Porcelain

Mouth Diameter 8 cm/ Bottom Diameter 4 cm/ Height 1 cm/ Weight 500 g

盘口，平底，盘内底施豆青釉，盘沿和底外
无釉。食器。完整。陕西省西安市八仙庵征集。

陕西医史博物馆藏

This dish has a plate-shaped mouth and a flat
bottom. And it is coated with a yellowish-
pea-green glaze on its interior bottom, while
the mouth rim and the exterior bottom are left
unglazed. It served as a food container and is
in good condition. The dish was collected from
Baxian Nunnery, Xi'an, Shaanxi Province.
Preserved in Shaanxi Museum of Medical History

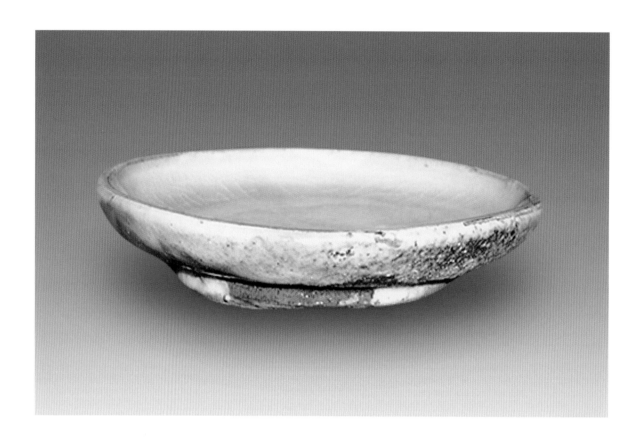

小瓷碟

宋

瓷质

口径 7 厘米，底径 4.5 厘米，高 1.1 厘米，重 40g

Small Porcelain Dish

Song Dynasty

Porcelain

Mouth Diameter 7 cm/ Bottom Diameter 4.5 cm/ Height 1.1 cm/ Weight 40 g

盘口，浅圈足，豆青色。食器。完整。2001
年9月入藏。陕西省西安市古玩市场八仙庵
征集。

陕西医史博物馆藏

Coated with a yellowish-pea-green glaze, the
dish has a plate-shaped mouth and a shallow
ring foot. It served as a food container and was
well preserved. The dish was collected from the
antique market of Xi'an, Shaanxi Province, in
September 2001.

Preserved in Shaanxi Museum of Medical History

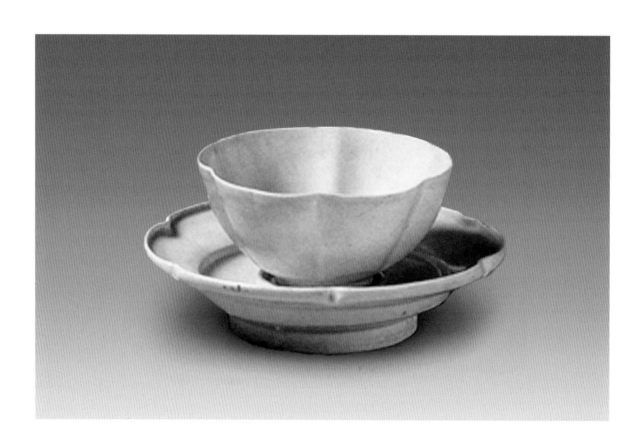

青白瓷带托茶盏

北宋

瓷质

高 6.5 厘米

Greenish-white-glazed Cup and Saucer

Northern Song Dynasty

Porcelain

Height 6.5 cm

由茶盏和盏托组成，敞口，呈六瓣莲蓬形，弧腹，圈足，底无釉，茶托形若小盘，圈足，底露胎。托座从盘内底凸起，矮于周边，中凹成平台，略大干盏足。这套带托茶盏胎质洁白细腻，釉色青白，盏、托底部均有渣饼垫烧遗留的浅褐色，是景德镇湖田窑烧制的产品。溧水区物资局宿舍工地宋墓出土。

溧水区博物馆藏

This vessel is made up of a cup and a saucer. The cup has a flared mouth in the shape of a six-petalled lotus seedpod, a curved belly and a ring foot, while the saucer looks like a small plate and has a ring foot as well. The bottoms of both the cup and the saucer are unglazed. The convex interior bottom of the saucer is lower than the saucer rim, forming a concave platform which is slightly larger than the cup's foot. This set of cup and saucer has an exquisite and pure white body coated with greenish-white glaze. Beige marks caused by the cushioning tool during the firing process can be seen on the bottoms of both the cup and the saucer. The vessel was produced by Hutian kiln in Jingdezhen Township and was unearthed from a tomb of the Song Dynasty in the dormitory construction site of Commodities Bureau of Lishui District, Jiangsu Province.

Preserved in Lishui Museum

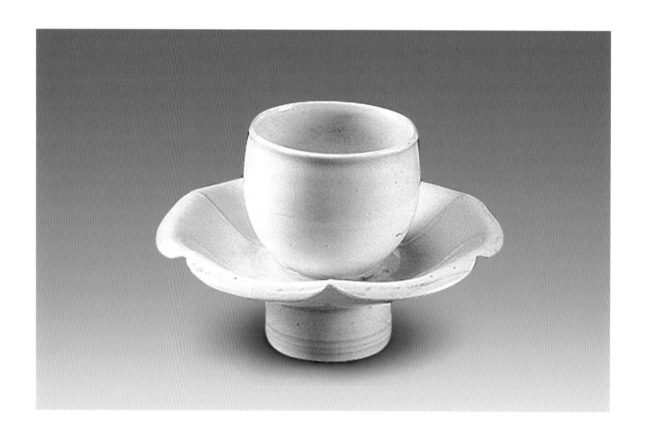

景德镇窑青白釉荷叶形托盏

北宋

瓷质

盏径 7.8 厘米，托径 13.8 厘米，底径 4.8 厘米，高 8.7 厘米

Greenish-white-glazed Cup and Saucer with Lotus-leaf-shaped Saucer, Jingdezhen Ware

Northern Song Dynasty

Porcelain

Cup Diameter 7.8 cm/ Saucer Diameter 13.8 cm/ Bottom Diameter 4.8 cm/ Height 8.7 cm

盏为小唇口，弧壁较深，下连六出荷叶形盏托，高圈足微外撇，圈足内可见垫烧痕，釉色青白滋润，胎体致密轻薄。

常州博物馆藏

The cup has a small lip-shaped mouth and a deep curved wall with its bottom connecting to the saucer which is in the shape of a six-lobed lotus leaf. The saucer has a tall ring foot with a slightly flared rim. Marks caused by cushioning tools during the firing process can be seen inside the foot ring. The vessel has a light and compact body coated with smooth greenish white glaze.

Preserved in Changzhou Museum

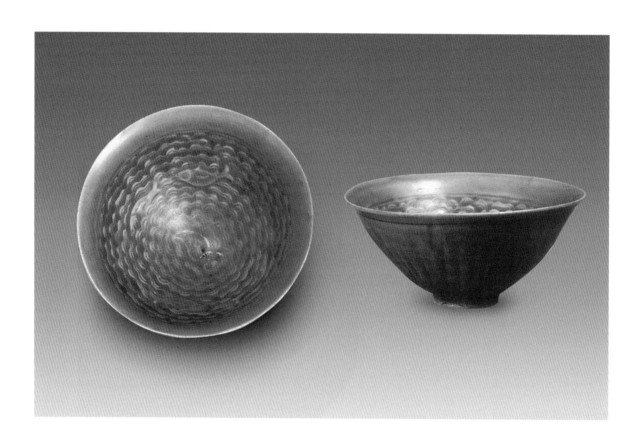

青釉水波鱼纹盏

北宋

瓷质

口径 12.4 厘米，底径 3.6 厘米，高 5.8 厘米

Celadon-glazed Cup with Ripple and Fish Patterns

Northern Song Dynasty

Porcelain

Mouth Diameter 12.4 cm/ Bottom Diameter 3.6 cm/ Height 5.8 cm

整器成斗笠形，敞口外撇，小弧腹，矮圈足，青灰薄胎，碗内剔刻 11 圈水波纹，中部刻饰四条腹向上背向下的鱼纹，外壁刻饰扇骨纹。水波纹起伏自然，鱼纹生动活泼，盏内外满施青绿色釉，透明莹润。1995 年宝应北宁墓群出土，系临汝窑产品。

宝应博物馆藏

Resembling a bamboo hat, the cup has a flared mouth, a slightly curved belly and a short ring foot. It has a celadon-grey thin body with eleven circles of ripple patterns scraped and carved on its interior wall and four belly-up fish patterns in the middle of them. The exterior of the cup is decorated with fan rib patterns. The ripple patterns look natural and the fish patterns vivid. Both the interior and the exterior of the cup are celadon-green-glazed, translucent and smooth. The cup was produced by Linru kiln and was unearthed from Beining tombs, Baoying County, Jiangsu Province, in 1995. Preserved in Baoying Museum

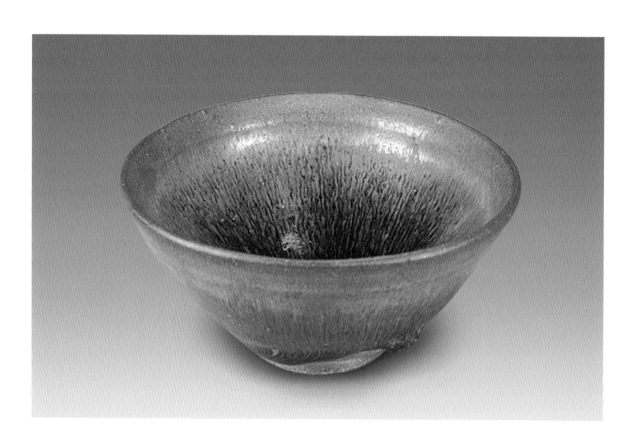

建窑黑釉兔毫盏

宋

瓷质

口径 12.5 厘米，底径 4.2 厘米，高 6 厘米

Black-glazed Small Cup with Cony-hair Pattern, Jian Ware

Song Dynasty

Porcelain

Mouth Diameter 12.5 cm/ Bottom Diameter 4.2 cm/ Height 6 cm

敞口，内沿以下一周微凸，斜壁深腹，小圈
足较浅。釉面显现兔毫结晶斑纹。外壁釉不
及底，并有聚釉、炸釉现象。胎体厚重，呈
铁褐色。

常州博物馆藏

The cup has a flared mouth, a sloping wall, a deep belly, and a shallow small ring foot with the part under the interior rim protruding slightly. Crystallized cony-hair patterns can be seen on the glaze. Its bottom is left unglazed and reveals coagulated glaze and crackles. The cup has a heavy body in iron brown.

Preserved in Changzhou Museum

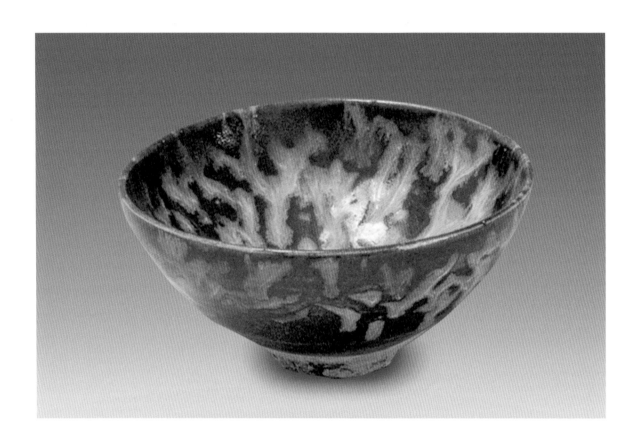

吉州窑玳瑁天目盏

宋

瓷质

口径 10.7 厘米，底径 3.5 厘米，高 5 厘米

Small Tianmu Cup with Hawksbill-coloured Glaze, Jizhou Ware

Song Dynasty

Porcelain

Mouth Diameter 10.7 cm/ Bottom Diameter 3.5 cm/ Height 5 cm

敛口，内壁满施褐釉，外壁施釉不到底。不
同色泽的釉面装饰出于天然，奇巧美丽，由
此可见宋人的生活审美情趣。南京市区出土。

南京博物院藏

This cup has a contracted mouth. Both its
interior and the exterior are brown-glazed,
but the bottom is left unglazed. Hawksbill-
coloured glaze decorates the cup in a natural
and ingenious way. It reveals the aesthetic taste
of the people in the Song Dynasty. The cup
was unearthed in downtown Nanjing, Jiangsu
Province.

Preserved in Nanjing Museum

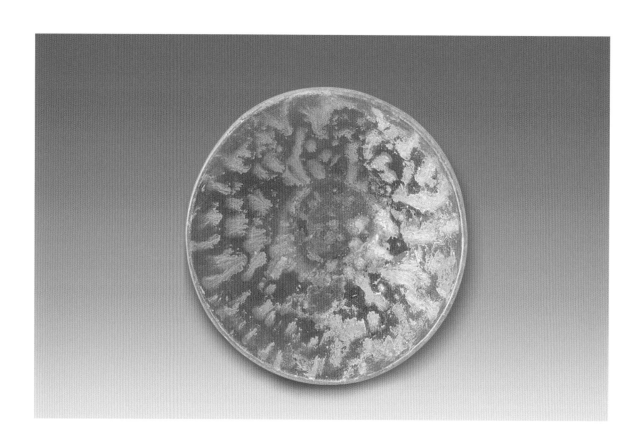

吉州窑玳瑁釉盏

宋

瓷质

口径 12 厘米

Small Cup with Hawksbill-coloured Glaze, Jizhou Ware

Song Dynasty

Porcelain

Mouth Diameter 12 cm

敛口，至足渐收，小浅圈足，里外施玳瑁釉，
圈足无釉，胎呈浅黄色，挖足草率。玳瑁釉
是宋代江西吉州窑代表品种之一。

林存义藏

The cup has a contracted mouth which gradually tapers down to the foot and a shallow small ring foot. The interior and the exterior of the cup are coated with Hawksbill-coloured glaze, but the ring foot is unglazed. The body of the cup is in pale yellow and its foot is shaped curtly. Hawksbill-coloured glaze is one of the representative glazes of Jizhou ware of Jiangxi Province in the Song Dynasty.

Collected by Lin Cunyi

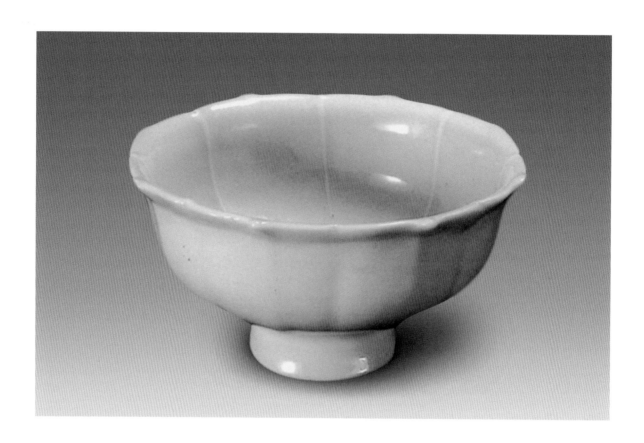

青白釉印龙纹菱花口盏

元

瓷质

口径 8.1 厘米，底径 3 厘米，盏高 4 厘米

Bluish-white-glazed Small Cup with Stamped Dragon Pattern and Water-chestnut-shaped Mouth

Yuan Dynasty

Porcelain

Mouth Diameter 8.1 cm/ Bottom Diameter 3 cm/ Height 4 cm

胎体轻薄，胎质洁白坚硬而致密，青白釉，釉面莹润光亮。盏为八瓣菱花形，弧腹，小圈足微外撇，足端露胎，内壁八条出筋，均匀的将腹部分为八个花瓣。

河北博物院藏

The purely white thin body of the cup is of hard and compact texture. The cup is coated with smooth bluish-white glaze. It is in the shape of an eight-petalled water-chestnut flower, and has a curved belly and a small slightly flared ring foot. The foot rim is unglazed. Eight ridge lines can be seen on the interior wall of the cup and they evenly divide the belly into eight petals.

Preserved in Hebei Museum

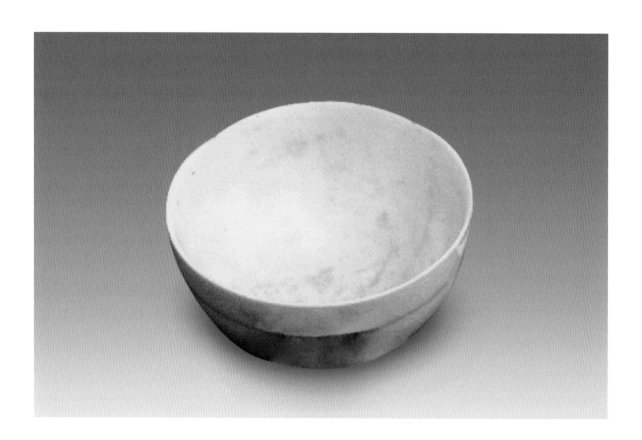

影青窑杯

宋

瓷质

口外径 7.3 厘米，底径 3.3 厘米，通高 3.9 厘米，腹深 3.5 厘米，重 61 克

Misty-blue-glazed Cup

Song Dynasty

Porcelain

Mouth Diameter 7.3 cm/ Bottom Diameter 3.3 cm/ Height 3.9 cm/ Depth 3.5 cm/ Weight 61 g

形似今小碗，平底，有瓜裂纹饰。饮水、酒等器皿。

广东中医药博物馆藏

The cup resembles a small bowl with a flat bottom. It has crackles which look like cracks in a melon. It served as a drinking and wine vessel. Preserved in Guangdong Chinese Medicine Museum

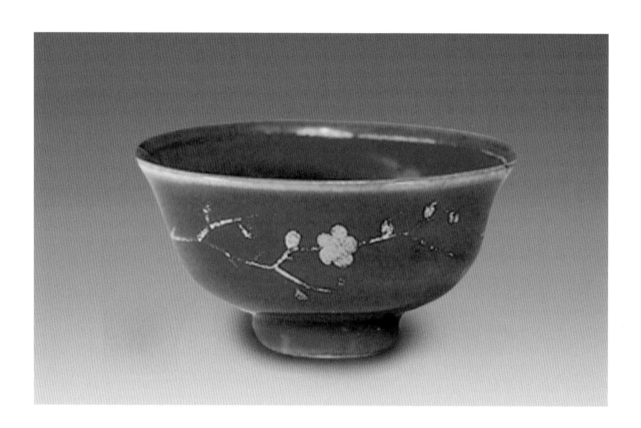

蓝釉金彩月影梅杯

元

瓷质

口径 8 厘米，底径 3 厘米，高 4 厘米

Blue-glazed Cup with Crescent and Plum Blossom Designs Painted in Gold Colour

Yuan Dynasty

Porcelain

Mouth Diameter 8 cm/ Bottom Diameter 3 cm/ Height 4 cm

胎洁白致密，内外满施蓝釉，施釉均匀，釉面柔和润泽，釉上以金彩描绘纹饰。口微敞，深腹，下腹微鼓，圈足。内口沿施弦纹一周，内底绘折枝花卉。外壁绘梅花一枝和新月一牙，笔法简洁流畅。

河北博物院藏

The cup has a white and compact body with its interior and the exterior coated evenly with blue glaze. The glaze is soft and mellow and has golden decorations painted on it. The cup has a slightly flared mouth, a deep belly which is slightly swollen on the lower part and a ring foot. One circle of string pattern is painted on the interior wall right under the mouth rim and floral patterns on the interior bottom. The exterior wall is decorated with a spray of plum blossoms and a crescent in a simple and smooth style.

Preserved in Hebei Museum

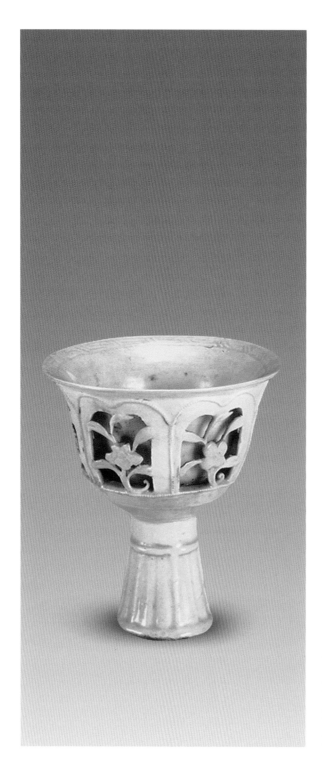

青白釉镂空折枝花高足杯

元

瓷质

口径 11.7 厘米，底径 5 厘米，高 12.7 厘米

Bluish-white-glazed Goblet with Openwork Design of Flower Branches

Yuan Dynasty

Porcelain

Mouth Diameter 11.7 cm/ Bottom Diameter 5 cm/

Height 12.7 cm

杯口外撇，深腹，喇叭形高圈足，挖足较深，杯身与圈足分
帛粘接。杯身为双层结构，内口沿印回纹图案，外壁腹部镂
雕牡丹、梅花、菊花等折枝花卉图案。镂雕部位外侧堆贴由
联珠纹组成的纹饰。圈足中部有一道横弦纹，其下至底饰一
周竖弦纹，排列规整，精细匀称。施白色釉，釉色莹润，胎
质细密洁白，此杯系景德镇窑烧制精品。1984 年扬州市老
虎山西路出土。

扬州博物馆藏

The cup has a flared mouth and a deep belly stuck on a tall
trumpet-shaped ring foot. The body of the cup has a two-layer
structure. Under the interior rim of the mouth are stamped a
ring of rectangular spiral pattern while on the exterior wall are
engraved openwork floral patterns, including patterns of peony,
plum blossom, chrysanthemum, etc. And these openworks are
surrounded by stamped bead strings in the shape of floral petals.
In the middle of the ring foot is placed one circle of transverse
string patterns which is linked to the bottom by one circle of
vertical string patterns that are arranged neatly and evenly. The
cup has an exquisite and white body coated with bright and
smooth white glaze. The cup is a masterpiece of Jingdezhen kiln
and was unearthed from the West Laohushan Road, Yangzhou,
Jiangsu Province, in 1984.

Preserved in Yangzhou Museum

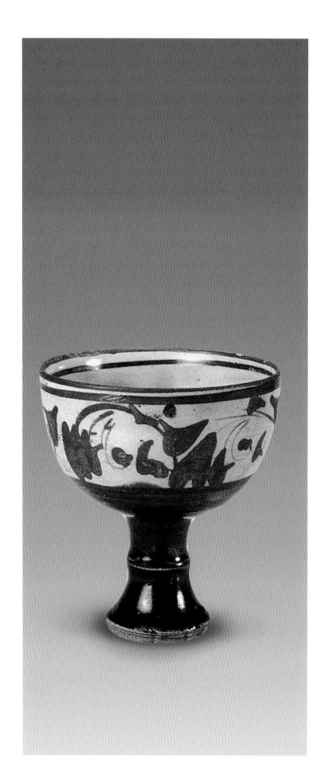

高足杯

元

瓷质

口径 8.8 厘米，足径 3.8 厘米，足高 4 厘米

Stem Cup

Yuan Dynasty

Porcelain

Mouth Diameter 8.8 cm/ Foot Diameter 3.8 cm/

Foot Height 4 cm

造型完美，纹饰简练。酒具。陕西澄城善化

出土。

陕西医史博物馆藏

This simply emblazoned stem cup is well
designed and was used as a wine vessel.
It was unearthed from Shanhua Township,
Chengcheng County, Shaanxi Province.
Preserved in Shaanxi Museum of Medical History

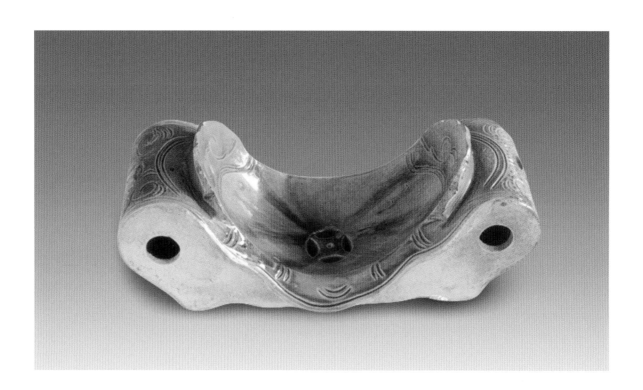

刻荷叶纹卷书形枕

辽

瓷质

长 35 厘米，高 16 厘米

Scrolled-book-shaped Pillow with Patterns of Lotus Leaves

Liao Dynasty

Porcelain

Length 35 cm/ Height 16 cm

两端卷书形。中间凹槽，形似荷叶，恰好容头部枕觚，刻荷叶纹。枕上镂一币孔，供枕者侧卧时搁耳。枕面平滑。

刘玉贤藏

The two ends are shaped like a scrolled book. The grooving middle part, suited for a resting head, is in the shape of lotus leaf with lotus leaf patterns. On the pillow is engraved a coin hole, on which the sleeper can rest his ear while lying on the side. The face of the pillow is flat and smooth.

Collected by Liu Yuxian

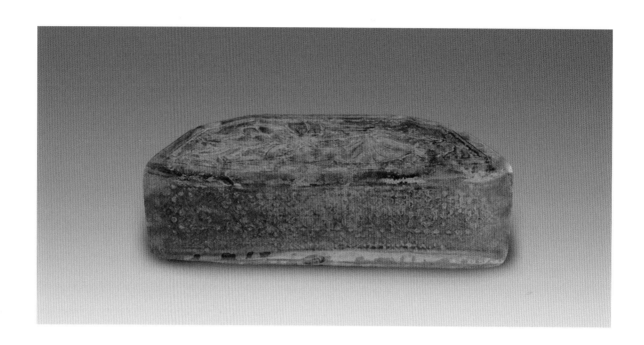

绿釉荷花纹枕

辽

瓷质

长 30 厘米，宽 14 厘米，高 9.3 厘米

Celadon-glazed Pillow with Lotus Design

Liao Dynasty

Porcelain

Length 30 cm/ Width 14 cm/ Height 9.3 cm

枕为抹角梯形，前低后高。枕面周沿排列边框，框内刻画折枝荷花一枝。枕面和侧面上部施青绿色釉，无釉处可看到白色化妆土流至底部。半陶半瓷胎，平底无釉。

罗浩权藏

The pillow is in the shape of a trapezoid with rounded corners. Its front side is lower than its back side. Around the edges of the pillow face are arranged a circle of frame, in which a lotus branch is incised. The pillow face and the upper part of its vertical sides are coated with turquoise glaze. White engobe can be seen from the unglazed part to its bottom. Half of the pillow body is pottery with the other half porcelain. Its flat bottom is unglazed.

Collected by Luo Haoquan

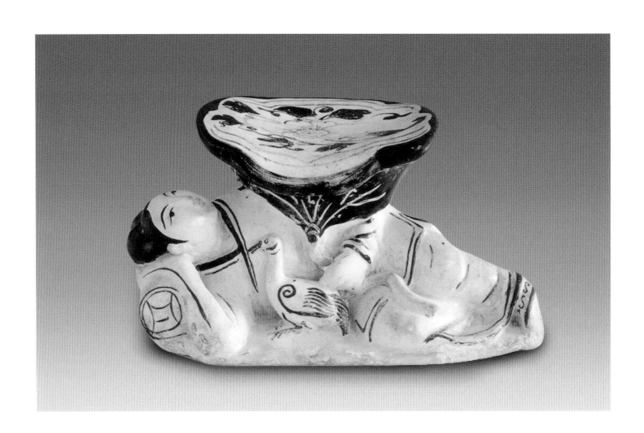

瓷州窑仕女枕

宋

瓷质

面长 12 厘米，面宽 26 厘米，高 12 厘米

Maid-shaped Pillow, Cizhou Ware

Song Dynasty

Porcelain

Surface Length 12 cm/ Surface Width 26 cm/ Height 12 cm

一仕女伏枕侧身而卧，身负海棠式枕面，头
梳发髻，着睡衣，一手垂于胸前，持握花柄，
胸前还雕画一小鸟，枕面黑彩绘花卉图案，
仕女画褐色彩衣纹，施灰黄色透明釉。雕塑、
绘画粗放简练，白色化妆粉打地，流至底部，
底有通气孔，为磁州窑的产品。

周振武藏

The pillow is shaped into a maid lying on her
side with one hand on the pillow. The maid in
pyjamas, with her hair in a bun, is covered by
the begonia-shaped pillow face. One of her
hand, holding the flower stalk, hangs down
on her breast, where is sculpted a little bird.
On the pillow face is painted a black floral
design. The maid, wearing clothes with brown
lines, is coated with transparent greyish-yellow
glaze. The style of the sculpture and drawing
is concise and free. Under the glaze is a layer
of white engobe, which extends to the pillow's
bottom, and there are pores on the bottom. The
pillow was produced in Cizhou kiln.
Collected by Zhou Zhenwu

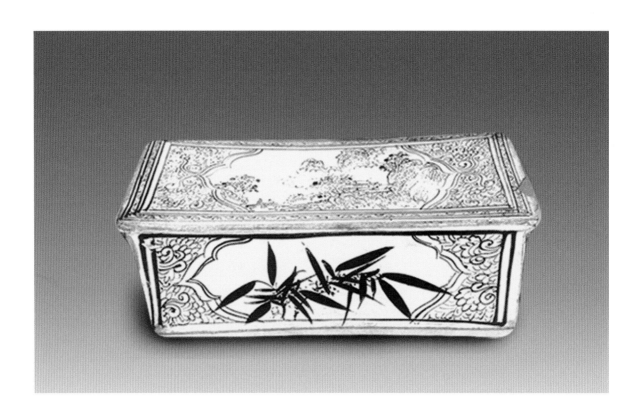

长方形白地褐花山水人物枕

宋

瓷质

长 32.5 厘米，宽 15.9 厘米，前高 10.4 厘米，后高 13.8 厘米

Rectangular Pillow with Brown Designs of Landscapes and Figures on a White Ground

Song Dynasty

Porcelain

Length 32.5 cm/ Width 15.9 cm/ Anterior Height 10.4 cm/ Posterior Height 13.8 cm

胎质硬坚灰褐，施化妆土、透明釉，底部无釉，背面上缘有气孔。枕面绘山水人物、深山古寺，山间有一座小桥，两人在桥上行进，前立面绘竹，后立面绘牡丹，两端面有并蒂牡丹图纹。底部有竖式双栏上莲叶、下荷花"张家造"戳记。

天津博物馆藏

The body of the pillow is taupe in colour and firm in texture. It is covered with a layer of engobe. The whole body except the bottom is coated with transparent glaze. There are pores on the upper edge of its back. On the pillow face are painted landscapes, ancient temples in mountains and two people walking on a bridge in the mountains. On the front wall of the pillow are drawn bamboo branches, while on the back wall are painted peonies, and patterns of double peonies decorate the pillow's side walls. The bottom is stamped with avertical double-column seal of "Zhang Jia Zao" (Made by Zhang's), with decorations of a lotus leaf motif on the upper edge and a lotus blossom motif on the lower edge.

Preserved in Tianjin Museum

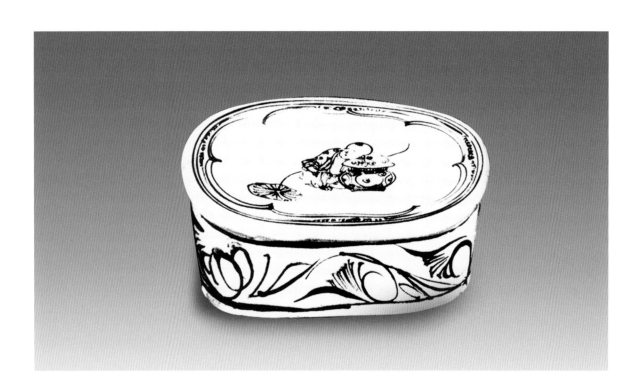

腰圆形白地黑花睡童枕

宋

瓷质

长 22.8 厘米，宽 17.1 厘米，高 9.6 厘米

Round-waisted Pillow with Black Designs of a Sleeping Child on a White Ground

Song Dynasty

Porcelain

Length 22.8 cm/ Width 17.1 cm/ Height 9.6 cm

胎质细而坚，呈灰白色，施化妆土、透明釉，底部无釉。枕面绘一童子，依物熟睡。周壁有卷草纹饰。底部印竖式双栏上莲叶、下荷花"张家造"戳记。

杨永德藏

The greyish-white body of the pillow is smooth and hard in texture. A layer of engobe is applied beneath a transparent glaze that coats the pillow. The bottom is left unglazed. A soundly-sleeping child, leaning on an object, is painted on the pillow face. All the peripheral walls of the pillow are decorated with patterns of rolled grass. The bottom is stamped with a vertical double-column seal of "Zhang Jia Zao" (Made by Zhang's), with decorations of a lotus leaf motif on the upper edge and a lotus blossom motif on the lower edge.

Collected by Yang Yongde

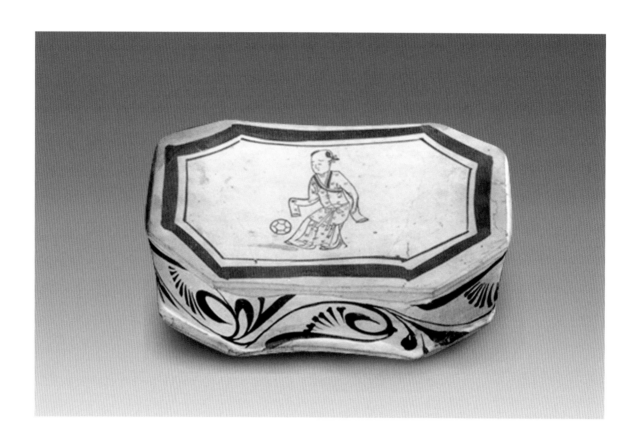

磁州窑白地黑花孩儿鞠球枕

北宋

瓷质

长 30 厘米，宽 18.5 厘米，高 10.8 厘米

Pillow with Black Cuju-playing-child Designs on a White Ground, Cizhou Ware

Northern Song Dynasty

Porcelain

Length 30 cm/ Width 18.5 cm/ Height 10.8 cm

胎质粗松，呈浅灰色，乳白色釉。枕作长八棱状，周边出檐，中间微内凹，两边翘起。周边绘有两道粗细不等的墨线，内绘孩儿蹴鞠图。孩儿头梳双丫辫，上穿左衽交领窄袖花衣，下着肥腿长裤，腰系带，左脚着地，右脚将球踢起。枕的四周绘卷草纹，底有阳文横书"张家造"印戳。

河北博物院藏

The pillow's body is pale-grey, rough and flaky in texture. It is coated with ivory-coloured glaze. With protruding brims around the pillow face and the bottom, it is in a long octagonal shape, which is slightly concave in the middle and cocked at the side walls. Two inked lines, one thick, the other thin, surround its edge, and inside the lines is a picture of a child playing Cuju. The child with two braids wears pied clothes with a cross-collar, a left-lapel and narrow-sleeves. His trousers are loose and long, tied by a belt at the waist. He stands on his left foot, kicking a ball with his right foot. The peripheral walls of the pillow are embellished with patterns of rolled grass. The pillow's bottom is stamped with a horizontal seal in relief fashion, "Made by Zhang's".

Preserved in Hebei Museum

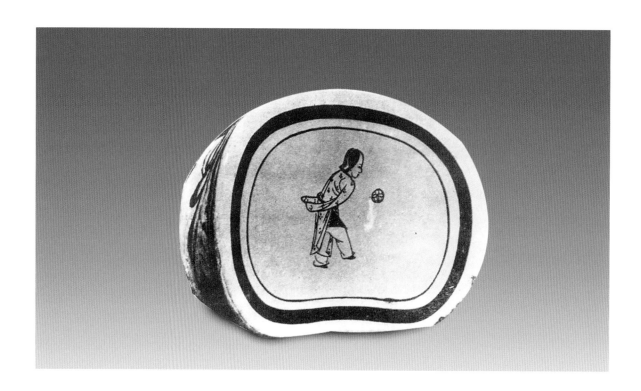

蹴鞠图陶枕

宋

陶质

Pottery Pillow with Design of Cuju

Song Dynasty

Pottery

蹴鞠图绘于陶枕的枕面中心，画中的人物为一活泼的少女，脑后梳髻，身着长裙，正步态轻盈地表演蹴鞠。画面效果朴素单纯，活泼清新。

故宫博物院藏

A design of Cuju is painted in the middle of the pottery pillow face, where a lovely girl in long skirt with hairs in a bun is playing Cuju skillfully. The picture is simple, fresh and lively.

Preserved in the Palace Museum

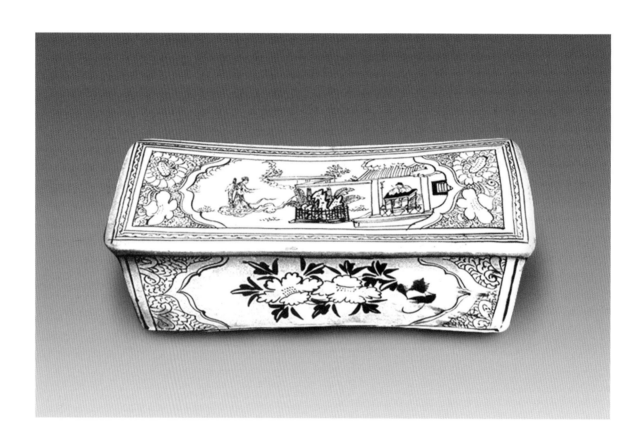

长方形白地黑花人物故事枕

金

瓷质

长 41.5 厘米，宽 17.5 厘米，高 14.5 厘米

Rectangular Pillow with Black Designs of Figure and Scene on a White Ground

Jin Dynasty

Porcelain

Length 41.5 cm/ Width 17.5 cm/ Height 14.5 cm

胎质灰白坚硬，施化妆土、透明釉，底部无釉，背面上缘有气孔。枕面绘人物故事，前后立面绘折枝牡丹，两端面绘荷花，背立面右边有墨书"滏源王家造"五字。磁县城北大营村出土。

The firm Greyish-white body is covered with a layer of engobe, and the whole body except the bottom is coated with transparent glaze. There are pores on the upper edge of the back wall of the pillow. Designs of figures and scenes are painted on the pillow face, designs of peony branches on the front and the back walls, and lotus designs on the side walls. Along the right edge of the back wall are an ink inscription of five Chinese characters "Fu Yuan Wang Jia Zao" (Made by the Wang family in Fuyuan). It was unearthed in Daying Village of the north of Ci County, Hebei Province.

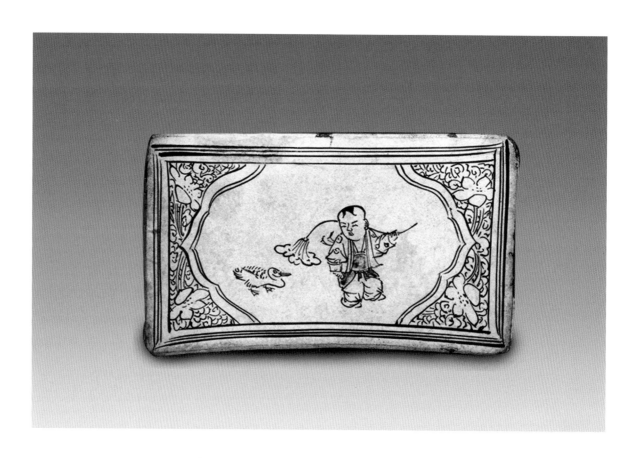

长方形白地黑花婴戏枕

宋

瓷质

长 28.5 厘米，宽 16.7 厘米，高 13.3 厘米

Rectangular Pillow with Black Design of a Playing Boy on a White Ground

Song Dynasty

Porcelain

Length 28.5 cm/ Width 16.7 cm/ Height 13.3 cm

胎质灰白坚硬，施化妆土和透明釉，底部无釉，背面上缘有气孔。枕面有一童子肩背荷叶，引鸭前行。前后立面绘折枝牡丹。两端面绘荷花。底部印有竖式双栏上莲叶、下荷花"张家造"戳记。磁县观台镇出土。

中国磁州窑博物馆藏

The greyish-white body of the pillow is firm and hard in texture. And it is covered with a layer of engobe beneath and a transparent glaze, while the bottom of it is left unglazed. There are pores on the upper edge of its back. On the pillow face is painted a boy with a lotus leaf on his shoulder, leading a duck to move forward. The front and the back walls of the pillow are decorated with designs of peony branches, while the side walls with lotus flowers. The bottom is stamped with a vertical double-column seal of "Zhang Jia Zao" (Made by Zhang's), with decorations of a lotus leaf motif on the upper edge and a lotus blossom motif on the lower edge. It was unearthed from Guantai Township, Ci County, Hebei Province.
Preserved in China Cizhou Kiln Museum

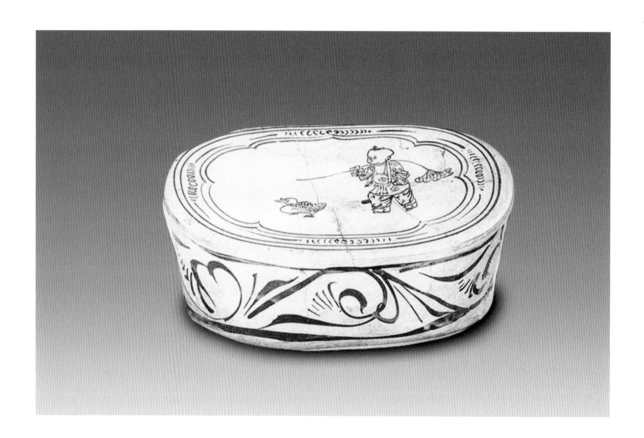

腰圆形白地黑花婴戏枕

宋

瓷质

长 24.3 厘米，宽 18.1 厘米，前高 7.2 厘米，后高 9.5 厘米

Round-waisted Pillow with Black Design of a Playing Child on a White Ground

Song Dynasty

Porcelain

Length 24.3 cm/ Width 18.1 cm/ Front Height 7.2 cm/ Back Height 9.5 cm

胎质灰褐坚硬，通体白釉，施化妆土、透明釉，底部无釉，背面上缘有气孔。枕面绘一童子，肩扛长茎荷叶，面前有一只鸭子向前行进，周壁有卷草纹饰。底部印有竖式双栏上莲叶、下荷花"张家造"戳记。

天津博物馆藏

This taupe hard body of the pillow except its bottom is fully coated with engobe and transparent glaze. There are pores on the upper edge of its back. On the pillow face is painted a boy, with a lotus leaf on his shoulder, leading a duck to move forward, while on peripheral walls are patterns of rolled grass. The bottom is stamped with a vertical double-column seal of "Zhang Jia Zao" (Made by Zhang's), with decorations of a lotus leaf motif on the upper edge and a lotus blossom motif on the lower edge.

Preserved in Tianjin Museum

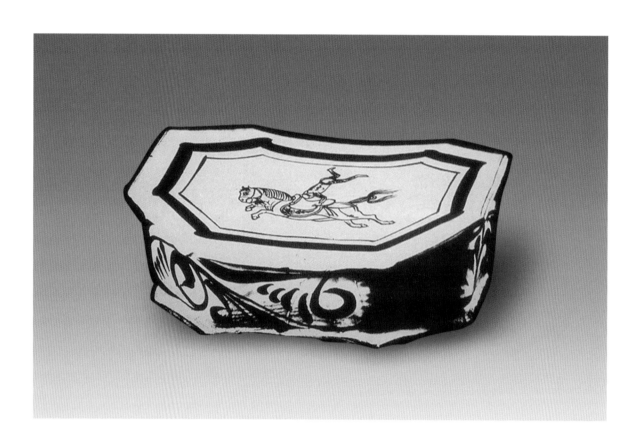

磁州窑马戏图瓷枕

北宋

瓷质

长 29 厘米，宽 21 厘米，高 12 厘米

Pottery Pillow with Design of Circus Performance, Cizhou Ware

Northern Dynasty

Porcelain

Length 29 cm/ Width 21 cm/ Height 12 cm

枕长方委角形。枕面中心绘一马疾驰，马鞍
上倒立一人，在做精彩的马戏表演。画面中
马技艺人的神情意态，具有浓厚的生活气息。

故宫博物院藏

The pillow is in the shape of a rectangle with
indented corners. On the centre of the pillow
face is painted a galloping horse on which rides
a man with his head on the saddle doing a circus
performance. The circus performer's expression
and manners are vivid, showing a strong flavour
of life.

Preserved in the Palace Museum

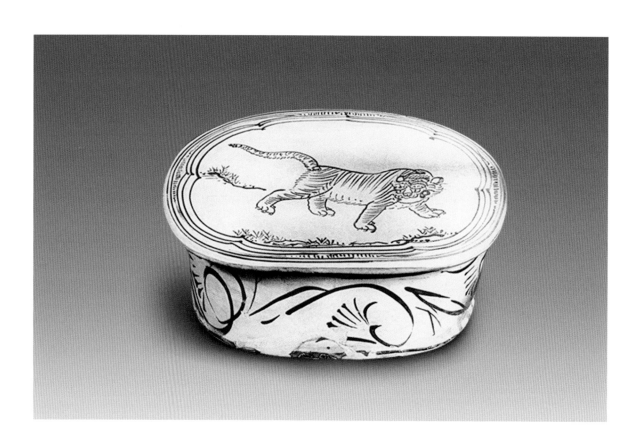

腰圆形白地黑花虎纹枕

宋

瓷质

长 27 厘米，宽 21.5 厘米，高 12.2 厘米

Round-waisted Pillow with Black Tiger Design on a White Ground

Song Dynasty

Porcelain

Length 27 cm/ Width 21.5 cm/ Height 12.2 cm

胎质坚硬，施化妆土、透明釉，底部无釉，背面上缘有气孔。枕面绘虎一只，周壁饰卷草纹。底部印有竖式双栏上莲叶、下荷花连排三个"张家造"戳记。磁县都党乡冶子村出土。

中国磁州窑博物馆藏

The pillow has a hard body, which is covered with engobe and transparent glaze, and its bottom is unglazed. There are pores on the upper edge of its back side. On the pillow face is painted a tiger, while its peripheral walls are embellished with patterns of rolled grass. The bottom is stamped with three vertical double-column seals of "Zhang Jia Zao" (Made by Zhang's), with decorations of a lotus leaf motif on the upper edge and a lotus blossom motif on the lower edge. It was unearthed in Yezi Village, Dudang Township, Ci County, Hebei Province. Preserved in China Cizhou Kiln Museum

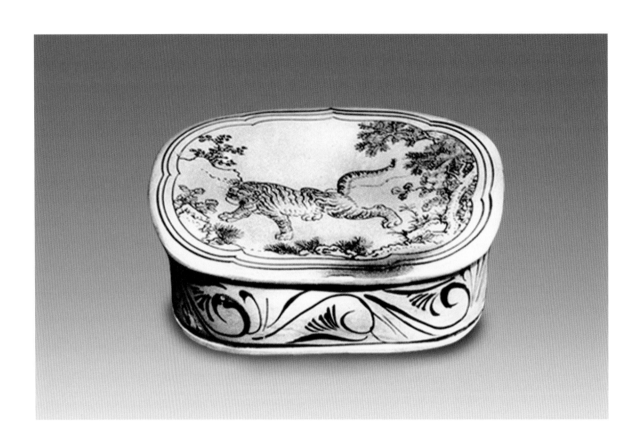

腰圆形白地黑花虎纹枕

宋

瓷质

长 28.2 厘米，宽 21.5 厘米，高 12.4 厘米

Round-waisted Pillow with Black Tiger Design on a White Ground

Song Dynasty

Porcelain

Length 28.2 cm/ Width 21.5 cm/ Height 12.4 cm

胎质灰白坚硬，施化妆土、透明釉，底部无
釉，背面上缘有气孔。枕面绘一猛虎和松石，
周壁有卷草纹饰。磁县观台镇东艾口村出土。

中国磁州窑博物馆藏

The pillow has a hard white body, which is
covered with engobe and transparent glaze, and
its bottom is unglazed. There are pores on the
upper edge of its back side. The pillow face is
embellished with a wild tiger, pine trees and
stones, while its peripheral walls are decorated
with patterns of rolled grass. It was unearthed in
the Dong'aikou Village, Guantai Township, Ci
County, Hebei Province.
Preserved in China Cizhou Kiln Museum

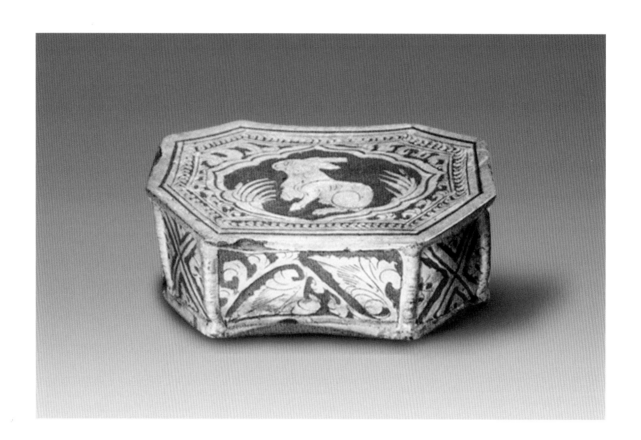

八角形白地剔花兔纹枕

宋

瓷质

长 31.9 厘米，宽 23.5 厘米，前高 8.8 厘米，后高 12.8 厘米

Octagonal Pillow with Carved Design of a Rabbit on a White Ground

Song Dynasty

Porcelain

Length 31.9 cm / Width 23.5 cm / Front Height 8.8 cm / Back Height 12.8 cm

胎质灰褐坚硬，施化妆土、透明釉。通体白釉，底部无釉，背面上缘有气孔。枕面有两条刻线为边框，向内卷草纹饰，开光内剔刻白兔一只，兔子前后各有一簇小草，周壁有叶纹和十字纹交替装饰。底部无戳记，有刻画"长命枕一只"字迹。

天津博物馆藏

This pillow has a greyish-brown and firm body, which is covered with engobe and a transparent glaze, but its bottom is left unglazed. There are pores on the upper edge of its back. Along the edge of the pillow face are carved two lines as the frame of the face, and along the inner side of the frame are motifs of rolled grass. Within this decorative frame is scraped and carved a white rabbit, in front of and behind which is painted a bunch of grass respectively. The peripheral walls of the pillow are alternatively embellished with leaf patterns and cross designs. Its bottom is incised with Chinese characters "Chang Ming Zhen Yi Zhi" (One pillow of longevity) instead of a seal.

Preserved in Tianjin Museum

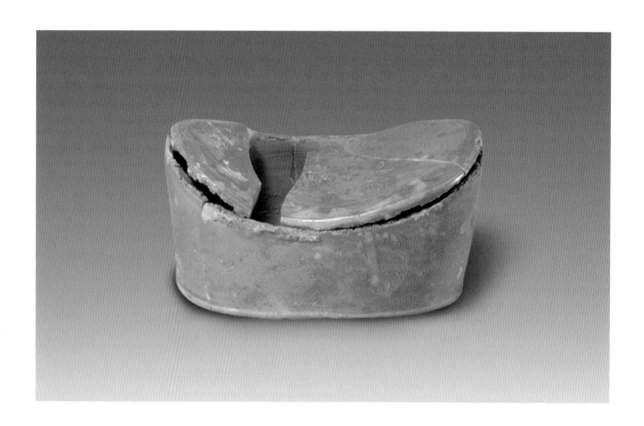

枕

北宋

瓷质

长 19 厘米，高 9.5 厘米

Pillow

Northern Song Dynasty

Porcelain

Length 19 cm/ Height 9.5 cm

整器俯视呈椭圆形，枕面凹弧，后侧略高于
前侧，两端上翘。其中一端面与腹接处有一
孔，枕身画有团菊，枕面画凤凰，全器满施
青釉。

浙江省文物考古研究所藏

The pillow on the whole is in the shape of an
oval via overlooking view. It has a concave face
with its front side lower than its rear and the
left and the right two edges cock up. There is a
hole in the junction between its side wall and its
belly. The pillow body is incised with rosettes,
while the pillow face with a phoenix. It is fully
celadon glazed.
Preserved in Institute of Cultural Relics and
Archaeology of Zhejiang Province

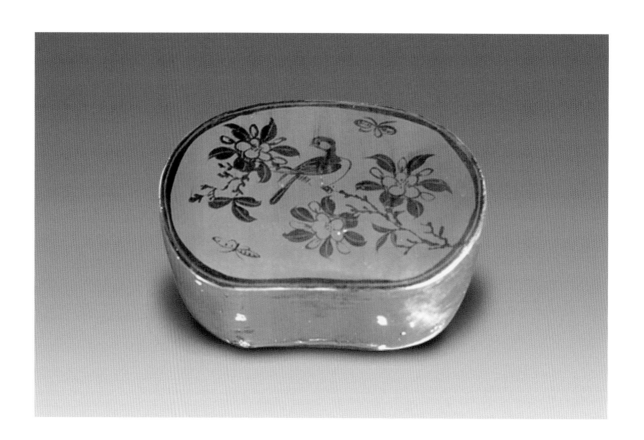

腰圆形绿釉黑花喜鹊踏枝枕

宋

瓷质

长 35 厘米，宽 25 厘米，前高 10.2 厘米，后高 12.4 厘米

Round-waisted Pillow with Black Magpie Design on a Green-glazed Ground

Song Dynasty

Porcelain

Length 35 cm/ Width 25 cm/ Front Height 10.2 cm/ Back Height 12.4 cm

胎质黄白较硬，釉深绿润泽。底部无釉，有
气孔，前后两壁有四个支钉痕迹。枕面绘喜
鹊闹枝，枝干上有盛开的花朵，花繁叶茂，
生意盎然，上右下左绘蝴蝶各一只，用墨饱
满；画法娴熟；笔意流畅，周壁无饰。河北
省望都县西堤乡沈家庄村出土。

河北省文物研究所藏

This pillow's body is firm and yellowish-
white, and is coated with glossy dark-green
glaze. There are pores on its unglazed bottom,
and four nail marks on its front and back
walls. The pillow face is incised with design
of a magpie perching on a branch of a tree in
full blossom and a butterfly flying on the top
right corner and on the bottom left corner of
the face respectively. All of the designs show
craftsman's marvelous skills of painting. There
is no decoration on the peripheral walls. The
pillow was unearthed from Shenjiazhuang
Village, Xidi Township, Wangdu County, Hebei
Province.
Preserved in Cultural Relics Institute of Hebei
Province

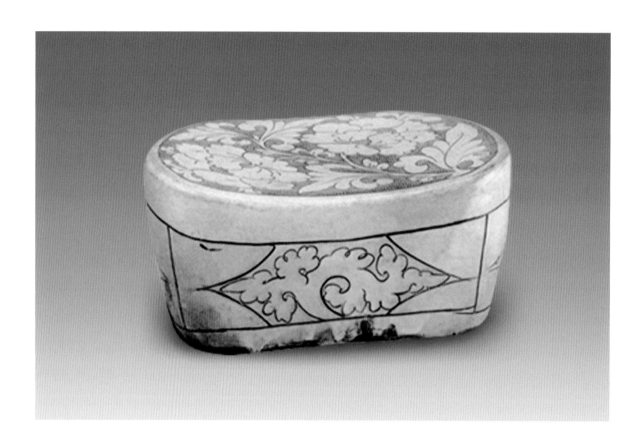

珍珠地划花折枝牡丹纹枕

宋

瓷质

长 25.8 厘米，宽 18.4 厘米，高 12 厘米

Pillow Incised with Peony Design on a Pearl-pattern Ground

Song Dynasty

Porcelain

Length 25.8 cm/ Width 18.4 cm/ Height 12 cm

枕呈腰圆形，黄褐色胎，整体敷洁白化妆土后，在枕面上刻画折枝牡丹纹，隙地以圆管戳印出密集的小圆圈，俗称"珍珠地"。四周划出菱形开光，开光内刻画卷草纹。

故宫博物院藏

This pillow has a round waist and a tawny body, which is covered with white engobe. On the pillow face are carved designs of penoy branches, and the vacant spaces are stamped with dense small circles, commonly called "Pearl-pattern Ground". The peripheral walls of the pillow are incised with a decorative rhombus shape, within which are engraved a design of scrolled grass.

Preserved in the Palace Museum

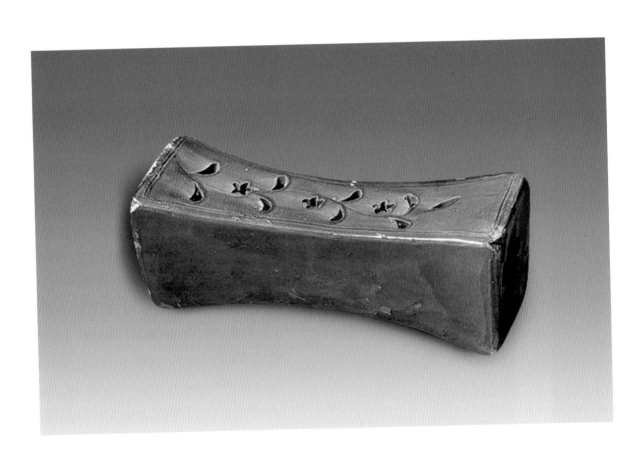

钽   **绿釉镂空花卉纹瓷枕**

宋   宋

瓷   瓷质

长   长 35 厘米，高 12 厘米

Si   **Celadon-glazed Porcelain Pillow with Openwork Floral Patterns**

Gl

So   Song Dynasty

Por   Porcelain

Ler   Length 35 cm/ Height 12 cm

翠绿色瓷质，枕面色泽光润，青翠欲滴，形微凹，呈现出自然的枕面状态。瓷枕两侧是镂空的菊花，枕身对称为镂空缠枝花，两侧四角均有露胎现象，推测为烧制时坚向叠放所致。

江宁博物馆藏

This pillow is in a lush emerald colour, which looks lustrous and smooth.The front and back walls are concave slightly, turning out a natural shape of the pillow face. Both the side walls of the pillow are incised with patterns of openwork chrysanthemum. On the pillow face are carved two symmetrical openwork interlocking floral designs. The corners of its side walls all expose the unglazed body, supposedly caused by being stacked up vertically in the process of firing.

Preserved in Jiangning Museum

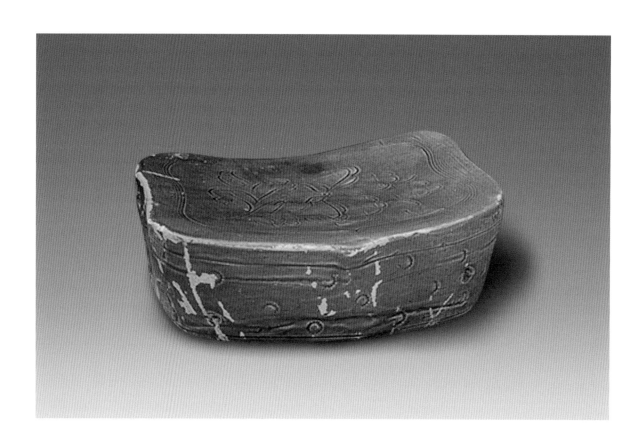

刻花瓷枕

宋

瓷质

长 25.5 厘米，宽 19.5 厘米，高 8.5 厘米

Porcelain Pillow Incised with Floral Patterns

Song Dynasty

Porcelain

Length 25.5 cm/ Width 19.5 cm/ Height 8.5 cm

枕作椭圆形、微凹，枕面施绿色釉，底部模印花押款，枕面纹饰简练，胎釉之间施化妆土，釉色绿中微微闪黄。高淳区鸿门寺遗址出土。

高淳博物馆藏

This pillow is in the shape of an oval, and its face, simply decorated, is slightly concave. The bottom of the pillow is stamped with a floral pattern. The pillow is fully covered with green glaze with a hint of yellow. A layer of engobe is applied between its body and the glaze. It was unearthed in the ruins of Hongmen Temple in Gaochun County.

Preserved in Gaochun Museum

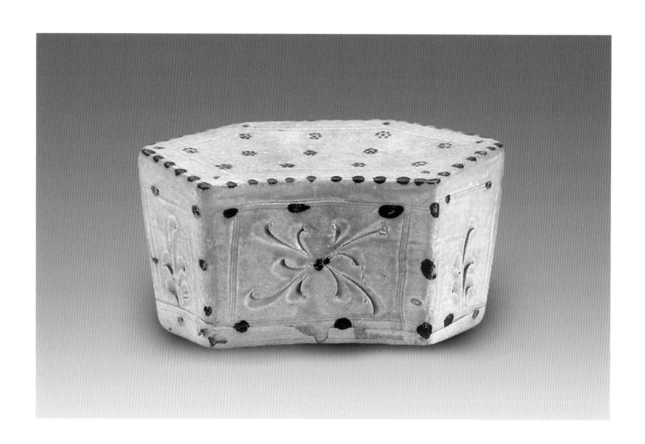

白釉褐彩刻花六角枕

北宋

瓷质

长 19.9 厘米，宽 10 厘米，高 10.4 厘米

Hexagonal White-glazed Pillow with Carved Brown Floral Patterns

Northern Song Dynasty

Porcelain

Length 19.9 cm/ Width 10 cm/ Height 10.4 cm

枕为传世品。枕作扁六角形，枕面前倾。枕面以弦纹刻六角边框，内点 12 个圈点褐彩花瓣纹。侧壁分别刻方边框，前后面剔刻两朵菊花，其余侧面剔刻兰草纹，刻花刀锋较深。边角皆以褐彩点装饰，胎灰白，满施白釉，底露胎。

扬州博物馆藏

This pillow is handed down from the ancient times. And it is in the shape of a flat hexagon with its face tilting forward and framed with string patterns around. Within the frame on the face are dotted twelve brown floral petal designs. There is a square frame on the side walls of the pillow. On the front and the back walls are scraped and carved chrysanthemum patterns while on the side walls are fragrant thoroughwort designs with deep carving lines. Each corner and rim is embellished with brown speckles. The pillow's body is greyish white and is fully glazed white, with its bottom left unglazed.

Preserved in Yangzhou Museum

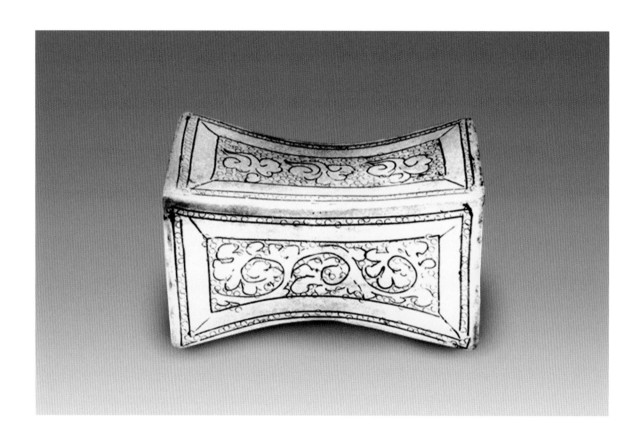

束腰形白釉珍珠地纹枕

宋

瓷质

长 19.9 厘米，宽 8.7 厘米，高 11.9 厘米

Waist-contracted White-glazed Pillow on a Pearl-pattern Ground

Song Dynasty

Porcelain

Length 19.9 cm/ Width 8.7 cm/ Height 11.9 cm

胎质灰白坚硬，施化妆土、透明釉，一端面
有气孔。枕面有珍珠地卷花纹，前后立面有
珍珠花朵，两端面绘珍珠十字叶形图纹。磁
县岳城水库出土。

峰峰矿区文物保管所藏

This pillow has a firm greyish-white body,
covered with engobe and transparent glaze.
There are pores on one of its flank side. Its
pillow face is incised with scrolled floral
designs on a pearl-pattern ground, and its front
and back walls are embellished with floral
designs on a pearl-pattern ground, and its side
walls are decorated with cross-shaped floral
patterns on a pearl-pattern ground. It was
unearthed in Yuecheng reservoir of Ci County,
Hebei Province.
Preserved in the Department of Cultural Relics
Conservation of Fengfeng Mining District

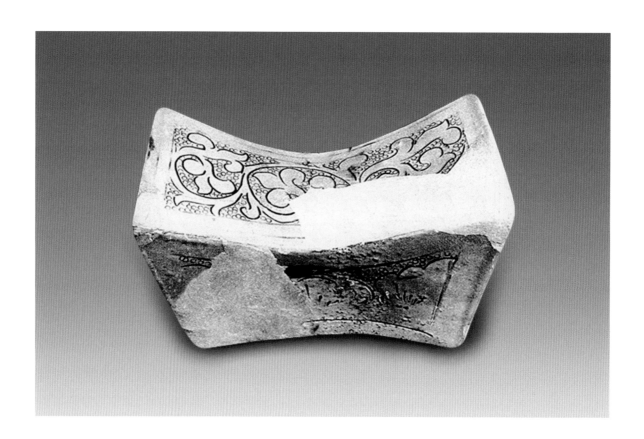

元宝形白釉珍珠地纹枕

宋

瓷质

长 22.3 厘米，宽 10 厘米，高 9 厘米

Sycee-shaped White-glazed Pillow with a Pearl-pattern Ground

Song Dynasty

Porcelain

Length 22.3 cm/ Width 10 cm/ Height 9 cm

胎质灰白坚硬，施化妆土、透明釉，底部无釉。
枕面及前后立面和两端均有珍珠地刻花卷勾
纹图案。磁县观台镇出土。

中国磁州窑博物馆藏

The pillow has a firm body in a greyish-white
colour, coated with engobe and transparent
glaze. Its bottom is unglazed. The pillow face
and its four walls are all incised with scrolled
floral designs on a pearl-pattern ground. It was
unearthed in Guantai Township, Ci County,
Hebei Province.

Preserved in China Cizhou Kiln Museum

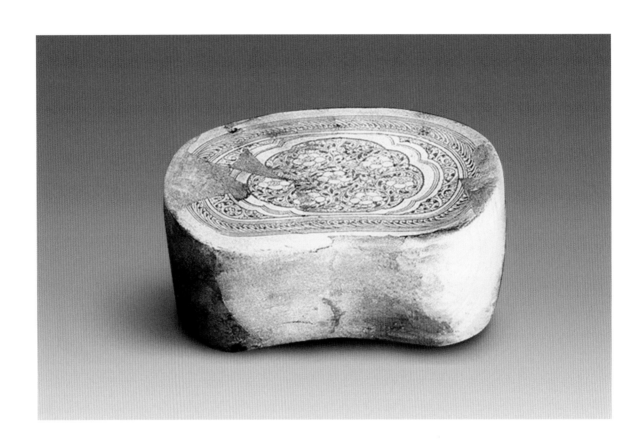

腰圆形白地刻剔花枕

宋

瓷质

长 35.5 厘米，宽 23 厘米，高 16.5 厘米

Round-waisted Pillow with Carved Floral Patterns on a White Ground

Song Dynasty

Porcelain

Length 35.5 cm/ Width 23 cm/ Height 16.5 cm

胎质灰白坚硬，施化妆土、透明釉，底部无釉。
枕面刻缠枝牡丹，周壁白釉无饰，背面上缘
有气孔。磁县观台镇出土。

中国磁州窑博物馆藏

This pillow has a firm greyish-white body,
coated with engobe and transparent glaze, and
its bottom is unglazed. On the pillow face are
carved motifs of interlocking peonies, and the
peripheral walls of the pillow are just white-
glazed with no decoration. There are pores on
the upper edge of its back. It was unearthed in
Guantai Township, Ci County, Hebei Province.
Preserved in China Cizhou Kiln Museum

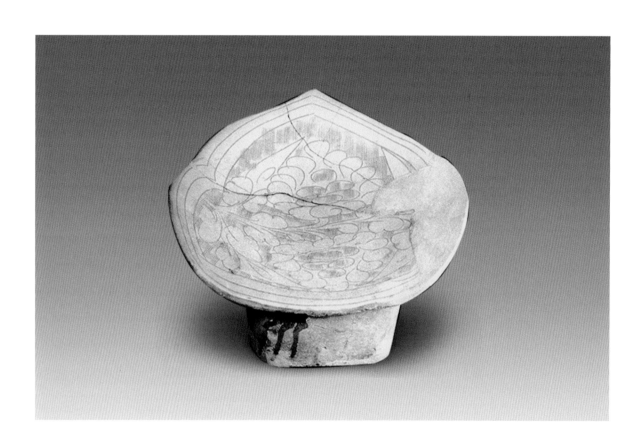

叶形白釉刻花枕

宋

瓷质

长 29.3 厘米，宽 28.5 厘米，高 18.5 厘米

Leaf-shaped White-glazed Pillow with Carved Floral Patterns

Song Dynasty

Porcelain

Length 29.3 cm/ Width 28.5 cm/ Height 18.5 cm

胎质灰白坚硬，施化妆土、透明釉，底部无

釉，枕残。枕面刻画有花卉，背面白釉无饰。

磁县观台镇出土。

中国磁州窑博物馆藏

The pillow, damaged, has a firm body in a
greyish-white colour, covered with engobe
and a layer of transparent glaze, and its bottom
is unglazed. The pillow face is incised with
flowers, and the bottom is covered with white
glaze without any decorations. The damaged
pillow was unearthed in Guantai Township, Ci
County, Hebei Province.

Preserved in China Cizhou Kiln Museum

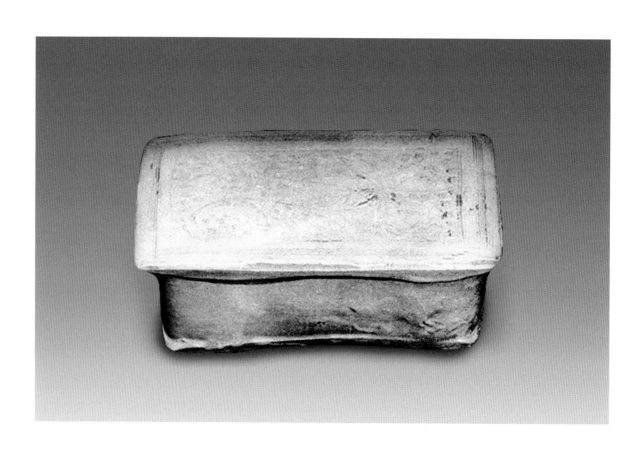

长方形白釉刻花纪年枕

金

瓷质

长 28 厘米，宽 16.5 厘米，高 9.5 厘米

Rectangular White-glazed Commemorative Pillow with Carved Floral Patterns

Jin Dynasty

Porcelain

Length 28 cm/ Width 16.5 cm/ Height 9.5 cm

胎质灰白坚硬，施化妆土、透明釉，底部无釉，背面上缘有气孔。枕面刻折枝花，四周皆是素面白釉。枕底部有墨书"金明昌六年六月……"。底部印有横式"张家造"戳记。磁县观台镇出土。

中国磁州窑博物馆藏

This pillow has a firm body in greyish white, covered with engobe and transparent glaze, and its bottom is unglazed. There are pores on the upper edge of its back wall. The pillow face is incised with flower branches, and the peripheral walls are all covered with white glaze. On its bottom are stamped a horizontal seal of "Zhang Jia Zao" (Made by Zhang's) and an inscription in black ink indicating the production date. It was unearthed in Guantai Township, Ci County, Hebei Province.

Preserved in China Cizhou Kiln Museum

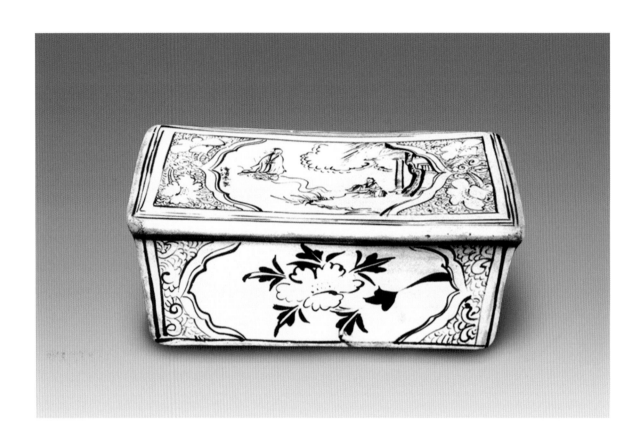

长方形白地黑花人物枕

金

瓷质

长 29 厘米，宽 16.5 厘米，高 13.2 厘米

Rectangular Pillow with Black Figure Design on a White Ground

Jin Dynasty

Porcelain

Length 29 cm/ Width 16.5 cm/ Height 13.2 cm

胎质灰白坚硬，施化妆土、透明釉，底部无釉，背面上缘有气孔。枕面上绘有一少年，双膝跪地祝祷先人徐徐升天，前后两立面绘折枝牡丹，两端面绘荷花。枕面左边刻画有"漳滨逸人制"五字。磁县都党乡冶子村出土。

中国磁州窑博物馆藏

This pillow has a firm body in greyish white, coated with engobe and a layer of transparent glaze, and its bottom is unglazed. There are pores on the upper edge of its back wall. On the pillow face is painted a boy on his knees praying for his ancestor's ascension to the heaven. Its front and back walls are embellished with peony branches, and the side walls lotus flowers. On the left side of the pillow face are carved five Chinese characters, meaning "made by Yiren living along the Zhang riverside". It was unearthed in Yezi Village, Dudang Township, Ci County, Hebei Province.
Preserved in China Cizhou Kiln Museum

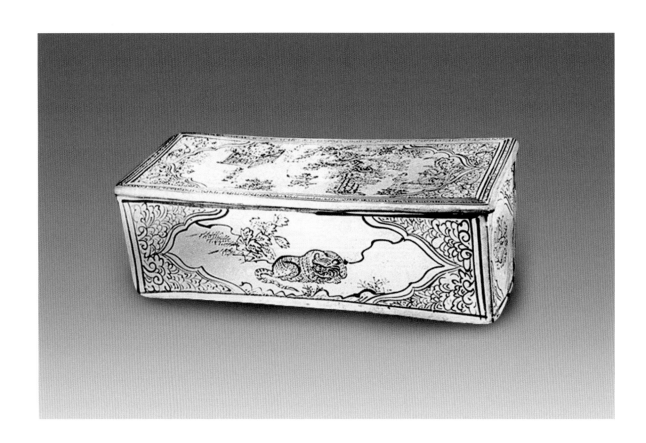

长方形白地黑花人物故事枕

金

瓷质

长 43.5 厘米，宽 16.7 厘米，高 13 厘米

Rectangular Pillow with Design of Black Figure and Scene on a White Ground

Jin Dynasty

Porcelain

Length 43.5 cm/ Width 16.7 cm/ Height 13 cm

胎质灰白坚硬，施化妆土、透明釉，底部无釉，
背面上缘有气孔。枕面有两人舞剑，前立面
绘一只卧虎，后立面绘凤凰，两端面绘荷花。
底部印有"张家造"戳记。河南省林州市出土。

林州文物保管所藏

The pillow has a firm greyish-white body,
covered with engobe and a layer of transparent
glaze, and its bottom is unglazed. There are
pores on the upper edge of its back wall.
The pillow face is incised with two figures
performing sword dance. On the front wall of
the pillow is painted a crouching tiger, while on
the back wall is drawn a phoenix, and on its side
walls lotus flowers. On the bottom is stamped a
seal of "Zhang Jia Zao" (Made by Zhang's). It
was unearthed in Linzhou.

Preserved in Linzhou Museum

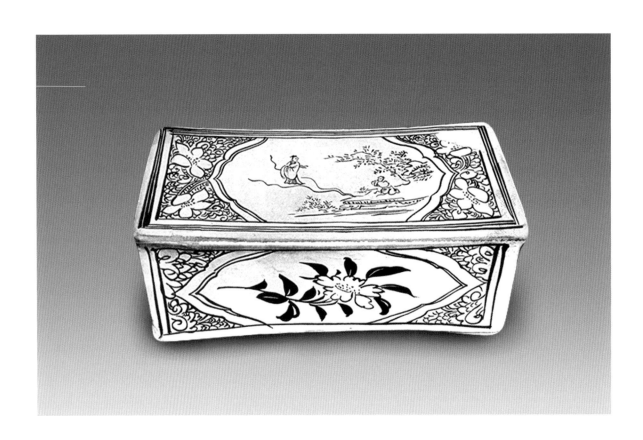

长方形白地黑花人物故事文字枕

金

瓷质

长 29.5 厘米，宽 15.5 厘米，高 14.5 厘米

Rectangular Pillow with Black Designs of Figure, Scene and Inscription on a White Ground

Jin Dynasty

Porcelain

Length 29.5 cm/ Width 15.5 cm/ Height 14.5 cm

胎质灰白坚硬，施化妆土、透明釉，底部无釉，背面上缘有气孔。枕面绘一少年双膝跪地，祝祷先人徐徐升天。前立面绘折枝花，后立面书杨大元诗一首，两端面绘荷花。底部印有竖式双栏上莲叶、下荷花"张家造"戳记。磁县观台镇出土。

中国磁州窑博物馆藏

The pillow has a firm and greyish-white body, covered with engobe and a transparent glaze, and its bottom is left unglazed. There are pores on the upper edge of its back. The pillow face is painted with a boy on his knees praying for his ancestors's ascension to the heaven. On the front wall of the pillow are drawn flower branches, while on the back is inscribed a poem written by Yang Dayuan. Lotus flowers are painted on its side walls. On the bottom is stamped a vertical seal of "Zhang Jia Zao" (Made by Zhang's), with decorations of a lotus leaf motif on the upper edge and a lotus blossom motif on the lower edge. It was unearthed in Guantai Township, Ci County, Hebei Province.
Preserved in China Cizhou Kiln Museum

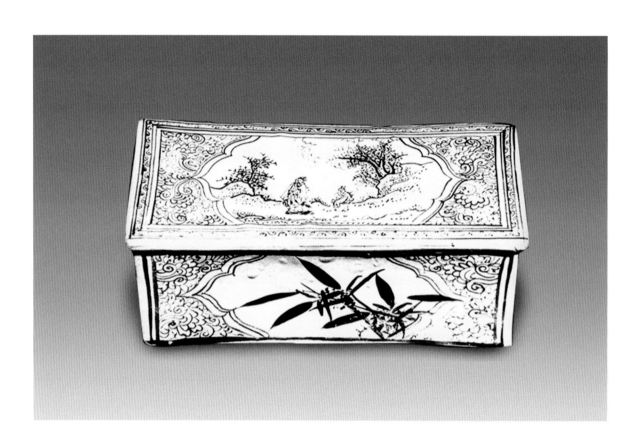

长方形白地黑花人物故事枕

金

瓷质

长 32.5 厘米，宽 15.5 厘米，高 12.2 厘米

Rectangular Pillow with Black Designs of Figure, Scene and Inscription on a White Ground

Jin Dynasty

Porcelain

Length 32.5 cm/ Width 15.5 cm/ Height 12.2 cm

胎质灰白坚硬，施化妆土、透明釉，底部无釉，背面上缘有气孔。枕面绘人物故事，前立面绘竹，后立面绘折枝牡丹，两端面绘花卉。底部印有竖式双栏上莲叶、下荷花"张家造"戳记。磁县观台镇东艾口村出土。

The pillow has a firm and greyish-white body, covered with engobe and a layer of transparent glaze, and its bottom is left unglazed. There are pores on the upper edge of its back. The pillow face is painted with design of figures and scenes. On the front wall of the pillow are drawn bamboo branches, while on the back wall are painted peony branches, with floral designs on its side walls. On the bottom is stamped a vertical double column seal of "Zhang Jia Zao" (Made by Zhang's), with decorations of a lotus leaf motif on the upper edge and a lotus blossom motif on the lower edge. It was unearthed in the Dong'aikou Village, Guantai Township, Ci County, Hebei Province.

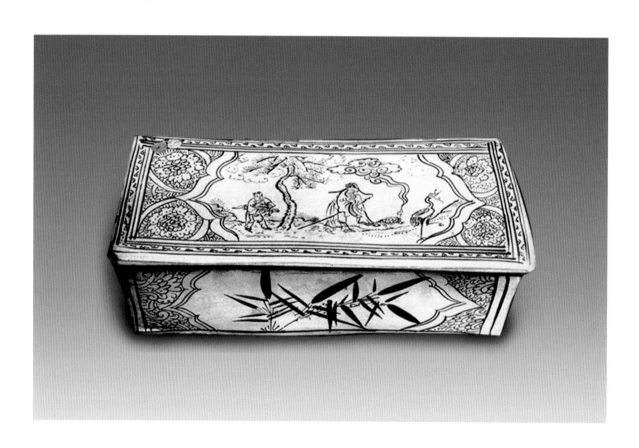

长方形白地黑花人物故事枕

金

瓷质

长 40.5 厘米，宽 18.5 厘米，高 12 厘米

Rectangular Pillow with Black Design of Figure and Scene on a White Ground

Jin Dynasty

Porcelain

Length 40.5 cm/ Width 18.5 cm/ Height 12 cm

胎质灰白坚硬，施化妆土、透明釉，底部无釉，背面上缘有气孔。枕面绘人物故事，前立面绘竹，后立面绘折枝牡丹，两端面绘花卉。底部印有竖式双栏上莲叶、下荷花 "古相张家造" 戳记。磁县观台镇东艾口村出土。

中国磁州窑博物馆藏

This pillow has a firm greyish-white body covered with engobe and a layer of transparent glaze, and its bottom is left unglazed. There are pores on the upper edge of its back. The pillow face is painted with design of figures and scenes. On the front wall of the pillow are drawn bamboo branches, while on the back wall are painted peony branches, with floral designs on its side walls. On the bottom is stamped a vertical double column seal of "Gu Xiang Zhang Jia Zao" (Made by Zhang's in ancient Xiangzhou), with decorations of a lotus leaf motif on the upper edge and a lotus blossom motif on the lower edge. It was unearthed in the Dong'aikou Village, Guantai Township, Ci County, Hebei Province.

Preserved in China Cizhou Kiln Museum

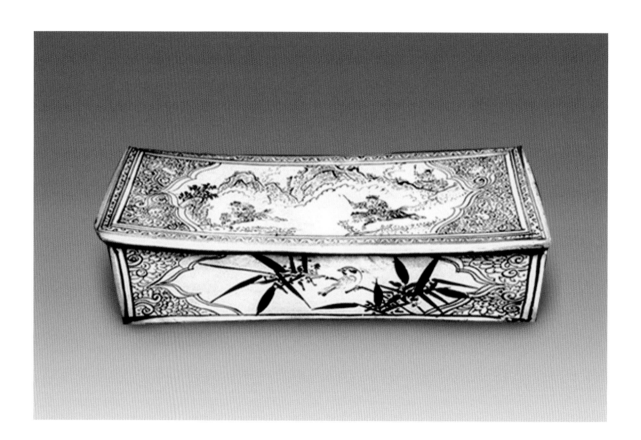

长方形白地黑花人物故事枕

金

瓷质

长 31 厘米，宽 15 厘米，高 13 厘米

Rectangular Pillow with Black Designs of Figure and Scene on a White Ground

Jin Dynasty

Porcelain

Length 31 cm/ Width 15 cm/ Height 13 cm

胎质灰白坚硬，施化妆土、透明釉，底部无
釉，背面上缘有气孔。枕面绘人物故事，前
立面绘竹鸟，后立面绘山水，两端面绘花卉。
底部印有竖式双栏上莲叶、下荷花"张家造"
戳记。磁县观台镇出土。

安阳博物馆藏

This pillow has a firm and greyish-white body
covered with engobe and a layer of transparent
glaze, and its bottom is unglazed. There are
pores on the upper edge of its back. The
pillow face is painted with design of figures
and scenes. On the front wall of the pillow
are drawn bamboo branches and birds, while
on the back wall are painted landscapes, with
floral designs on its side walls. On the bottom is
stamped a vertical double column seal of "Zhang
Jia Zao" (Made by Zhang's), with decorations
of a lotus leaf motif on the upper edge and a
lotus blossom motif on the lower edge. It was
unearthed in Guantai Township, Ci County,
Hebei Province.

Preserved in Anyang Municipal Museum

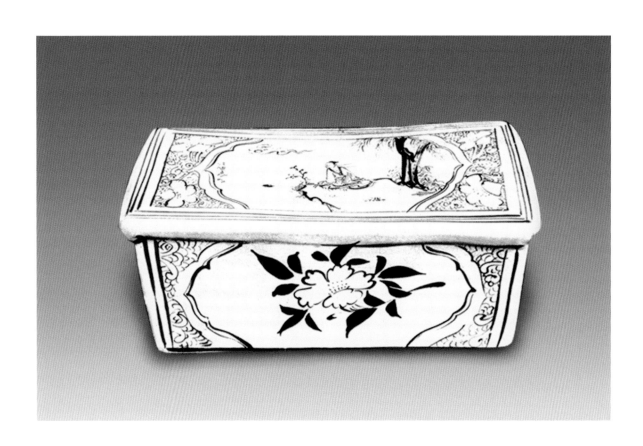

长方形白地黑花人物故事枕

金

瓷质

长 29 厘米，宽 16.4 厘米，高 13 厘米

Rectangular Pillow with Black Designs of Figure and Scene on a White Ground

Jin Dynasty

Porcelain

Length 29 cm/ Width 16.4 cm/ Height 13 cm

胎质灰白坚硬，施化妆土、透明釉，底部无釉，背面上缘有气孔。枕面绘一人跪坐在河边的一块大石上，前立面绘折枝花，后立面绘牡丹，两端面绘荷花。枕面左边刻画有"漳滨逸人制"五字。磁县城北孟庄村南口出土。

中国磁州窑博物馆藏

This pillow has a firm and greyish-white body covered with engobe and a layer of transparent glaze, and its bottom is unglazed. There are pores on the upper edge of its back. The pillow face is painted with a figure kneeling on a boulder by the river. On the front wall of the pillow is drawn a flower branch, while on the back wall peonies, with lotus flowers on its side walls. On the left side of the pillow face are incised five Chinese characters, meaning "made by Yiren living along the Zhang riverside". It was unearthed around the south gate of Mengzhuang Village in the north of Ci County, Hebei Province.

Preserved in China Cizhou Kiln Museum

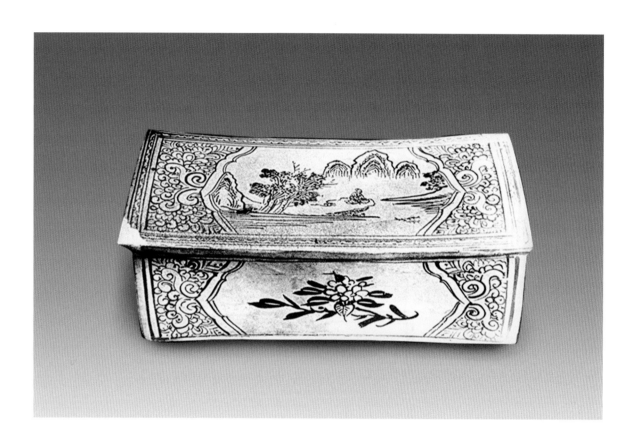

长方形白地黑花山水人物故事枕

金

瓷质

长 32 厘米，宽 15.7 厘米，高 14 厘米

Rectangular Pillow with Black Designs of Landscape and Figure on a White Ground

Jin Dynasty

Porcelain

Length 32 cm/ Width 15.7 cm/ Height 14 cm

胎质灰白坚硬，施化妆土、透明釉，底部无釉，背面上缘有气孔。枕面绘山水人物，前立面绘折枝花，后立面有墨书文字："寒食少天色，春风多柳花。倚楼心绪乱，不觉见栖鸦"。底部印有单栏竖式"张家造"戳记。磁县观台镇出土。

This pillow has a firm and greyish-white body, covered with engobe and a transparent glaze, and its bottom is unglazed. There are pores on the upper edge of its back. The pillow face is painted with design of landscapes and figures. On the front wall of the pillow are drawn flower branches, while on the back wall an ink inscription of a poem in Chinese. On the bottom is stamped a vertical single-coumn seal of "Zhang Jia Zao" (Made by Zhang's). It was unearthed in Guantai Township, Ci County, Hebei Province.

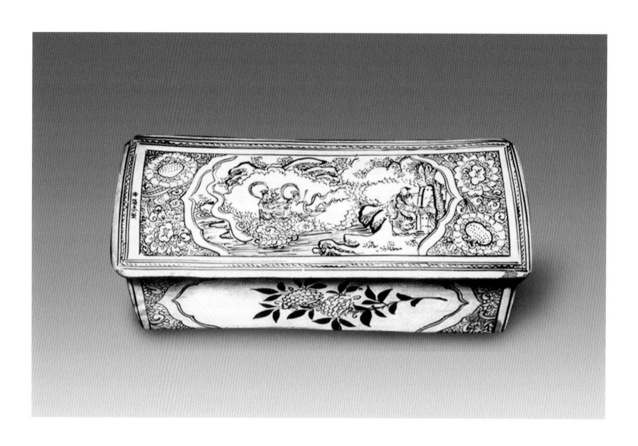

长方形白地黑花人物故事枕

金

瓷质

长 37.1 厘米，宽 15.8 厘米，高 12.4 厘米

Rectangular Pillow with Black Designs of Figure and Scene on a White Ground

Jin Dynasty

Porcelain

Length 37.1 cm/ Width 15.8 cm/ Height 12.4 cm

胎质灰白坚硬，施化妆土、透明釉，底部无釉，背面上缘有气孔。枕面绘人物故事，前立面绘折枝花，后立面绘牡丹，两端面绘荷花。枕面左边刻画有"漳滨逸人制"五字。磁县岳城水库出土。

峰峰矿区文物保管所藏

This pillow has a firm and greyish-white body, covered with engobe and a layer of transparent glaze, and its bottom is unglazed. There are pores on the upper edge of its back. The pillow face is painted with designs of a figure and scenes. On the front wall of the pillow is drawn a flower branch, while on the back wall peonies, with lotus flowers on its side walls. On the left side of the pillow face are incised five Chinese characters, meaning "Made by Yiren living along the Zhang riverside". It was unearthed in Yuecheng Reservoir in Ci County, Hebei Province.

Preserved in the Department of Cultural Relics Conservation of Fengfeng Mining District

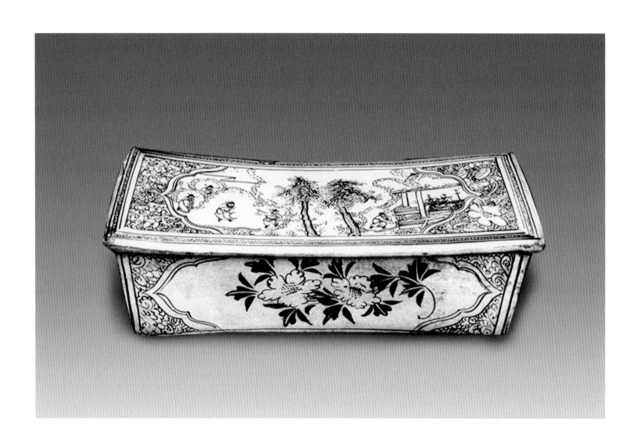

长方形白地黑花人物故事枕

金

瓷质

长 43.5 厘米，宽 18.3 厘米，高 15.8 厘米

Rectangular Pillow with Black Designs of Figure and Scene on a White Ground

Jin Dynasty

Porcelain

Length 43.5 cm/ Width 18.3 cm/ Height 15.8 cm

胎质灰白坚硬，施化妆土、透明釉，底部无釉，背面上缘有气孔，背右残补，局部有开片。枕面绘人物故事，前立面绘折枝花，后立面绘孔雀牡丹，两端面绘荷花。磁县都党乡冶子村出土。

中国磁州窑博物馆藏

This pillow has a firm body in greyish white and is covered with engobe and a layer of transparent glaze. Its bottom is unglazed. There are pores on the upper edge of its back wall, and the right part of its back wall is damaged. Crackles can be found on some parts. The pillow face is painted with designs of figures and scenes. On the front wall of the pillow are drawn flower branches, while on the back wall are painted a peacock and peonies, with lotus flower on its side walls. It was unearthed in Yezi Village, Dudang Township in Ci County, Hebei Province.

Preserved in China Cizhou Kiln Museum

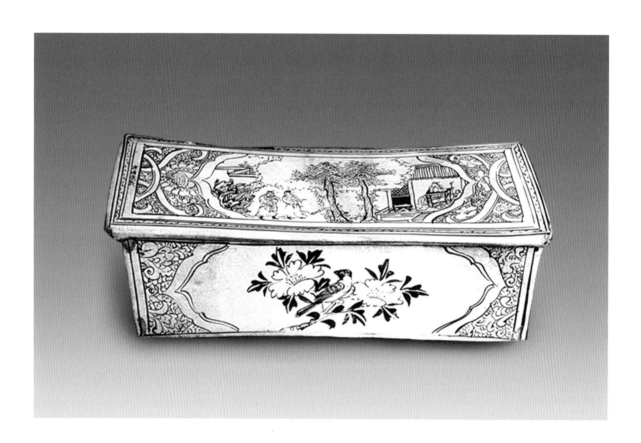

长方形白地黑花人物故事枕

金

瓷质

长 42.7 厘米，宽 17.3 厘米，高 16.6 厘米

Rectangular Pillow with Black Designs of Figure and Scene on a White Ground

Jin Dynasty

Porcelain

Length 42.7 cm/ Width 17.3 cm/ Height 16.6 cm

胎质灰白坚硬，施化妆土、透明釉，底部无釉，背面上缘有气孔。枕面绘人物故事，前立面绘花鸟，后立面绘折枝牡丹，两端面绘荷花。底部印有钟形"王氏寿明"戳记。枕面左边刻画有"漳滨逸人制"五字。磁县观台镇出土。

The pillow has a firm body in greyish white and is covered with engobe and a layer of transparent glaze, and its bottom is unglazed. There are pores on the upper edge of its back. The pillow face is painted with designs of figures and scenes. On the front wall of the pillow are drawn flowers and a bird, while on the back wall peony branches, with lotus flower designs on its side walls. On the bottom of the pillow is stamped a bell-shaped seal of "Wang Shi Shou Ming" (Shouming of the Wang family), and on the left side of the pillow face are incised five Chinese characters, meaning "made by Yiren living along the Zhang riverside". It was unearthed in Guantai Township, Ci County, Hebei Province.

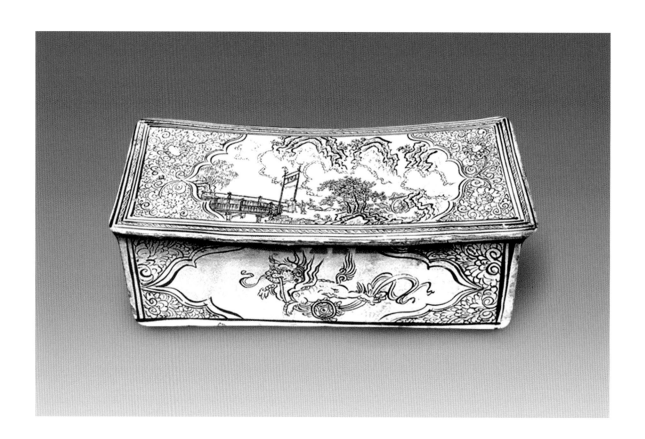

长方形白地黑花人物故事枕

金

瓷质

长 44 厘米，宽 18 厘米，高 10 厘米

Rectangular Pillow with Black Designs of Figure and Scene on a White Ground

Jin Dynasty

Porcelain

Length 44 cm/ Width 18 cm/ Height 10 cm

胎质灰白坚硬，施化妆土、透明釉，底部无釉，背面上缘有气孔。枕面绘山水人物故事，前立面绘狮子绣球，后立面绘猛虎，两端绘花卉。底部有竖式双栏上莲叶、下荷花"张家造"戳记。磁县南来村西岗古墓出土。

中国磁州窑博物馆藏

The firm greyish-white body of the pillow is covered with engobe and a layer of transparent glaze. The upper edge of the back wall has pores. The face of the pillow is embellished with a motif of figures and scenes. On the front wall is painted a lion playing with a ball with floral designs on the side walls. The bottom is stamped with a vertical double column seal of "Zhang Jia Zhao" (Made by Zhang's), with decorations of a lotus leaf motif on the upper edge and a lotus blossom motif on the lower edge. It was unearthed from the ancient Xigang tomb in Nanlai Village, Ci County, Hebei Province.

Preserved in China Cizhou Kiln Museum

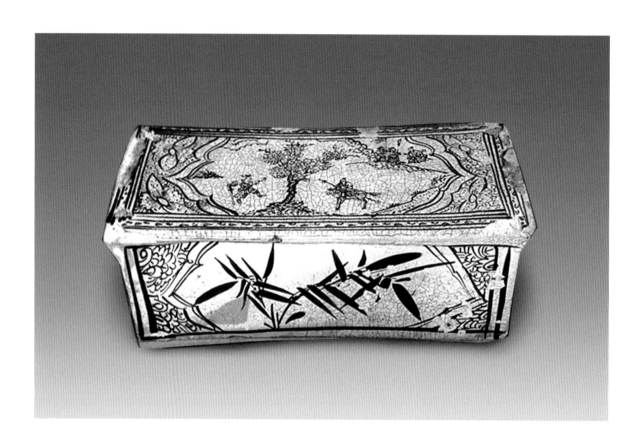

长方形白地褐花人物故事枕

金

瓷质

长 31.3 厘米，宽 16 厘米，前高 10 厘米，后高 13.5 厘米

Rectangular Pillow with Brown Designs of Figure and Scene on a White Ground

Jin Dynasty

Porcelain

Length 31.3 cm/ Width 16 cm/ Front Height 10 cm/ Back Height 13.5 cm

胎质灰白粗坚，施化妆土、透明釉，有开片，呈酱色釉彩，背面上缘有气孔，底部无釉。枕面绘人物故事，前立面绘竹，后立面绘折枝牡丹，端面各绘牡丹一朵。底部印有竖式双栏上莲叶、下荷花"古相张家造"戳记。

天津博物馆藏

The greyish-white body of the pillow is rough and firm in texture. It is covered with a layer of engobe, on which is transparent glaze with crackles, showing a caramel tint. There are pores on the upper edge of the back wall of the pillow. The bottom of it is unglazed. The pillow face is decorated with designs of figures and scenes, the front wall with bamboo branches, the back wall with peony branches, with a peony flower on each of the side walls. The bottom is stamped with a vertical double column seal of "Gu Xiang Zhang Jia Zhao" (Made by Zhang's in ancient Xiangzhou), with decorations of a lotus leaf motif on the upper edge and a lotus blossom motif on the lower edge.

Preserved in Tianjin Museum

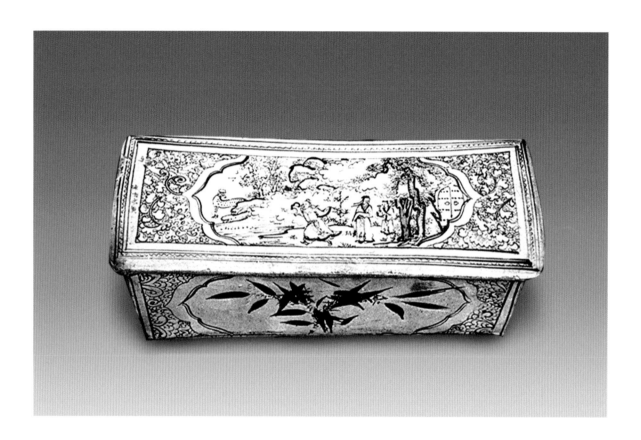

长方形白地黑花人物故事枕

金

瓷质

长 41.5 厘米，宽 16.6 厘米，高 15.6 厘米

Rectangular Pillow with Black Designs of Figure and Scene on a White Ground

Jin Dynasty

Porcelain

Length 41.5 cm/ Width 16.6 cm/ Height 15.6 cm

胎质灰白坚硬，施化妆土、透明釉，底部无釉，背面上缘有气孔。枕面绘人物故事，前立面绘竹，后立面绘凤凰，两端面绘荷花。底部印有钟形"王氏寿明"戳记。枕面左边刻画有"漳滨逸人制"五字。磁县南开河乡小侯召村出土。

中国磁州窑博物馆藏

The pillow has a firm body in greyish white and is covered with engobe and a layer of transparent glaze, and its bottom is unglazed. There are pores on the upper edge of its back wall. The pillow face is painted with designs of figures and scenes. On the front wall of the pillow are drawn bamboos, while on the back wall a phenix, with lotus flower designs on its side walls. On the bottom of the pillow is stamped a bell-shaped seal of "Wang Shi Shou Ming" (Shouming of the Wang family), and on the left side of the pillow face are incised five Chinese characters, meaning "made by Yiren living along the Zhang riverside". It was unearthed in Xiaohouzhao Village, Nankaihe Township, Ci County, Hebei Province.

Preserved in China Cizhou Kiln Museum

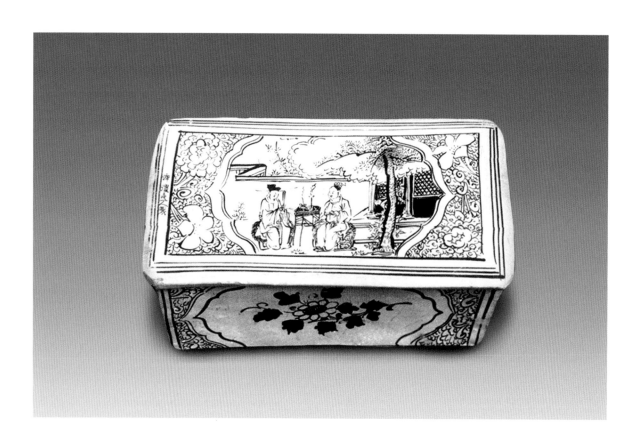

长方形白地黑花人物故事枕

金

瓷质

长 29.5 厘米，宽 17 厘米，高 14.5 厘米

Rectangular Pillow with Black Designs of Figure and Scene on a White Ground

Jin Dynasty

Porcelain

Length 29.5 cm/ Width 17 cm/ Height 14.5 cm

胎质灰白坚硬，施化妆土、透明釉，底部无釉，背面上缘有气孔。枕面绘人物故事，前立面绘折枝花，后立面绘牡丹，两端面绘花卉。底部印有钟形"王氏寿明"戳记。枕面左边刻画有"漳滨逸人制"五字。磁县观台镇出土。

中国磁州窑博物馆藏

The pillow has a firm body in greyish white and is covered with engobe and a layer of transparent glaze, and its bottom is unglazed. There are pores on the upper edge of its back wall. The pillow face is painted with designs of figures and scenes. On the front wall of the pillow are drawn flower branches, while on the back wall peony designs, with floral designs on its side walls. On the bottom of the pillow is stamped a bell-shaped seal of "Wang Shi Shou Ming" (Shouming of the Wang family), and on the left side of the pillow face are incised five Chinese characters, meaning "made by Yiren living along the Zhang riverside". It was unearthed in Guantai Township, Ci County, Hebei Province.

Preserved in China Cizhou Kiln Museum

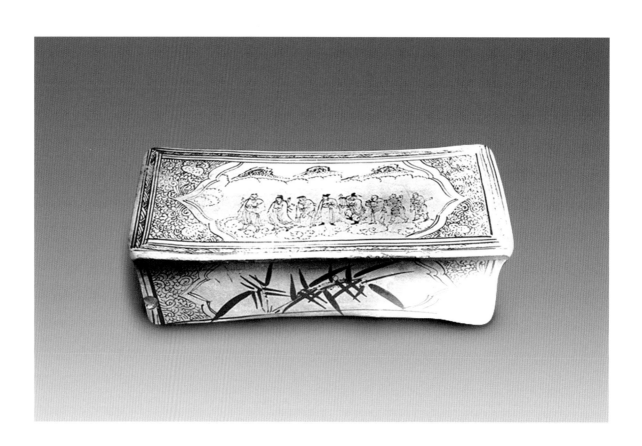

长方形白地黑花人物故事枕

金

瓷质

长 41.2 厘米，宽 19 厘米，高 14.6 厘米

Rectangular Pillow with Black Designs of Figure and Scene on a White Ground

Jin Dynasty

Porcelain

Length 41.2 cm/ Width 19 cm/ Height 14.6 cm

胎质灰白坚硬，施化妆土、透明釉，底部无釉，背面上缘有气孔。枕面绘8个人物在云上行走，前立面绘竹，后立面绘折枝牡丹，两端面绘花卉。底部印有"张家造"戳记。磁县岳城水库出土。

峰峰矿区文物保管所藏

A layer of engobe is applied to the firm greyish-white body of the pillow. The whole body except the bottom is covered with transparent glaze. There are pores on the upper edge of the back wall of the pillow. The pillow face is decorated with designs of eight figures walking on the clouds. Bamboos are painted on the front wall, and branches of peonies on the back wall, with floral designs on the side walls. On the bottom is inscribed a seal of "Zhang Jia Zhao" (Made by Zhang's). It was unearthed in Yuecheng Reservior in Ci County, Hebei Province.

Preserved in the Department of Cultural Relics Conservation of Fengfeng Mining District

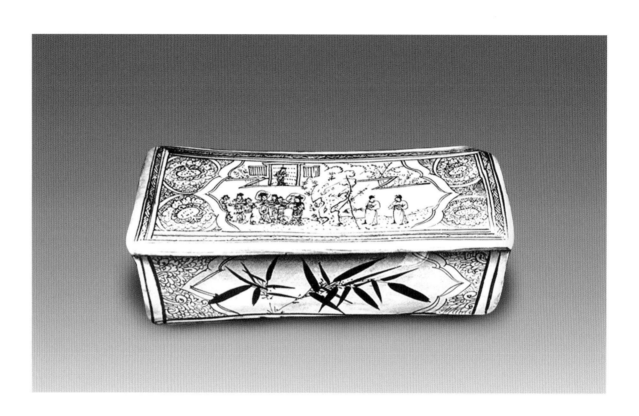

长方形白地黑花人物故事枕

金

瓷质

长 39.3 厘米，宽 17.8 厘米，高 15 厘米

Rectangular Pillow with Black Designs of Figure and Scene on a White Ground

Jin Dynasty

Porcelain

Length 39.3 cm/ Width 17.8 cm/ Height 15 cm

胎质灰白坚硬，施化妆土、透明釉，底部无釉，背面上缘有气孔。枕面绘人物故事，前立面绘竹，后立面绘折枝牡丹，两端面绘花卉。磁县岳城水库出土。

峰峰矿区文物保管所藏

The firm greyish-white body is covered with a layer of engobe, and the whole body except the bottom is coated with a transparent glaze. There are pores on the upper edge of the back wall of the pillow. The pillow face is decorated with designs of figures and scenes, the front wall with bamboo branches, the back wall with peony branches, and the side walls with floral designs. It was unearthed in Yuecheng Reservoir in Ci County, Hebei Province.

Preserved in the Department of Cultural Relics Conservation of Fengfeng Mining District

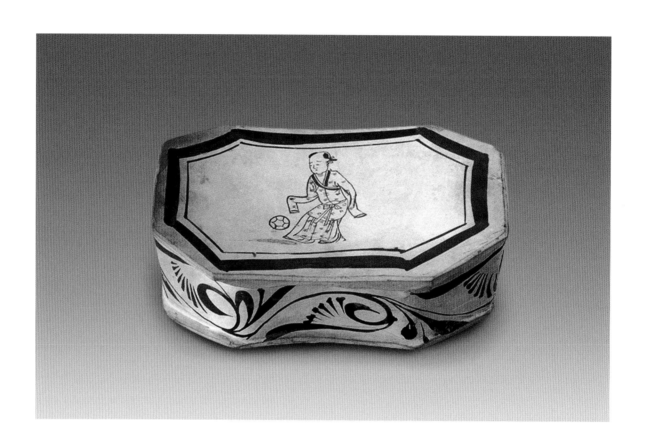

八角形白地黑花童子蹴鞠枕

金

瓷质

长 30 厘米，宽 18.5 厘米，高 10.8 厘米

Octagonal Pillow with Black Cuju-playing-boy Design of on a White Ground

Jin Dynasty

Porcelain

Length 30 cm/ Width 18.5 cm/ Height 10.8 cm

胎质灰白坚硬，施化妆土、透明釉，底部无釉，背面上缘有气孔。枕面绘一童子踢球，周壁有卷草纹饰。底部印有横书阳文"张家造"戳记。邢台市出土。

河北博物院藏

The firm greyish-white body is covered with engobe and a layer of transparent glaze. The bottom is left unglazed. There are pores on the upper edge of the back wall of the pillow. A motif of a child playing Cuju is painted on the pillow face. A pattern of rolled grass embellishes the four peripheral walls. The pillow's bottom is stamped with a horizontal seal in relief of "Zhang Jia Zhao" (Made by Zhang's). It was unearthed in Xingtai, Hebei Province.

Preserved in Hebei Museum

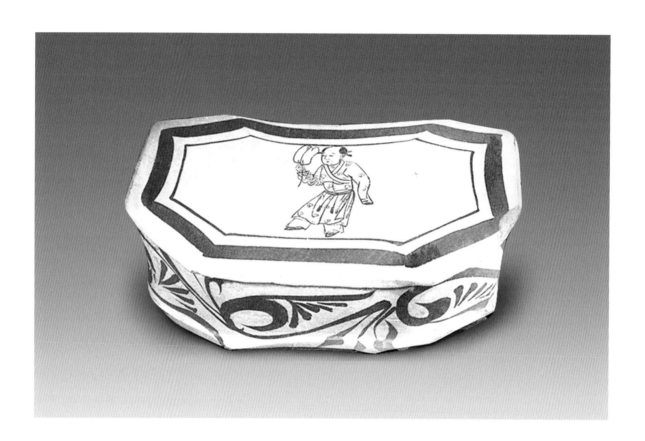

八角形白地黑花童子执扇枕

金

瓷质

长 31.2 厘米，宽 19.3 厘米，高 11.3 厘米

Octagonal Pillow with Black Design of a Boy Holding a Fan on a White Ground

Jin Dynasty

Porcelain

Length 31.2 cm/ Width 19.3 cm/ Height 11.3 cm

胎质灰白坚硬，施化妆土、透明釉，底部无釉，背面上缘有气孔。枕面绘一执扇童子，周壁有卷草纹饰。底部印有竖式"张家造"戳记。磁县观台镇出土。

安阳博物馆藏

The firm greyish-white body is covered with a layer of engobe, and the body except the bottom is coated with a transparent glaze. There are pores on the upper edge of the back wall of the pillow. The pillow face is decorated with designs of a boy holding a fan, while the four peripheral walls are embellished with patterns of rolled grass. The pillow's bottom is stamped with a vertical seal of "Zhang Jia Zhao" (Made by Zhang's). It was unearthed in Guantai Township, Ci County, Hebei Province.
Preserved in Anyang Municipal Museum

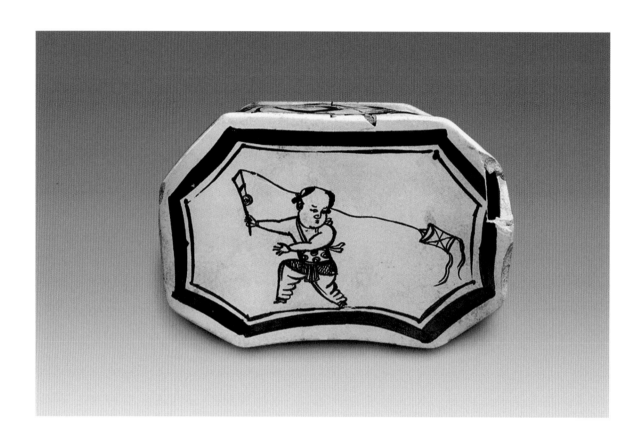

八角形白地黑花婴戏风筝枕

金

瓷质

长 28.7 厘米，宽 20 厘米，高 10 厘米

Octagonal Pillow with Black Kite-flying-child Design on a White Ground

Jin Dynasty

Porcelain

Length 28.7 cm/ Width 20 cm/ Height 10 cm

胎质灰白坚硬，施化妆土、透明釉，彩绘呈深褐色，底部无釉，背面上缘有气孔。枕面绘一童子戏风筝图，周壁有卷草纹饰。磁县都党乡冶子村出土。

中国磁州窑博物馆藏

The firm greyish-white body is covered with a layer of engobe. The body except the bottom is coated with a transparent glaze and decorated with dark-brown paintings. There are pores on the upper edge of the back wall of the pillow. The pillow face is decorated with a picture of a child flying a kite. The four peripheral walls are embellished with patterns of rolled grass. It was unearthed in Yezi Village in Dudang Township, Ci County, Hebei Province.

Preserved in China Cizhou Kiln Museum

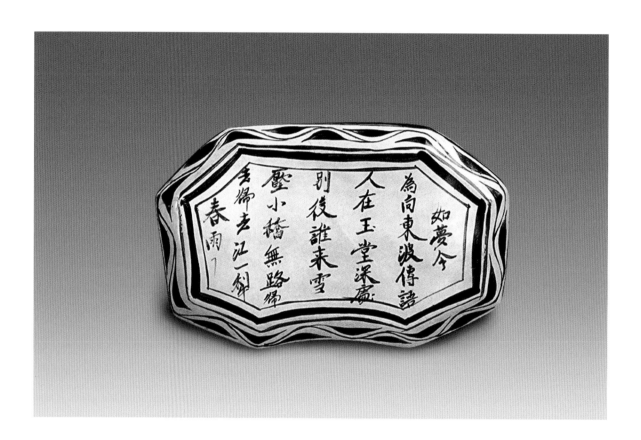

八角形白地黑花文字枕

金

瓷质

长 34 厘米，宽 21 厘米，高 13 厘米

Octagonal Pillow with Black Chinese Characters on a White Ground

Jin Dynasty

Porcelain

Length 34 cm/ Width 21 cm/ Height 13 cm

胎质灰白坚硬，施化妆土、透明釉，底部无釉，背面上缘有气孔。枕面墨书苏轼《如梦令》词一首。周壁有卷草纹饰。底部印有竖式"张家造"戳记。磁县都党乡冶子村出土。

中国磁州窑博物馆藏

The firm greyish-white body is covered with a layer of engobe, and the body except the bottom is coated with transparent glaze. There are pores on the upper edge of the back wall of the pillow. On the pillow face are an ink inscription of a Ci-poem named Rumengling by Su Shi. The four peripheral walls are embellished with patterns of rolled grass. The bottom is stamped with a vertical seal of "Zhang Jia Zhao" (Made by Zhang's). It was unearthed in Yezi Village in Dudang Township, Ci County, Hebei Province. Preserved in China Cizhou Kiln Museum

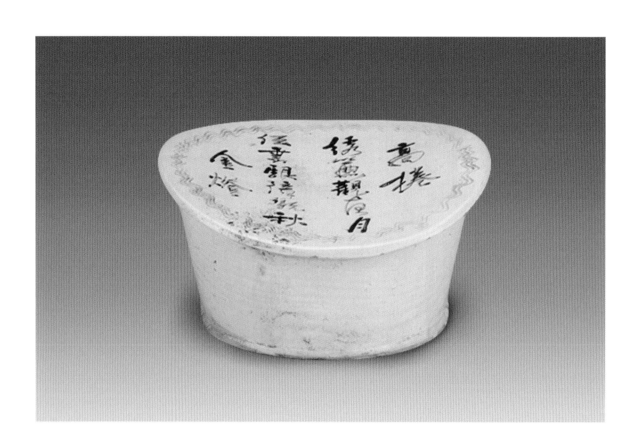

白釉褐彩诗句枕

金

瓷质

长 27 厘米，宽 24.2 厘米，高 14 厘米

White-glazed Pillow with a Poem in Brown

Jin Dynasty

Porcelain

Length 27 cm/ Width 24.2 cm/ Height 14 cm

腰圆形，两边翘起，中间微凹，胎灰白，有化妆土，除底外遍施白釉，釉色白中泛黄，枕面刻有三道曲线弦纹，中间褐彩书写"高捲绣帘观夜月，低垂银樟玩秋灯"七言诗。

山西博物院藏

This pillow has a round waist and a slightly concave face with the two ends cocking upward. The greyish-white body is covered with a layer of engobe, and the whole body except the bottom is coated with white glaze with a hint of yellow. On the pillow face are carved patterns of three curved strings, inside of which is written poem of seven-character octave in brown.

Preserved in Shanxi Museum

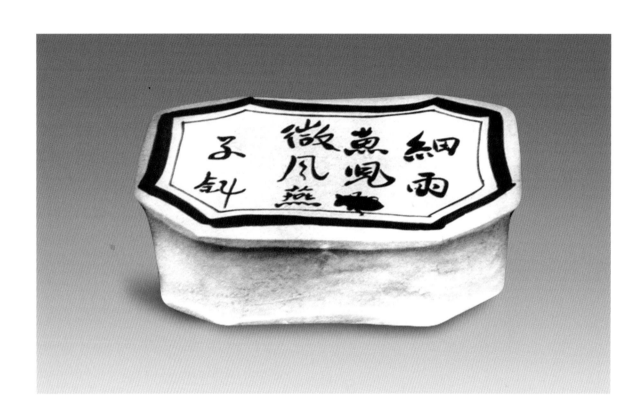

八角形白地文字枕

金

瓷质

长 27 厘米，宽 17.5 厘米，高 10 厘米

Octagonal Pillow with Black Inscription on a White Ground

Jin Dynasty

Porcelain

Length 27 cm/ Width 17.5 cm/ Height 10 cm

胎质灰白坚硬，施化妆土、透明釉，底部无釉，背面上缘有气孔。枕面墨书杜甫诗句"细雨鱼儿出，微风燕子斜"。周壁无饰。底部印有竖式单栏"张家造"戳记。河南省内黄县东庄乡渡店村出土。

河南省内黄县文物保管所藏

The firm greyish-white body is covered with engobe and a layer of transparent glaze, but the bottom is left unglazed. There are pores on the upper edge of the back wall. On the pillow face are written two lines of a poem by Du Fu in Chinese ink, while the peripheral walls are plain with no decoration. The bottom is stamped with a vertical single column seal of "Zhang Jia Zhao" (Made by Zhang's). It was unearthed in Dudian Village, Dongzhuang Township, Neihuang County, Henan Province.

Preserved in the Department of Cultural Relics Conservation, Neihuang County, Henan Province

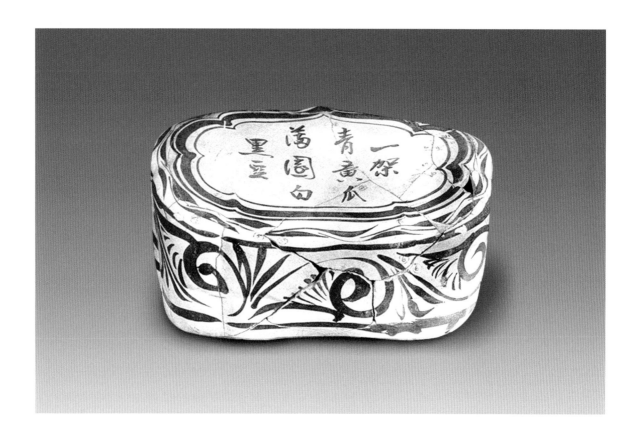

如意形白地黑花文字枕

金

瓷质

长 30.5 厘米，宽 23.5 厘米，高 14 厘米

Ruyi-shaped Pillow with Black Inscription on a White Ground

Jin Dynasty

Porcelain

Length 30.5 cm/ Width 23.5 cm/ Height 14 cm

胎质灰白坚硬，施化妆土、透明釉，底部无

釉，背面上缘有气孔，枕残。枕面墨书"一

架青黄瓜，满园白黑豆"。周壁有卷草纹饰。

磁县观台镇出土。

中国磁州窑博物馆藏

The firm greyish-white body is covered with
engobe and a layer of a transparent glaze, but
the bottom is left unglazed. There are pores on
the upper edge of the back wall of this pillow,
which is damaged so that cracks can be seen.
On the pillow face are written two Chinese
sentences in Chinese ink, while the peripheral
walls are embellished with designs of rolled
grass. It was unearthed in Guantai Township, Ci
County, Hebei Province.

Preserved in China Cizhou Kiln Museum

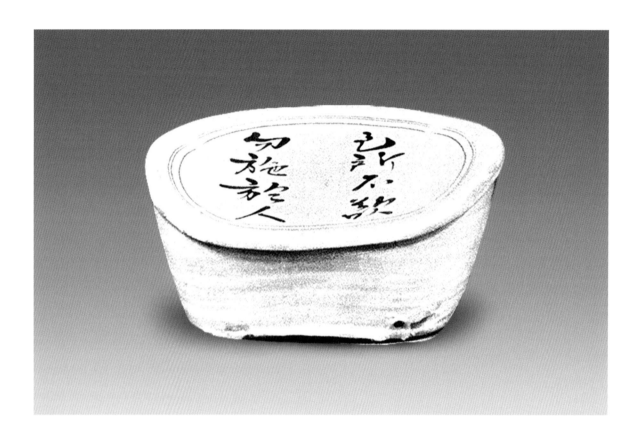

腰圆形白地文字枕

金

瓷质

长 26 厘米，宽 21.9 厘米，高 12.6 厘米

Round-waisted Pillow with Black Inscription on a White Ground

Jin Dynasty

Porcelain

Length 26 cm/ Width 21.9 cm/ Height 12.6 cm

胎质细而坚，呈深褐色，施化妆土、透明釉，底部无釉，背面有气孔。枕面墨书"己所不欲，勿施于人"。周壁白釉无饰。

杨永德藏

A layer of engobe is applied to the dark-brown body, which is fine and firm. The entire body except the bottom is covered with transparent glaze. There are pores on the back wall. On the pillow face is written a famous Chinese saying in Chinese ink, while the peripheral walls are only white-glazed without any decoration.

Collected by Yang Yongde

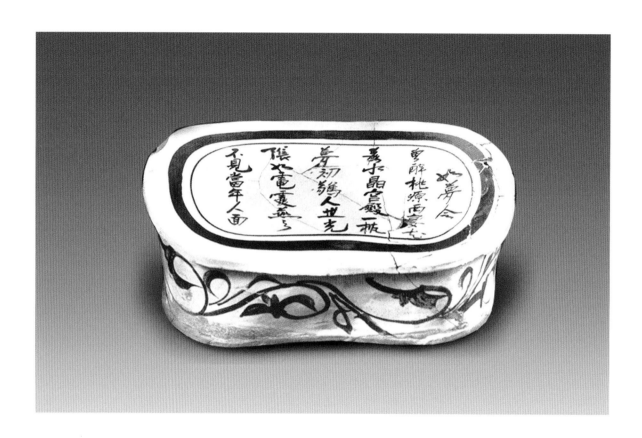

腰圆形白地黑花文字枕

金

瓷质

长 33.6 厘米，宽 21.6 厘米，高 12.5 厘米

Round-waisted Pillow with Black Inscription and Floral Design on a White Ground

Jin Dynasty

Porcelain

Length 33.6 cm/ Width 21.6 cm/ Height 12.5 cm

胎质灰白坚硬，施化妆土、透明釉，底部无釉，
背面上缘有气孔。枕面墨书《如梦令》词一首，
周壁饰卷草纹。磁县岳城水库出土。

峰峰矿区文物保管所藏

The firm greyish-white body of the pillow is
covered with engobe, and the body except
the bottom is coated with transparent glaze.
There are pores on the upper edge of the back
wall. On the pillow face is written a Ci-poem,
named Rumengling, in Chinese ink, while the
peripheral walls are embellished with designs
of rolled grass. It was unearthed in Yuecheng
Reservoir in Ci County, Hebei Province.
Preserved in the Department of Cultural Relics
Conservation of Fengfeng Ming District

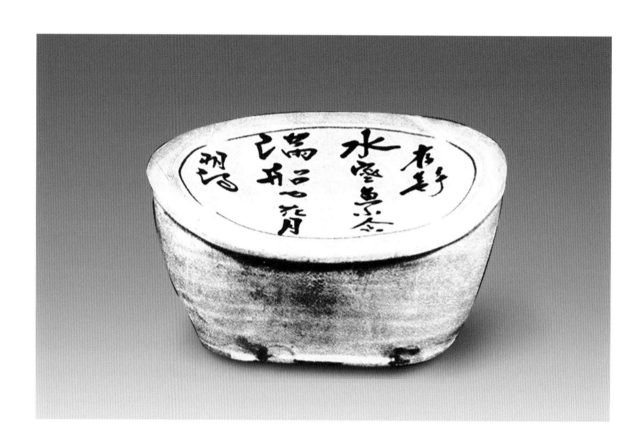

腰圆形白地诗文枕

金

瓷质

长 25.8 厘米，宽 22.5 厘米，高 12.6 厘米

Round-waisted Pillow with Poem on a White Ground

Jin Dynasty

Porcelain

Length 25.8 cm/ Width 22.5 cm/ Height 12.6 cm

胎质细而坚，呈灰白色，施化妆土、透明釉，底部无釉，气孔在背面下部。枕面墨书"水寒鱼小念存静，满船身在月明诗"。周壁白釉无饰。

杨永德藏

The greyish-white body is fine and firm and is covered with a layer of engobe. The whole body except the bottom is coated with transparent glaze. There are pores on the lower part of the back wall. On the pillow face are written two lines of a poem in Chinese ink, while the vertical sides are only glazed white without any decoration.

Collected by Yang Yongde

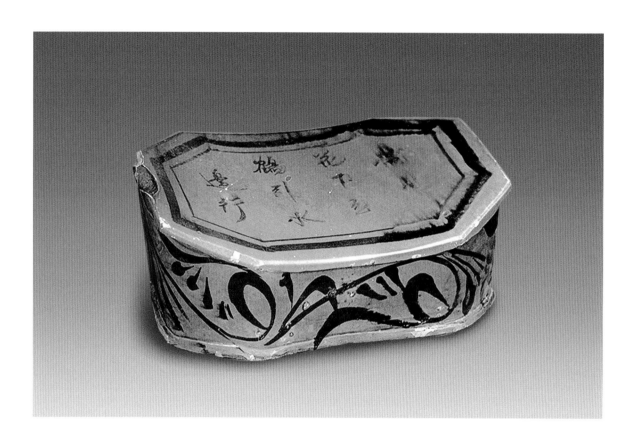

八角形绿釉文字枕

金

瓷质

长 30 厘米，宽 20 厘米，高 12 厘米

Octagonal Green-glazed Pillow with Inscription

Jin Dynasty

Porcelain

Length 30 cm/ Width 20 cm/ Height 12 cm

胎质松软，呈微红色，施绿釉和透明釉，底部无釉，背面上缘有气孔。枕面有黑框，框内墨书"蜂飞花下至，鹤引水边行"。周壁有卷草纹饰。磁县都党乡冶子村出土。

中国磁州窑博物馆藏

The slight-red body is of loose texture and coated with green and transparent glazes, with the bottom left unglazed. There are pores on the upper edge of the back wall. The pillow face has a black frame, inside of which are written two lines of a poem in Chinese ink. The peripheral walls are embellished with designs of rolled grass. It was unearthed in Yezi Village, Dudang Township, Ci County, Hebei Province. Preserved in China Cizhou Kiln Museum

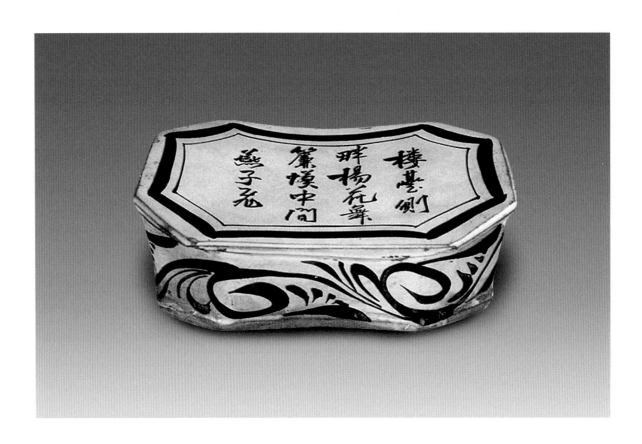

八角形白地黑花诗文枕

金

瓷质

长 28.5 厘米，宽 18.5 厘米，前高 7.5 厘米，后高 10.4 厘米

Octagonal Pillow with Black Poem and Floral Designs on a White Ground

Jin Dynasty

Porcelain

Length 28.5 cm/ Width 18.5 cm/ Front Height 7.5 cm/ Back Height 10.4 cm

胎质灰褐，釉色淡黄，施化妆土、透明釉，底部无釉，背面上缘有气孔。枕面有一粗一细两条直线作边框，中间抄录："楼台侧畔杨花过，帘幕中间燕子飞"诗文两句，周壁有卷草纹饰。底部印有竖式单栏"张大家枕"戳记。

天津博物馆藏

The greyish-brown body is coated with engobe and a layer of transparent glaze with a yellowish tint. The bottom is unglazed and there are pores on the upper edge of the back wall. The pillow face has a frame made by a thick and a thin lines, inside of which are written two lines of a poem. The peripheral walls are embellished with designs of rolled grass. The bottom is stamped a vertical single-coloum seal "Zhang Da Jia zhen" (Made by Zhang Da Jia).
Preserved in Tianjin Museum

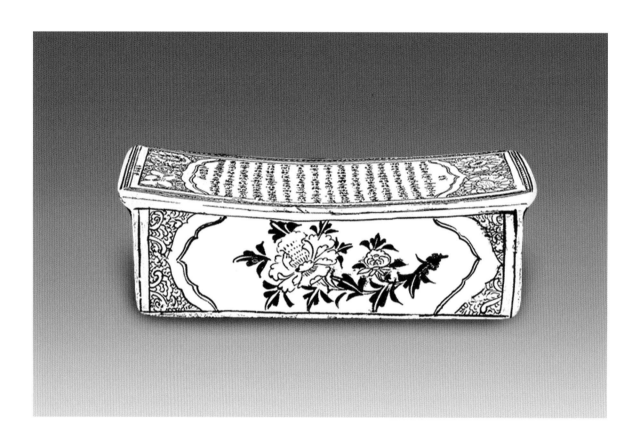

长方形白地黑花文字枕

金

瓷质

长 42 厘米，宽 15.7 厘米，高 14.4 厘米

Rectangular Pillow with Black Floral Design and Inscription on a White Ground

Jin Dynasty

Porcelain

Length 42 cm/ Width 15.7 cm/ Height 14.4 cm

胎质灰白坚硬，施化妆土、透明釉，底部无釉，背面上缘有气孔。枕面墨书"枕赋"。左端刻画有"漳滨逸人制"五字，前立面绘牡丹，端面绘荷花。底部有方形印款"王氏寿明"。

杨永德藏

The firm greyish-white body is coated with engobe and a layer of a transparent glaze. There on pores on the upper edge of the back wall. On the pillow face is written with a prose in Chinese ink, and on the left part of the face are incised five Chinese characters, meaning "made by Yiren living along the Zhang riverside". The front wall is decorated with peony designs, and lotus designs on the side walls. The bottom is stamped with a square seal of "Wang Shi Shou Ming" (Shouming of the Wang family).

Collected by Yang Yongde

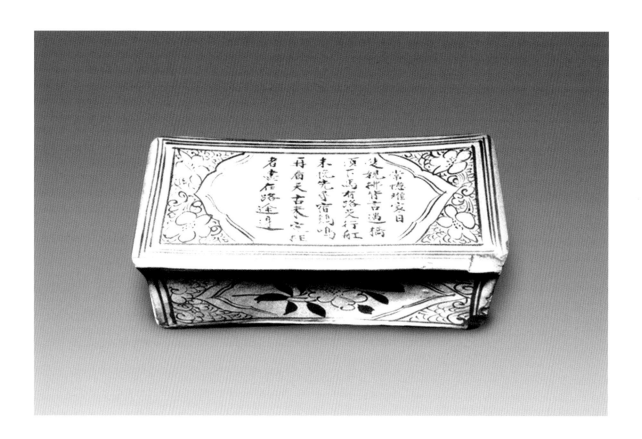

长方形白地黑花文字枕

金

瓷质

长 31 厘米，宽 15 厘米，高 13 厘米

Rectangular Pillow with Black Floral Design and Inscription on a White Ground

Jin Dynasty

Porcelain

Length 31 cm/ Width 15 cm/ Height 13 cm

胎质灰白坚硬，施化妆土、透明釉，底部无釉，背面上缘有气孔。枕面书"常忆离家日……"诗一首。前立面绘折枝花，后立面绘牡丹，两端面绘荷花。磁县岳城水库出土。

峰峰矿区文物保管所藏

The firm greyish-white body is covered with a layer of engobe. The entire body except the bottom is coated with transparent glaze. There are pores on the upper edge of the back wall. On the pillow face is written a poem. On the front wall is painted a flower branch design, and on the back wall peony motifs, with lotus design on the side walls. It was unearthed in the Yuecheng Reservoir in Ci County, Hebei province.

Preserved in the Department of Cultural Relics Conservation of Fengfeng Mining District

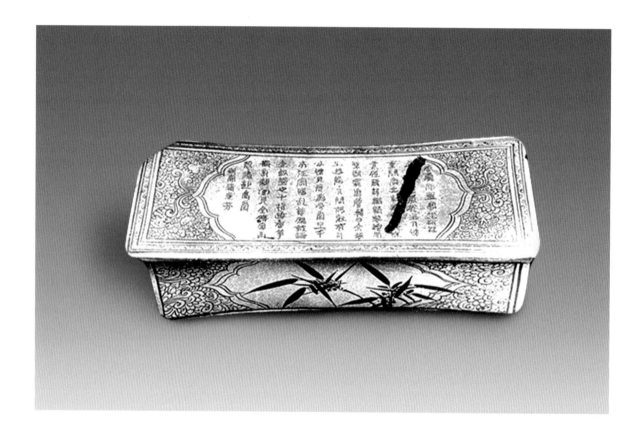

长方形白地黑花文字枕

金

瓷质

长 44.4 厘米，宽 18 厘米，高 14.5 厘米

Rectangular Pillow with Black Floral Design and Inscription on a White Ground

Jin Dynasty

Porcelain

Length 44.4 cm/ Width 18 cm/ Height 14.5 cm

胎质灰白坚硬，施化妆土、透明釉，底部无釉，背面上缘有气孔。枕面书苏东坡《满庭芳》词一首。前立面绘竹，后立面绘凤凰，两端面绘花卉。磁县岳城水库出土。

峰峰矿区文物保管所藏

The firm greyish-white body is coated with engobe and transparent glaze. The bottom is unglazed and there are pores on the upper edge of the back wall. On the pillow face is written a Ci-poem named "*Man Ting Fang*" by Su Dongpo; on the front wall are painted bamboo branches; on the back wall is a phoenix; on the side walls are floral design. It was unearthed in Yuecheng Reservoir in Ci County, Hebei Province.

Preserved in the Department of Cultural Relics Conservation of Fengfeng District

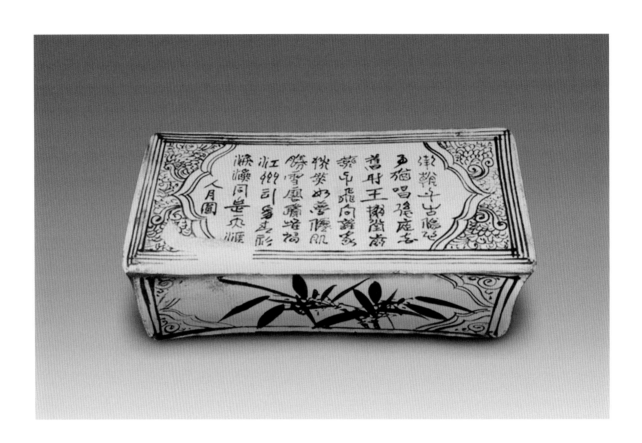

长方形白地黑花文字枕

金

瓷质

长 32 厘米，宽 15.5 厘米，高 12.5 厘米

Rectangular Pillow with Black Floral Design and Inscription on a White Ground

Jin Dynasty

Porcelain

Length 32 cm/ Width 15.5 cm/ Height 12.5 cm

胎质灰白坚硬，施化妆土、透明釉，底部无釉，背面上缘有气孔。枕面书吴激《人月圆》曲一首。前立面绘竹，后立面绘菊花，两端面绘花卉。底部印有竖式双栏上莲叶、下荷花"张家造"戳记。磁县牛尾岗村出土。

中国磁州窑博物馆藏

The firm greyish-white body is coated with engobe and transparent glaze. The bottom is unglazed and pores can be seen on the upper edge of the back wall. On the pillow face is written a verse named *"Ren Yue Yuan"* by Wu Ji. Bamboo branches are painted on the front wall; chrysanthemums on the back wall; floral designs on the side walls. On the bottom is inscribed a vertical double column seal of "Zhang Jia Zhao" (Made by Zhang's), with decorations of a lotus leaf motif on the upper edge and a lotus blossom motif on the lower edge. It was unearthed in Niuweigang Village, Ci County, Hebei Province.

Preserved in China Cizhou Kiln Museum

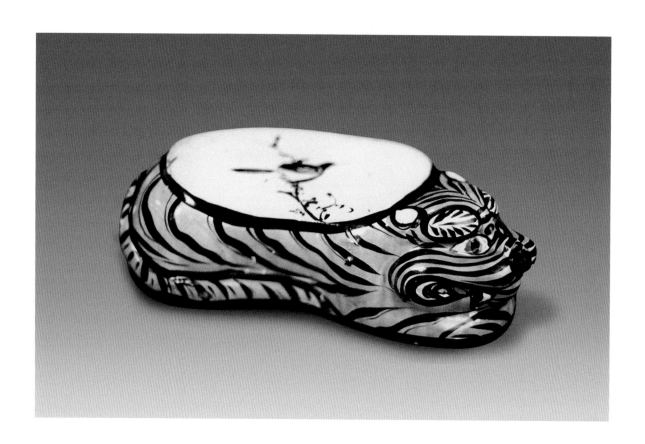

虎形彩色花鸟纹枕

金

瓷质

长 35 厘米，宽 13.2 厘米，高 11 厘米

Tiger-shaped Pillow with Designs of Colourful Flower and Bird

Jin Dynasty

Porcelain

Length 35 cm/ Width 13.2 cm/ Height 11 cm

胎质灰白坚硬，施化妆土、透明釉，底部无釉。
枕面绘雀鸟踏枝，周壁有虎纹饰。山西省长
治市出土。

长治市博物馆藏

The firm greyish-white body is covered with
a layer of engobe, and the whole body except
the bottom is coated with transparent glaze.
The pillow face is decorated with a design of a
bird perching on a branch, while the peripheral
walls are embellished with tiger stripes. It was
unearthed in Changzhi, Shanxi Province.

Preserved in Changzhi Museum

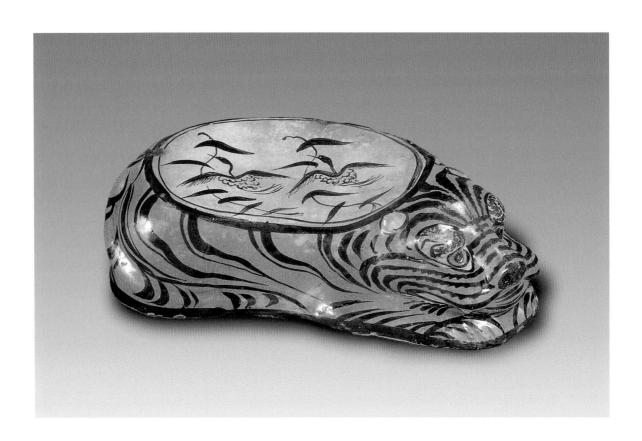

磁州窑黄褐釉芦雁图虎形枕

金

瓷质

长 34 厘米，宽 13.4 厘米，高 10.5 厘米

Yellowish-brown-glazed Pillow in the Shape of Tiger with Bulrush and Swan Goose Designs, Cizhou Ware

Jin Dynasty

Porcelain

Length 34 cm/ Width 13.4 cm/ Height 10.5 cm

胎质坚硬，上敷化妆土。枕作卧虎状。虎背为枕面，呈椭圆形，上施白釉，周边绘两条墨线作边框，内绘芦雁图，两只鸿雁口衔苇草，展翅飞翔于空中。虎身施赭黄釉，间以黄、褐色虎斑纹。

河北博物院藏

The body of the pillow is firm and covered with a layer of engobe. The pillow is in a shape of crouching tiger, and the back of the tiger serves as the ova-shaped pillow face, which is coated with white glaze. The edge of the face is decorated with two lines in Chinese ink as the frame, inside of which are painted two flying swan geese with bulrush in their mouths. The body of the tiger is coated with sienna glaze and decorated with tiger stripes.

Preserved in Hebei Museum

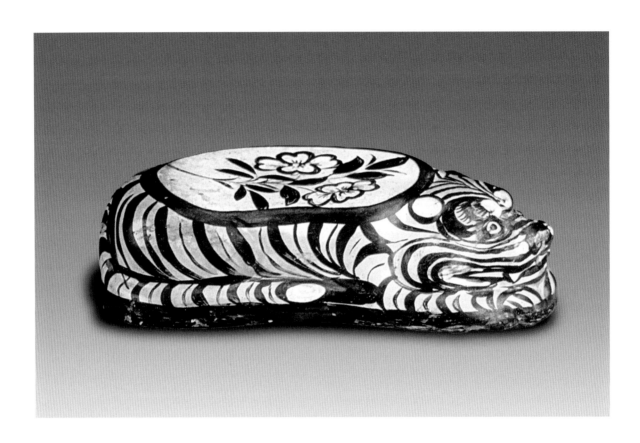

三彩虎枕

金

瓷质

长 32.5 厘米，高 8 厘米

Tricolour Tiger-shaped Pillow

Jin Dynasty

Porcelain

Length 32.5 cm/ Height 8 cm

枕呈卧虎状，一端为虎头，虎尾从另端盘至
前身，虎爪前伸微曲合于颔下，拱背前抵，
张口怒目，獠牙外露，虎背为椭圆形枕面，
微斜略凹，虎身以橘黄色黑彩虎纹，虎头为
白釉黑彩纹，枕面为白釉绘黑彩折枝花卉图，
画面着墨不多，生意盎然。

山西博物院藏

This pillow is in the shape of a crouching tiger, with the head on one side and the tail on the other. The tail of the tiger coils forward from the bottom of its body to the front, its claws stretching ahead and bending slightly under the jaw. Its back is arched and lean forward, its mouth opens with tusks outside, and its eyes stare full of anger. The back of the tiger, slightly sloping and concaving, functions as the ova-shaped face of the pillow. The tiger is orange-glazed while its head is white-glazed, but both are decorated with black stripes. The pillow face is white-glazed with a motif of a flowering branch in black. Though simple, the picture is vigorous and lively.

Preserved in Shanxi Museum

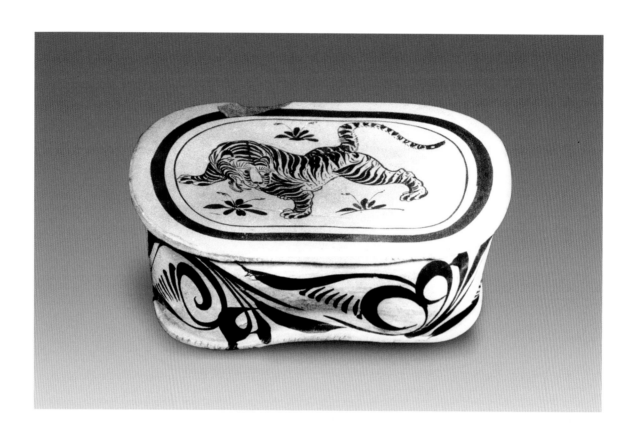

腰圆形白地黑花虎纹枕

金

瓷质

长 37.8 厘米，宽 27 厘米，高 14.8 厘米

Round-waisted Pillow with Black Tiger Design on a White Ground

Jin Dynasty

Porcelain

Length 37.8 cm/ Width 27 cm/ Height 14.8 cm

胎质灰白坚硬，施化妆土、透明釉，底部无釉，背面上缘有气孔。枕面绘猛虎，周壁饰卷草纹。底部印有竖式单栏上莲叶、下荷花"张家枕"戳记。磁县观台镇出土。

安阳博物馆藏

The firm greyish-white body is coated with engobe and a layer of transparent glaze. The bottom is unglazed and pores can be seen on the upper edge of the back wall. On the pillow face is painted a tiger, and the peripheral walls are embellished with designs of rolled grass. On the bottom is inscribed a vertical single-column seal of "Zhang Jia Zhen", with decorations of a lotus leaf motif on the upper edge and a lotus blossom motif on the lower edge. It was unearthed in Guantai Township, Ci County, Hebei Province.

Preserved in Anyang Municipal Museum

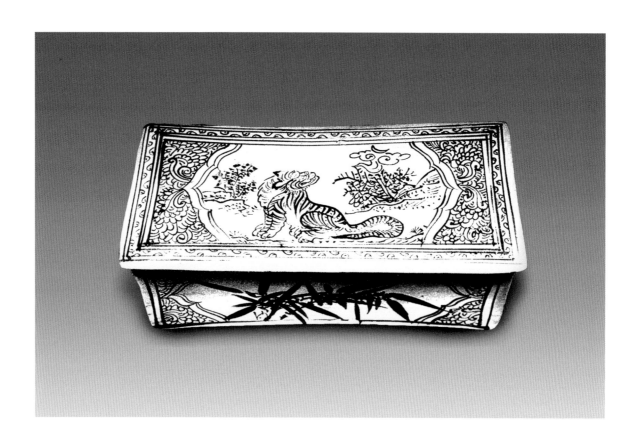

长方形白地黑花虎纹枕

金

瓷质

长 29 厘米，宽 15.2 厘米，高 12 厘米

Rectangular Pillow with Black Tiger Design on a White Ground

Jin Dynasty

Porcelain

Length 29 cm/ Width 15.2 cm/ Height 12 cm

胎质灰白坚硬，施化妆土、透明釉，底部无釉，背面上缘有气孔。枕面绘虎，前立面绘竹，后立面绘折枝牡丹，两端面绘花卉。底部印有竖式双栏上莲叶、下荷花"张家造"戳记。磁县观台镇出土。

峰峰矿区文物保管所藏

The firm greyish-white body is coated with engobe and transparent glaze. The bottom is unglazed and pores can be seen on the upper edge of back side. The pillow face is decorated with a tiger design; the front wall with bamboo branches; the back wall with peony branches; the side walls with floral designs. The bottom is is stamped with a vertical double column seal of "Zhang Jia Zhao" (Made by Zhang's). It was unearthed in Guantai Township in Ci County, Hebei Province.

Preserved in the Department of Cultural Relics Conservation of Fengfeng Mining District

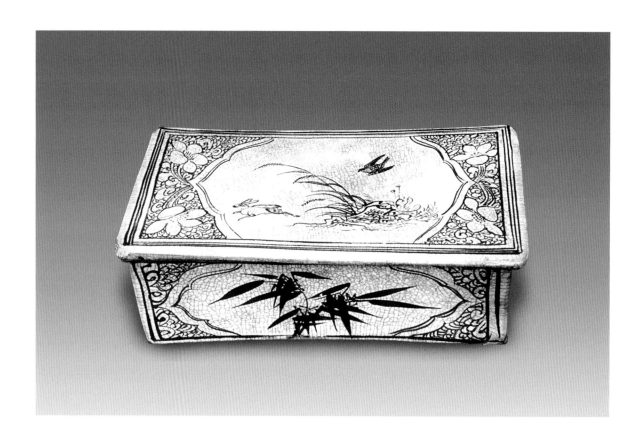

长方形白地黑花鹰兔纹枕

金

瓷质

长 30.3 厘米，宽 16.3 厘米，高 13 厘米

Rectangular Pillow with Black Designs of Eagle and Rabbit on a White Ground

Jin Dynasty

Porcelain

Length 30.3 cm/ Width 16.3 cm/ Height 13 cm

胎质灰白坚硬，施化妆土、透明釉，底部无釉，背面上缘有气孔，通体开片。枕面绘老鹰抓兔子，前立面绘竹，后立面绘折枝牡丹，两端面绘荷花。磁县南关石桥东南出土。

中国磁州窑博物馆藏

The firm greyish-white body is coated with engobe and transparent glaze with crackles. The bottom is unglazed, and pores can be seen on the upper edge of the back wall. A picture of an eagle catching a rabbit is painted on the pillow face, bamboo branches on the front wall, peony branches on the back wall, and lotus flowers on the side walls. It was unearthed from the place to the southeast of the Shiqiao Bridge in Nanguan of Ci County, Hebei Province.
Preserved in China Cizhou Kiln Museum

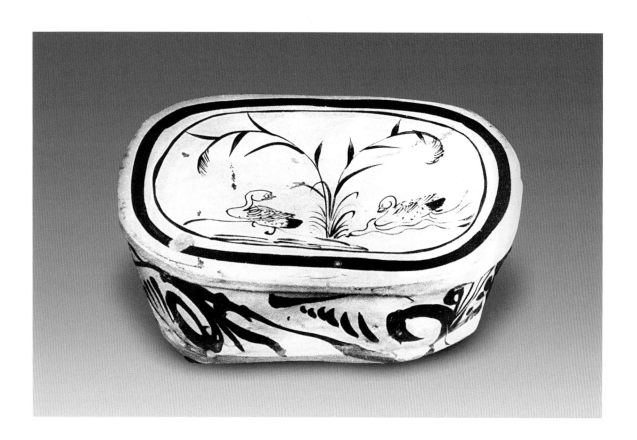

腰圆形白地黑花鸳鸯戏水枕

金

瓷质

长 29.3 厘米，宽 19.3 厘米，高 10 厘米

Round-waisted Pillow with Black Design of Two Mandarin Ducks Playing in Water on a White Ground

Jin Dynasty

Porcelain

Length 29.3 cm/ Width 19.3 cm/ Height 10 cm

胎质灰白坚硬，施化妆土、透明釉，底部无釉，背面上缘有气孔。枕面绘芦苇和鸳鸯戏水图，周壁卷草纹饰。底部印有横式阳文"张家造"戳记。磁县观台镇出土。

安阳博物馆藏

The firm greyish-white body is coated with engobe and transparent glaze. The bottom is unglazed, and pores can be seen on the upper edge of the back wall. The pillow face is decorated with designs of bulrushes and two mandarin ducks playing in water and the peripheral walls are embellished with designs of rolled grass. On the bottom is stamped a horizontal seal in relief of "Zhang Jia Zhao" (Made by Zhang's). It was unearthed in Guantai Township, Ci County, Hebei Province.

Preserved in Anyang Municipal Museum

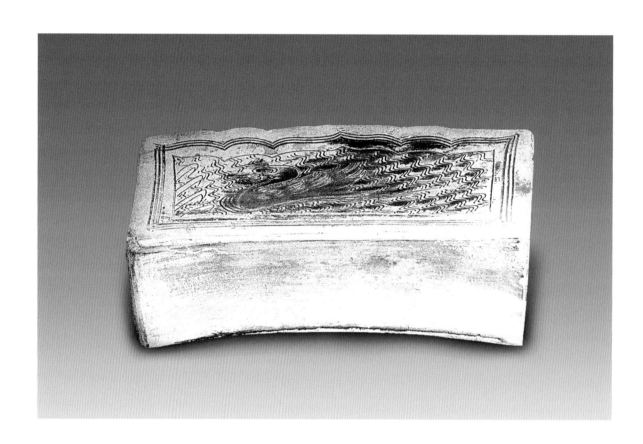

扇形绿釉鸭纹枕

金

瓷质

长 33 厘米，宽 16.8 厘米，高 10.8 厘米

Green-glazed and Fan-shaped Pillow with Duck Designs

Jin Dynasty

Porcelain

Length 33 cm/ Width 16.8 cm/ Height 10.8 cm

胎质松软，无化妆土，施绿釉，底部无釉，背面上缘有气孔。枕面刻画鸭子游水及水波纹，背面印有奔跑动物和花纹，前立面和两端面绿釉无饰。磁县白塔乡柳儿营村出土。

中国磁州窑博物馆藏

The body of the pillow is of loose texture and coated with green glaze except the bottom. There are pores on the upper edge of the back wall. The pillow face is incised with a design of a duck swimming in water and water ripple patterns; the back wall is decorated with patterns of running animals and floral designs; the front and the side walls are just coated with a green glaze without any decoration. It was unearthed in Liuerying Village, Baita Township, Ci County, Hebei Province.

Preserved in China Cizhou Kiln Museum

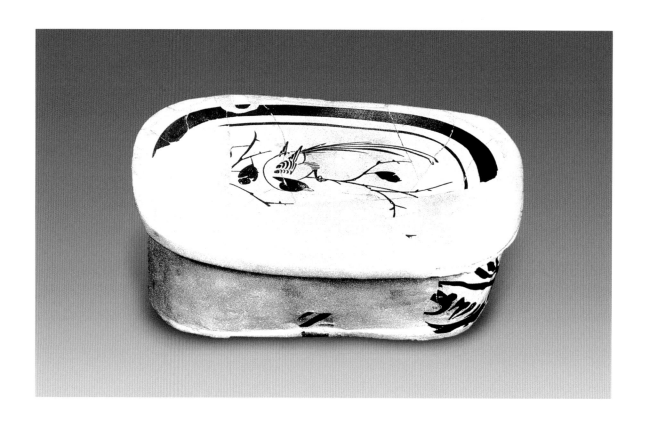

腰圆形白地黑花纪年枕

金

瓷质

长 30.1 厘米，宽 21.2 厘米，高 11 厘米

Round-waisted Commemorative Pillow with Black Floral Design on a White Ground

Jin Dynasty

Porcelain

Length 30.1 cm/ Width 21.2 cm/ Height 11 cm

胎质灰白坚硬，施化妆土、透明釉，底部无釉，背面上缘有气孔。枕面绘长尾鸟踏在一树枝上，周壁有卷草纹饰。印记破碎不清，有墨书"□定二年十……"。磁县观台镇出土。

中国磁州窑博物馆藏

The firm greyish-white body is coated with engobe and transparent glaze. The bottom is unglazed and pores can be seen on the upper edge of the back wall. The pillow face is decorated with a pattern of a reedling perching on a branch, while the peripheral walls are embellished with designs of rolled grass. As the pillow is not preserved well, the seal cannot be identified clearly, with only a few inked characters left indicating the date of production. It was unearthed in Guantai Township, Ci County, Hebei Province.

Preserved in China Cizhou Kiln Museum

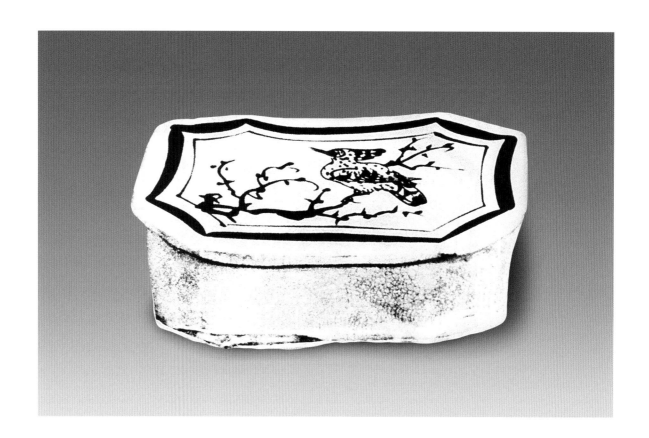

八角形白地黑花鸟纹枕

金

瓷质

长 28.4 厘米，宽 18.2 厘米，高 11 厘米

Octagonal Pillow with Black Floral and Bird Designs on a White Ground

Jin Dynasty

Porcelain

Length 28.4 cm/ Width 18.2 cm/ Height 11 cm

胎质细坚，呈深褐色，施化妆土、透明釉，
有粗开片，底部无釉，背面上缘有气孔。枕
面绘鸟踏树枝，周壁白釉无饰。底部印有竖
式"张家造"戳记。

杨永德藏

The dark brown body is fine and firm, and it is
coated with engobe and transparent glaze with
big crackles. The bottom is unglazed and pores
can be seen on the upper edge of the back wall.
The pillow face is decorated with a design of a
bird perching on a branch, while the peripheral
walls are just coated with white glaze with no
decoration. On the bottom is stamped a vertical
seal of "Zhang Jia Zhao" (Made by Zhang's).
Collected by Yang Yongde

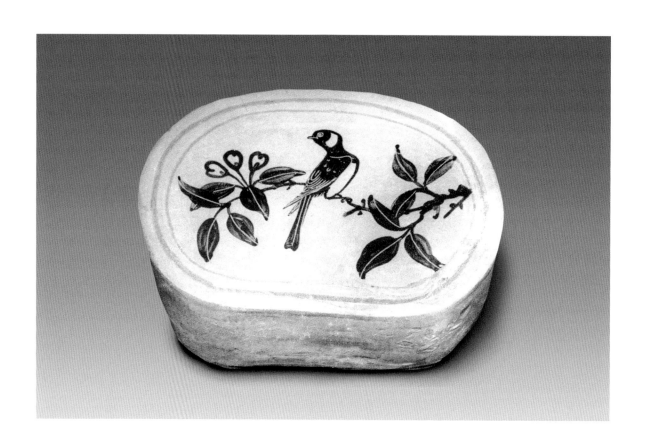

腰圆形白地黑花花鸟枕

金

瓷质

长 31 厘米，宽 22.7 厘米，高 12.7 厘米

Round-waisted Pillow with Black Designs of Bird and Flower on a White Ground

Jin Dynasty

Porcelain

Length 31 cm/ Width 22.7 cm/ Height 12.7 cm

胎质灰白坚硬，施化妆土、透明釉，底部无釉，有一扁气孔。枕面绘喜鹊踏枝，周壁白釉无饰。磁县都党乡冶子村出土。

中国磁州窑博物馆藏

The firm greyish-white body is coated with engobe and transparent glaze. The unglazed bottom has a flat pore. The pillow face is decorated with a design of a magpie perching on a branch, while the peripheral walls are coated only with white glaze with no decoration. It was unearthed in Yezi Village in Dudang Township, Ci County, Hebei Province.

Preserved in China Cizhou Kiln Museum

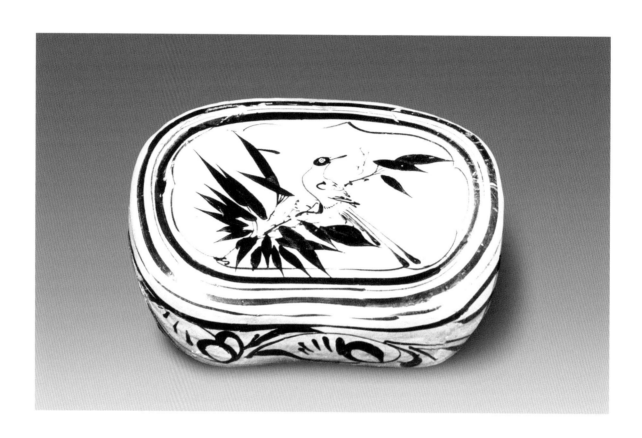

腰圆形白地黑花竹鸟枕

金

瓷质

长 30.5 厘米，宽 21.5 厘米，高 13 厘米

Round-waisted Pillow with Black Designs of Bamboo and Bird on a White Ground

Jin Dynasty

Porcelain

Length 30.5 cm/ Width 21.5 cm/ Height 13 cm

胎质灰白坚硬，施化妆土、透明釉，底部无釉，

背面上缘有气孔。枕面绘竹枝上踏一长尾鸟，

周壁有卷草纹饰。磁县观台镇东艾口村出土。

中国磁州窑博物馆藏

The firm greyish-white body is coated with engobe and transparent glaze. The bottom is unglazed, and pores can be seen on the upper edge of the back wall. The pillow face is decorated with a design of a reedling perching on a bamboo branch, while the peripheral walls are embellished with scrolled grass patterns. It was unearthed in the Dong'aikou Village, Guantai Township, Ci County, Hebei Province. Preserved in China Cizhou Kiln Museum

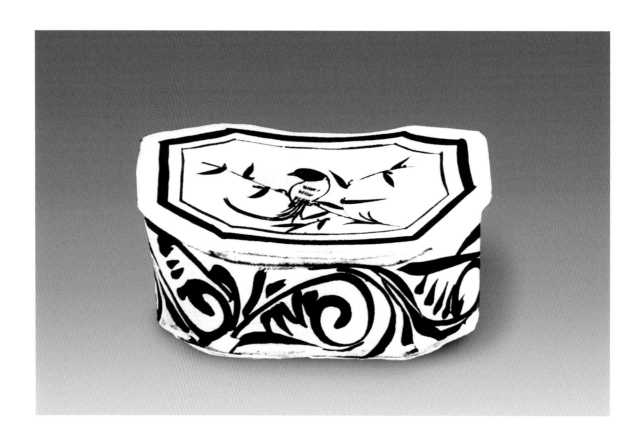

八角形白地黑花竹鸟图纹枕

金

瓷质

长 28.8 厘米，宽 20.9 厘米，高 12.3 厘米

Octagonal Pillow with Black Designs of Bamboo and Bird on a White Ground

Jin Dynasty

Porcelain

Length 28.8 cm/ Width 20.9 cm/ Height 12.3 cm

胎质较细坚硬，呈灰白色，施化妆土、透明釉，部分有开片，底部无釉，背面上缘有气孔。枕面绘竹篁和长尾鸟，周壁饰卷草纹。

杨永德藏

The greyish-white body is fine and firm, and it is coated with engobe and transparent glaze, parts of which have crackles. The bottom is unglazed and pores can be seen on the upper edge of the back wall. The pillow face is decorated with designs of bamboo grove and a reedling, and the peripheral walls are embellished with designs of scrolled grass.

Collected by Yang Yongde

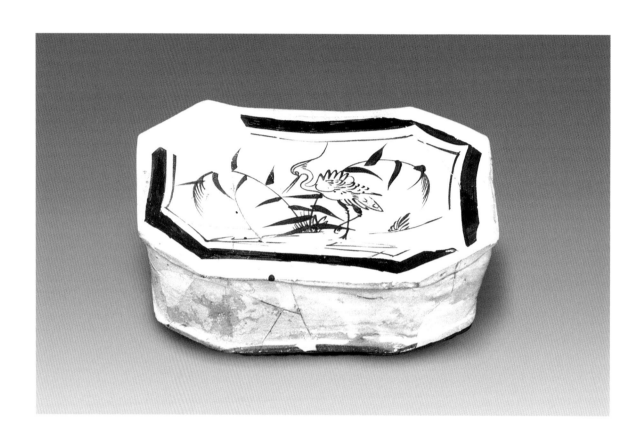

八角形白地黑花芦苇鹭鸶枕

金

瓷质

长 27 厘米，宽 17.8 厘米，高 11 厘米

Octagonal Pillow with Black Designs of Bulrushes and an Egret on a White Ground

Jin Dynasty

Porcelain

Length 27 cm/ Width 17.8 cm/ Height 11 cm

胎质灰白坚硬，施化妆土、透明釉，底部无釉，

背面上缘有气孔。枕面绘有两棵芦苇、一只

鹭鸶，周壁白釉无饰。磁县观台镇出土。

中国磁州窑博物馆藏

The firm greyish-white body is coated with
engobe and transparent glaze. The bottom is
unglazed and pores can be seen on the upper
edge of the back wall. On the pillow face are
painted two bulrushes and an egret, while
the peripheral walls are coated with white
glaze only and without any decoration. It was
unearthed in Guantai Township, Ci County,
Hebei Province.

Preserved in China Cizhou Kiln Museum

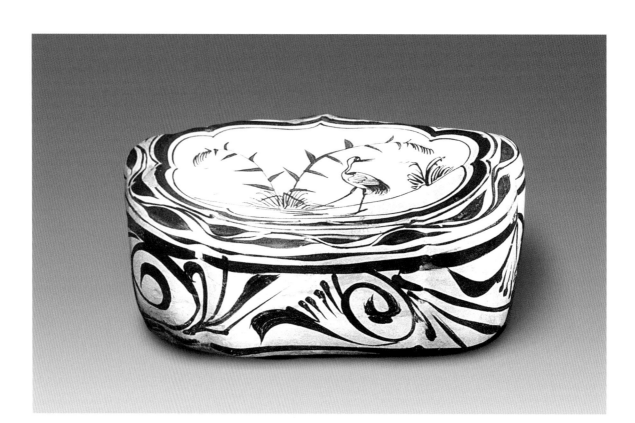

如意形白地黑花芦鹤枕

金

瓷质

长 32 厘米，宽 23 厘米，高 13 厘米

Ruyi-shaped Pillow with Black Designs of Bulrushes and Crane on a White Ground

Jin Dynasty

Porcelain

Length 32 cm/ Width 23 cm/ Height 13 cm

胎质灰白坚硬，施化妆土、透明釉，底部无釉，背面上缘有气孔。枕面绘有两棵芦苇，一只仙鹤，周壁有卷草纹饰。底部印有竖式"张家造"戳记。磁县观台镇东艾口村出土。

中国磁州窑博物馆藏

The firm greyish-white body is coated with engobe and transparent glaze. The bottom is unglazed and pores can be seen on the upper edge of the back wall. On the pillow face are painted two bulrushes and a crane, while on the peripheral walls designs of scrolled grass. On the bottom is stamped a vertical seal of "Zhang Jia Zhao" (Made by Zhang's). It was unearthed in the Dong'aikou Village, Guantai Township, Ci County, Hebei Province.

Preserved in China Cizhou Kiln Museum

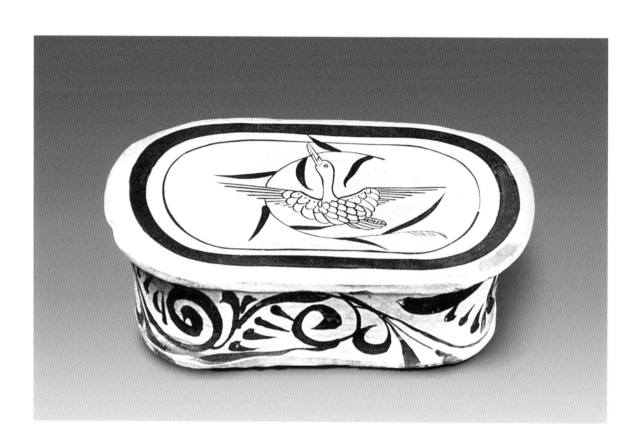

腰圆形白地黑花芦雁枕

金

瓷质

长 31 厘米，宽 20.5 厘米，高 11 厘米

Round-waisted Pillow with Black Designs of Bulrush and Crane on a White Ground

Jin Dynasty

Porcelain

Length 31 cm/ Width 20.5 cm/ Height 11 cm

胎质灰白坚硬，施化妆土、透明釉，底部无
釉，背面上缘有气孔。枕面绘一只大雁，嘴
里衔着一根芦苇向天空飞翔，周壁绘卷草纹。
磁县都党乡冶子村出土。

中国磁州窑博物馆藏

The firm greyish-white body is coated with
engobe and transparent glaze. The bottom is
unglazed and pores can be seen on the upper
edge of the back wall. The pillow face is
decorated with a design of a flying crane with a
bulrush in the mouth, while the peripheral walls
are embellished with design of scrolled grass.
It was unearthed in Yezi Village in Dudang
Township, Ci County, Hebei Province.
Preserved in China Cizhou Kiln Museum

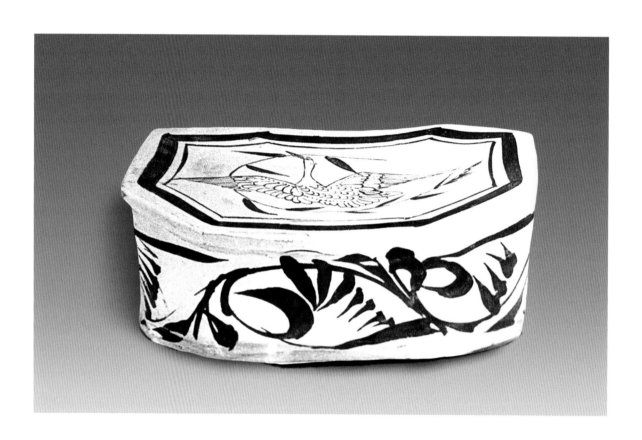

腰圆形白地黑花芦雁枕

金

瓷质

长 31 厘米，宽 20.5 厘米，高 11 厘米

Round-waisted Pillow with Black Designs of Bulrush and Crane on a White Ground

Jin Dynasty

Porcelain

Length 31 cm/ Width 20.5 cm/ Height 11 cm

胎质灰白坚硬，施化妆土、透明釉，底部无
釉，背面上缘有气孔。枕面绘一只大雁，嘴
里衔着一根芦苇向天空飞翔，周壁绘卷草纹。
磁县都党乡冶子村出土。

中国磁州窑博物馆藏

The firm greyish-white body is coated with
engobe and transparent glaze. The bottom is
unglazed and pores can be seen on the upper
edge of the back wall. The pillow face is
decorated with a design of a flying crane with a
bulrush in the mouth, while the peripheral walls
are embellished with designs of scrolled grass.
It was unearthed in Yezi Village in Dudang
Township, Ci County, Hebei Province.
Preserved in China Cizhou Kiln Museum

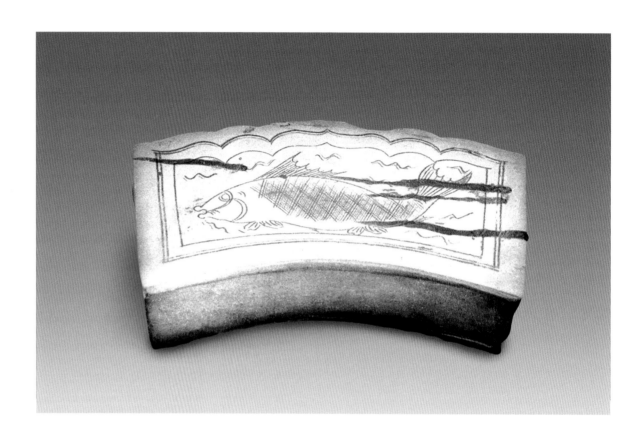

扇形无釉刻画鲤鱼纹枕

金

瓷质

长 36.5 厘米，宽 20.2 厘米，高 10.8 厘米

Unglazed Fan-shaped Pillow with Carp Design

Jin Dynasty

Porcelain

Length 36.5 cm/ Width 20.2 cm/ Height 10.8 cm

胎质灰白坚硬，无化妆土和透明釉，为素烧品。枕面刻画鲤鱼一条，略带水纹，面上有流釉痕迹四道。背面印有奔马和缠枝花卉图案，前立面和两端面无饰。磁县都党乡冶子村出土。

中国磁州窑博物馆藏

The greyish white body of the pillow is hard, and with no engobe or transparent glaze on. The pillow belongs to unglazed pottery. On the pillow face is curved a carp among waves, and four sagging marks can be seen on it as well. The front wall and two side walls are without any decoration, but on the back wall are impressed a galloping horse design and scrolling flower motifs. It was unearthed in Yezi Village, Dudang Township of Ci County, Hebei Province.

Preserved in China Cizhou Kiln Museum

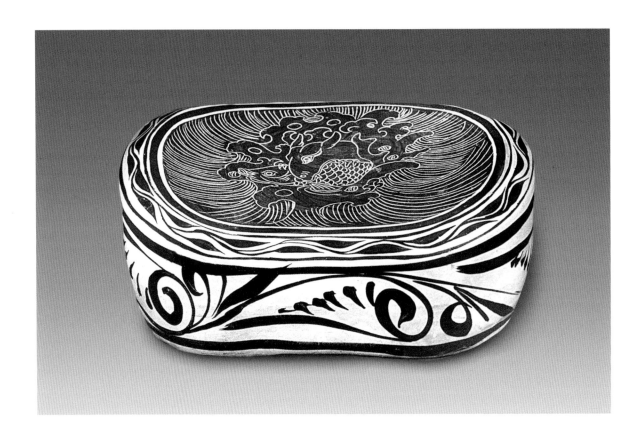

腰圆形白地黑花鱼纹纪年枕

金

瓷质

长 31 厘米，宽 20 厘米，高 11 厘米

Bean-shaped Commemorative Pillow with Black Fish Design on a White Ground

Jin Dynasty

Porcelain

Length 31 cm/ Width 20 cm/ Height 11 cm

胎质灰白坚硬，施化妆土、透明釉，底部无釉，背面上缘有气孔。枕面绘海兽吞鱼图，周壁饰卷草纹。

邯郸市文物保护研究所藏

The greyish white body of the pillow is hard and coated with engobe and transparent glaze except the bottom. There are pores on the upper edge of the back wall. On the pillow face is painted a design of a sea monster swallowing a fish, with floral scroll motifs incised around the peripheral walls.

Preserved in Handan Institute of cultural relics protection

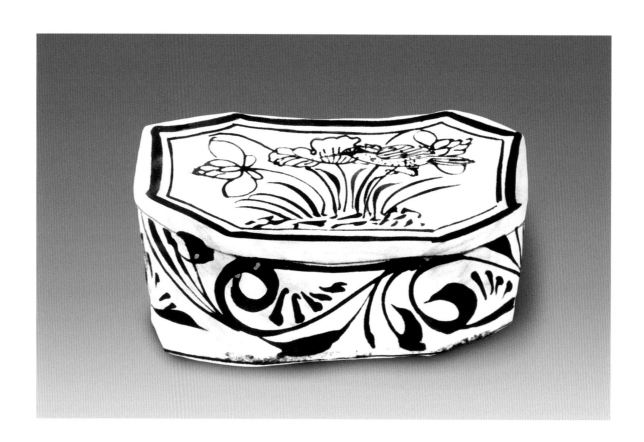

八角形白地黑花荷花纹枕

金

瓷质

长 26.9 厘米，宽 18.1 厘米，高 9.4 厘米

Octagonal Pillow with Black Lotus Design on a White Ground

Jin Dynasty

Porcelain

Length 26.9 cm/ Width 18.1 cm/ Height 9.4 cm

胎质灰白坚硬，施化妆土、透明釉，底部无釉，背面上缘有气孔。枕面绘荷花、翠鸟，周壁饰卷草纹。

杨永德藏

The greyish white body of the pillow is hard and coated with engobe and transparent glaze except the bottom. There are pores on the upper edge of the back wall. On the pillow face are painted designs of a lotus and a kingfisher, with floral scrolls motifs incised around the peripheral walls.

Collected by Yang Yongde

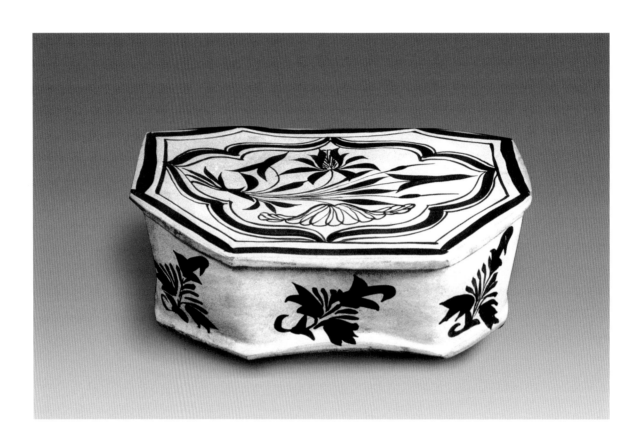

八角形白地黑花荷花纹枕

金

瓷质

长 30.5 厘米，宽 22.2 厘米，高 12.3 厘米

Octagonal Pillow with Black Lotus Design on a White Ground

Jin Dynasty

Porcelain

Length 30.5 cm/ Width 22.2 cm/ Height 12.3 cm

胎质灰白坚硬，施化妆土、透明釉，底部无釉，背面上缘有气孔。枕面绘荷花、水草，周壁有卷草纹饰。磁县都党乡冶子村出土。

中国磁州窑博物馆藏

The greyish white body of the pillow is hard and coated with engobe and transparent glaze except the bottom. There are pores on the upper edge of the back. On the pillow face are painted designs of lotus and aquatic weeds, with floral scroll motifs incised around the peripheral walls. It was unearthed in Yezi Village, Dudang Township of Ci County, Hebei Province. Preserved in China Cizhou Kiln Museum

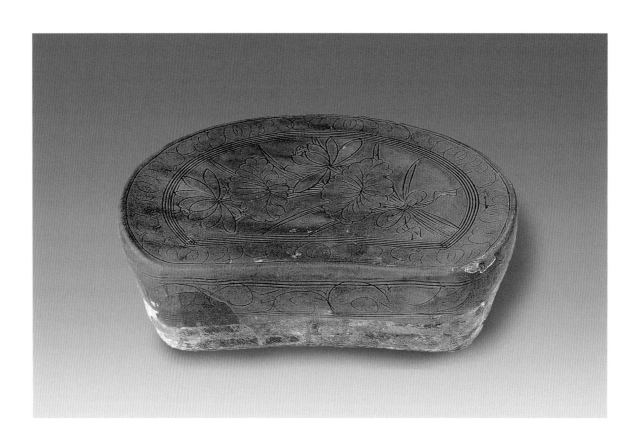

腰圆形绿釉荷花纹枕

金

瓷质

长 40.5 厘米，宽 26.5 厘米，高 13 厘米

Bean-shaped Pillow with Lotus Patterns in a Green Glaze

Jin Dynasty

Porcelain

Length 40.5 cm/ Width 26.5 cm/ Height 13 cm

胎质粗松，呈土黄色，周壁施绿釉不到底，底部无釉，局部有开片。枕面刻画荷花，周壁有卷钩纹饰。河北省河间市出土。

河北博物院藏

The khaki body of the pillow is of rough and loose texture. Green glaze stretches all over the peripheral walls but the unglazed bottom which is partially crackled. On the pillow face is painted a lotus design, with hook patterns incised around the peripheral walls. It was unearthed in Hejian City, Hebei Province.

Preserved in Hebei Museum

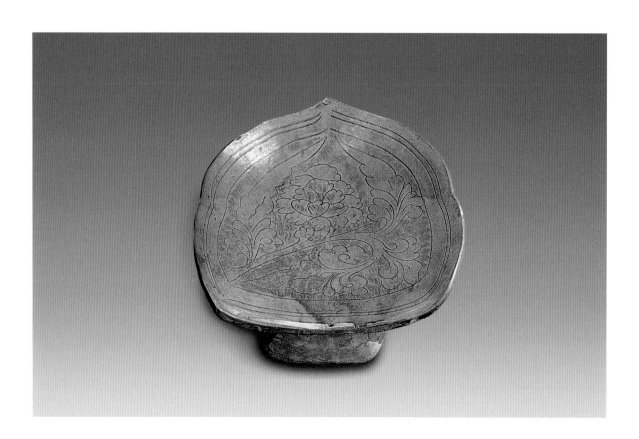

叶形绿釉牡丹纹枕

金

瓷质

长 30 厘米，宽 30 厘米，高 19.5 厘米

Green-glazed Pillow with Foiled Leaf-shaped Peony Patterns

Jin Dynasty

Porcelain

Length 30 cm/ Width 30 cm/ Height 19.5 cm

胎质灰白微红，施绿釉和透明釉，前面露胎，

其他面有绿釉，底部无釉。枕面稍凹，刻画

三条线作边框，框内为牡丹纹，其间有篦纹

点缀。磁县都党乡冶子村出土。

中国磁州窑博物馆藏

The greyish white body of the pillow, with a
tint of red, is coated with green and transparent
glazes. The body on the front wall is exposed
with the other sides glazed green and the bottom
unglazed. On the slightly concave pillow face
are incised peony patterns decorated with comb
marks and enclosed in three strings. It was
unearthed in Yezi Village, Dudang Township of
Ci County, Hebei Province.

Preserved in China Cizhou Kiln Museum

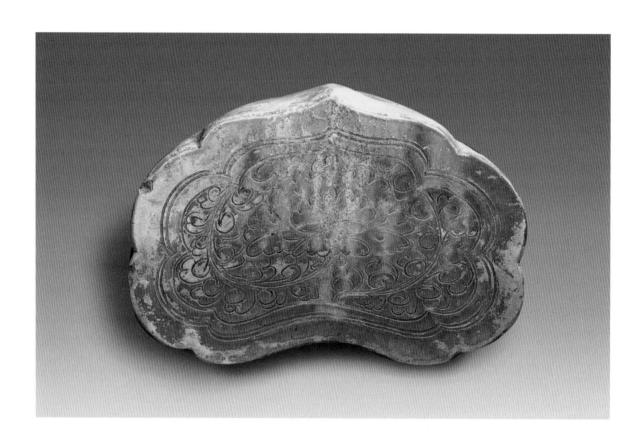

如意形绿釉缠枝牡丹花纹枕

金

瓷质

长 29.5 厘米，宽 20 厘米，高 11.5 厘米

Green-glazed Ruyi-shaped Pillow with Interlocking Branch Peony Patterns

Jin Dynasty

Porcelain

Length 29.5 cm/ Width 20 cm/ Height 11.5 cm

胎质松软微红，无化妆土，施绿釉，底部无釉，背面上缘有气孔。枕面刻缠枝牡丹，周壁绿釉无饰。磁县观台镇出土。

中国磁州窑博物馆藏

The slightly reddish soft body of the pillow is coated with green glaze with no engobe underneath. The bottom is unglazed. There are pores on the upper edge of the back. On the pillow face are carved the interlocking peony patterns with no decoration on the peripheral walls. It was unearthed in Guantai Township in Ci County, Hebei Province.

Preserved in China Cizhou Kiln Museum

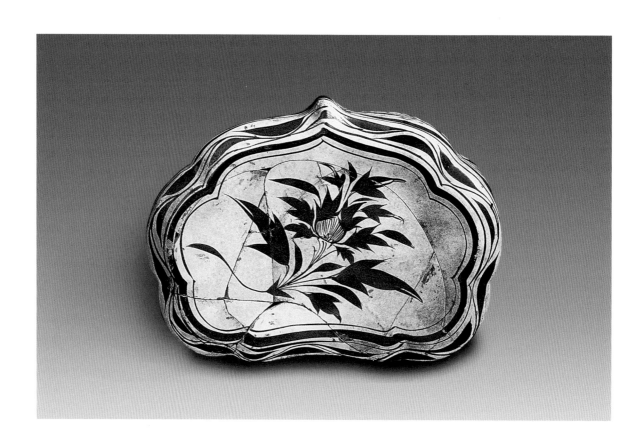

如意形白地黑花枕

金

瓷质

长 31 厘米，宽 23.4 厘米，高 13.1 厘米

Ruyi-shaped Pillow with Black Floral Design on a White Ground

Jin Dynasty

Porcelain

Length 31 cm/ Width 23.4 cm/ Height 13.1 cm

胎质灰白坚硬，施化妆土、透明釉，底部无釉，背上缘有气孔。枕面绘折枝花，周壁卷草纹无饰。底部印有竖式单栏"张家造"戳记。磁县观台镇东艾口村出土。

中国磁州窑博物馆藏

The greyish white body of the pillow is hard and coated with engobe and transparent glaze except the bottom. There are pores on the back. On the pillow face is painted a single flower, with floral scroll designs incised around the peripheral walls. The bottom is stamped with a single-vertical-column seal of "Zhang Jia Zao" (Made by Zhang's). It was unearthed in Dong'aikou Village, Guantai Township in Ci County, Hebei Province.

Preserved in China Cizhou Kiln Museum

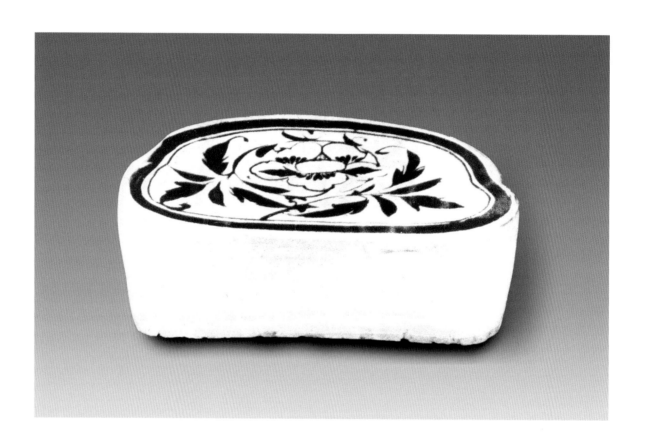

腰圆形白地黑花枕

金

瓷质

长 28.5 厘米，宽 18.7 厘米，高 9.8 厘米

Bean-shaped Pillow with Black Floral Patterns on a White Ground

Jin Dynasty

Porcelain

Length 28.5 cm/ Width 18.7 cm/ Height 9.8 cm

胎质细而坚，呈灰白色，施化妆土、透明釉，局部有开片，底部无釉，背面上缘有气孔。枕面绘折枝牡丹，周壁白釉无饰。

杨永德藏

The greyish white body of the pillow is of hard and fine texture and it is coated with engobe and transparent glaze except the bottom. Crackles can be found on some parts of the pillow. There are pores on the upper edge of the back. On the pillow face are painted peony patterns, while the peripheral walls are glazed white with no decoration.

Collected by Yang Yongde

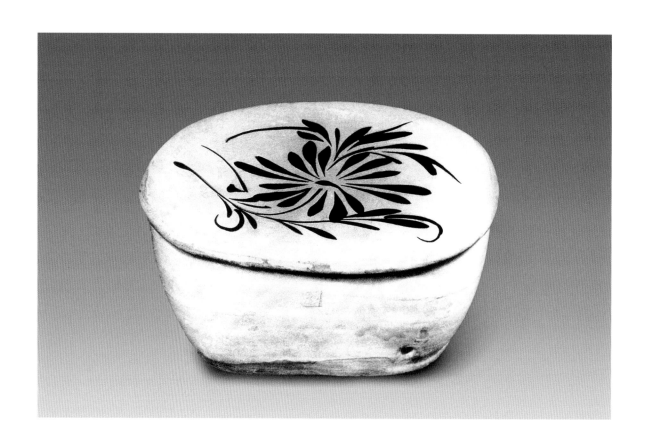

腰圆形白地黑花枕

金

瓷质

长 22.8 厘米，宽 18.5 厘米，高 11.7 厘米

Bean-shaped Pillow with Black Floral Patterns on a White Ground

Jin Dynasty

Porcelain

Length 22.8 cm/ Width 18.5 cm/ Height 11.7 cm

胎质灰白坚硬，施化妆土、透明釉，底部无釉。
枕面绘折枝花，周壁白釉无饰。山西省出土。

长治市博物馆藏

The greyish white body of the pillow is hard
and coated with engobe and transparent glaze
except the bottom. On the pillow face are
painted floral patterns, while the peripheral
walls are glazed white with no decoration. It
was unearthed in Shanxi Province.

Preserved in Changzhi Museum

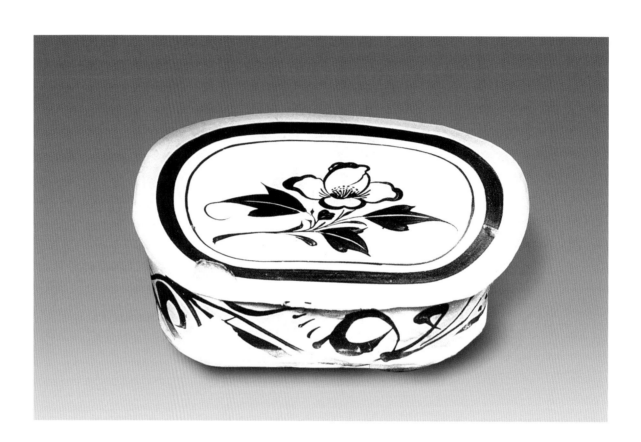

腰圆形白地黑花枕

金

瓷质

长 31.3 厘米，宽 22.4 厘米，高 11.1 厘米

Bean-shaped Pillow with Black Floral Patterns on a White Ground

Jin Dynasty

Porcelain

Length 31.3 cm/ Width 22.4 cm/ Height 11.1 cm

胎质灰白坚硬，施化妆土、透明釉，底部无釉，背面上缘有气孔。枕面绘折枝花，周壁有卷草纹饰。磁县岳城水库出土。

峰峰矿区文物保管所藏

The greyish white body of the pillow is hard and coated with engobe and transparent glaze except the bottom. There are pores on the upper edge of the back. A picture of a single flower is painted on the pillow face, with floral scroll designs incised around the peripheral walls. It was unearthed in the reservoir of Yuecheng, Ci County, Hebei Province.

Preserved in Department of Cultural Relics Conservation of Fengfeng Mine

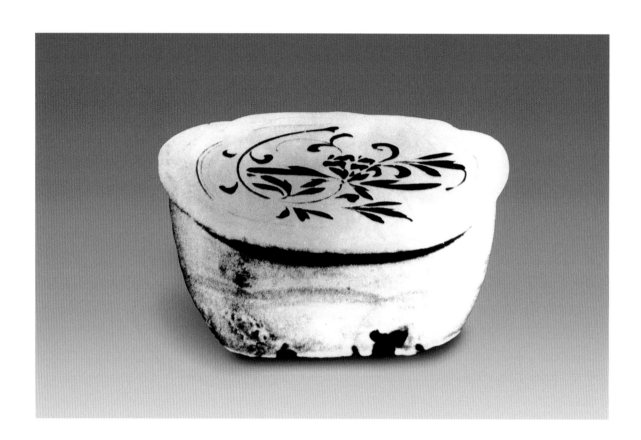

腰圆形白地黑花枕

金

瓷质

长 23.3 厘米，宽 19 厘米，高 11.6 厘米

Bean-shaped Pillow with Black Floral Patterns on a White Ground

Jin Dynasty

Porcelain

Length 23.3 cm/ Width 19 cm/ Height 11.6 cm

胎质细而坚,呈灰白色,施化妆土、透明釉,底部无釉,背面有气孔。枕面绘折枝花一枝,周壁白釉无饰。

杨永德藏

The greyish white body of the pillow is of fine and hard texture, and it is coated with engobe and transparent glaze except the bottom. There are pores on the upper edge of the back. On the pillow face is painted a flowering branch, while no decoration is found on the white-glazed peripheral walls.

Collected by Yang Yongde

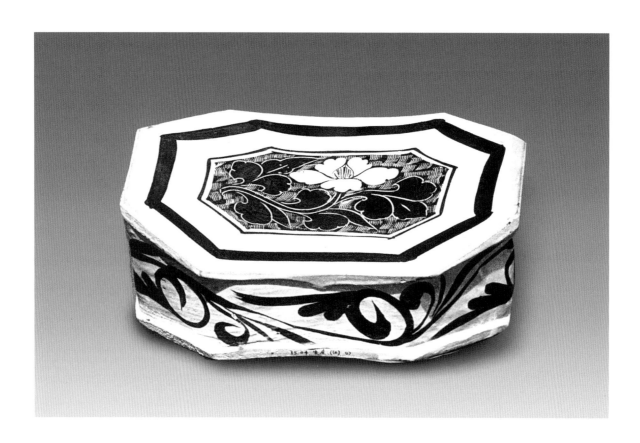

八角形白地黑花枕

金

瓷质

长 29 厘米，宽 20.5 厘米，高 11.4 厘米

Octagonal Pillow with Black Floral Patterns on a White Ground

Jin Dynasty

Porcelain

Length 29 cm/ Width 20.5 cm/ Height 11.4 cm

胎质灰白坚硬，施化妆土、透明釉，底部无釉，背面上缘有气孔。枕面绘牡丹花，花间有篦纹。周壁有卷草纹饰。底部印有横式"张家造"戳记。磁县南开河乡朱庄村出土。

中国磁州窑博物馆藏

The greyish white body of the pillow is hard and coated with engobe and transparent glaze except the bottom. There are pores on the upper edge of the back. On the pillow face is painted a peony motif decorated by comb patterns, with floral scroll designs incised around the peripheral walls. The bottom is stamped with a horizontal seal of "Zhang Jia Zao" (Made by Zhang's). It was unearthed in Zhuzhuang Village, Nankaihe Townshipship, Ci County, Hebei Province.

Preserved in China Cizhou Kiln Museum

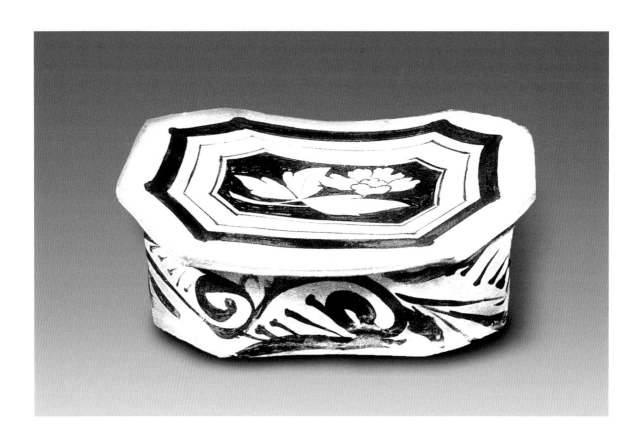

八角形白地黑花枕

金

瓷质

长 29.1 厘米，宽 20.5 厘米，高 10 厘米

Octagonal Pillow with Black Floral Patterns on a White Ground

Jin Dynasty

Porcelain

Length 29.1 cm/ Width 20.5 cm/ Height 10 cm

胎质灰白坚硬，施化妆土、透明釉，底部无
釉，背面上缘有气孔。枕面绘折枝花，周壁
有卷草纹饰。底部印有单栏"张家记"戳记。
磁县岳城水库出土。

峰峰矿区文物保管所藏

The greyish white body of the pillow is hard
and coated with engobe and transparent glaze
except the bottom. There are pores on the upper
edge of the back. On the pillow face is painted
a flowering branch, with floral scroll designs
incised around the peripheral walls. The bottom
is stamped with a single column seal of "Zhang
Jia Zao" (Made by Zhang's). It was unearthed
in the reservoir of Yuecheng, Ci County, Hebei
Province.

Preserved in Department of Cultural Relics
Conservation of Fengfeng Mine

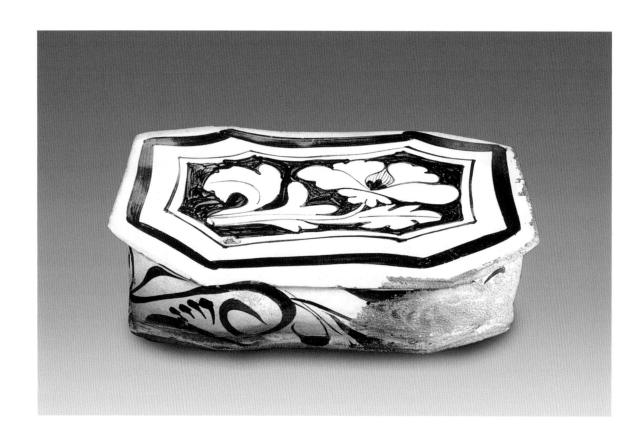

八角形白地黑花花卉枕

金

瓷质

长 28.5 厘米，宽 19 厘米，高 10 厘米

Octagonal Pillow with Black Floral Patterns on a White Ground

Jin Dynasty

Porcelain

Length 28.5 cm/ Width 19 cm/ Height 10 cm

胎质灰白坚硬，施化妆土、透明釉，底部无釉，背面上缘有气孔。枕面绘折枝花，周壁卷草纹饰。底部印有横式"张家造"戳记。磁县观台镇出土。

中国磁州窑博物馆藏

The greyish white body of the pillow is hard and coated with engobe and transparent glaze except the bottom. There are pores on the upper edge of the back. On the pillow face is painted a flowering branch, with floral scroll designs incised around the peripheral walls. The bottom is stamped with a horizontal seal of "Zhang Jia Zao" (Made by Zhang's). It was unearthed in Guantai Township, Ci County, Hebei Province. Preserved in China Cizhou Kiln Museum

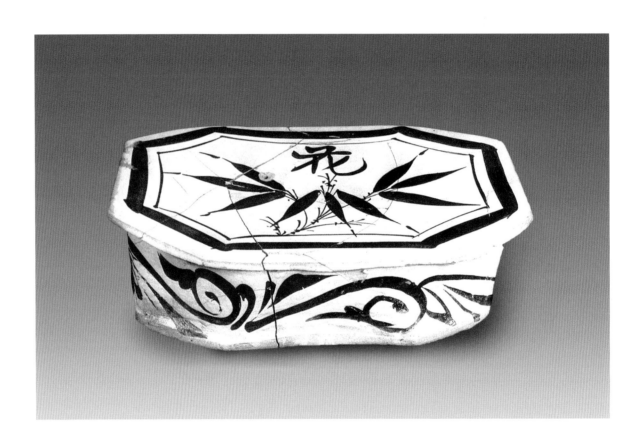

八角形白地黑花花竹枕

金

瓷质

长 28.5 厘米，宽 18 厘米，高 9 厘米

Octagonal Pillow with Black Floral and Bamboo Patterns on a White Ground

Jin Dynasty

Porcelain

Length 28.5 cm/ Width 18 cm/ Height 9 cm

胎质灰白坚硬，施化妆土、透明釉，底部无釉，背面上缘有气孔。枕面绘竹枝和墨书"花"字，组成"花竹（烛）"含意，周壁卷草纹饰。底部印有横式单栏"张家造"戳记。磁县观台镇东艾口村出土。

中国磁州窑博物馆藏

The greyish white body of the pillow is hard and coated with engobe and transparent glaze except the bottom. There are pores on the upper edge of the back. On the pillow face are painted bamboo branches and ink inscription "Hua" (Flower), symbolizing wedding candles, with floral scroll designs incised around the peripheral walls. The bottom is stamped with a single-horizontal-column seal of "Zhang Jia Zao" (Made by Zhang's). It was unearthed in Dong'aikou Village, Guantai Township, Ci County, Hebei Province.

Preserved in China Cizhou Kiln Museum

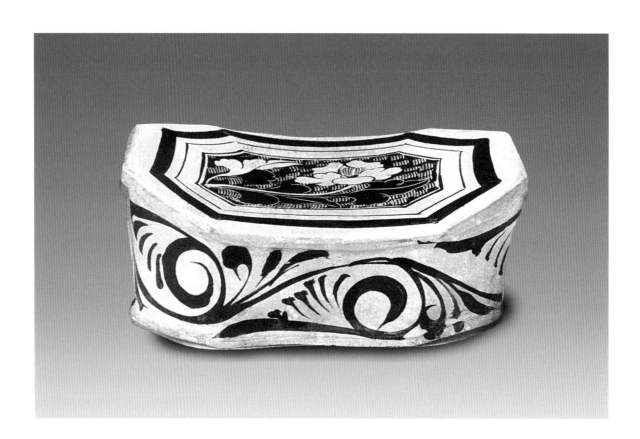

八角形白地黑花折枝花枕

金

瓷质

长 28 厘米，宽 20.4 厘米，高 11.2 厘米

Octagonal Pillow with Black Floral Patterns on a White Ground

Jin Dynasty

Porcelain

Length 28 cm/ Width 20.4 cm/ Height 11.2 cm

胎质细坚，呈浅褐黄色，施化妆土、透明釉，底部无釉，背面上缘有气孔。枕面绘一折枝花，花间有篦纹，周壁有卷草纹饰。底部印有竖式单栏上莲叶、下荷花"张家枕"戳记。

杨永德藏

The light yellowish brown body of the pillow is of fine and hard texture and coated with engobe and transparent glaze except the bottom. There are pores on the upper edge of the back. On the pillow face is painted a flowering branch decorated by comb patterns, with floral scroll design incised around the peripheral walls. The bottom is stamped with a single-vertical-column inscription of "Zhang Jia Zhen" (The pillow made by Zhang's), with the decoration of a lotus leaf motif on the upper edge and a lotus blossom motif on the lower edge.

Colleted by Yang Yongde

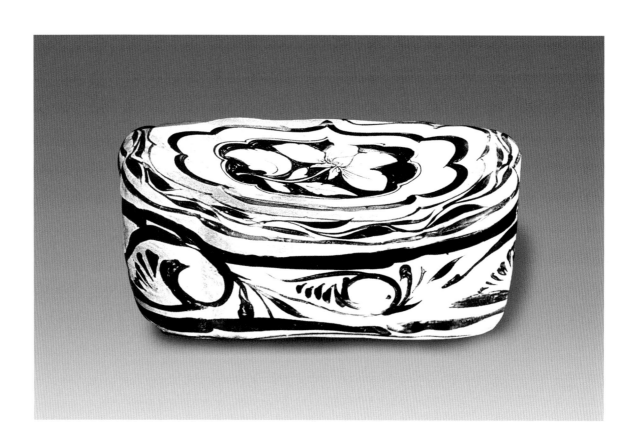

如意形白地黑花折枝花枕

金

瓷质

长 31 厘米，宽 22.5 厘米，高 13 厘米

Ruyi-shaped Pillow with Black Floral Patterns on a White Ground

Jin Dynasty

Porcelain

Length 31 cm/ Width 22.5 cm/ Height 13 cm

胎质灰白坚硬，施化妆土、透明釉，底部无釉，背面上缘有气孔。枕面绘折枝花卉，周壁有卷草纹饰。磁县都党乡冶子村出土。

中国磁州窑博物馆藏

The greyish white body of the pillow is hard and coated with engobe and transparent glaze except the bottom. There are pores on the upper edge of the back. A flowering branch is painted on the pillow face, with floral scroll design incised around the peripheral walls. It was unearthed in Yezi Village, Dudang Township, Ci County, Hebei Province.

Preserved in China Cizhou Kiln Museum

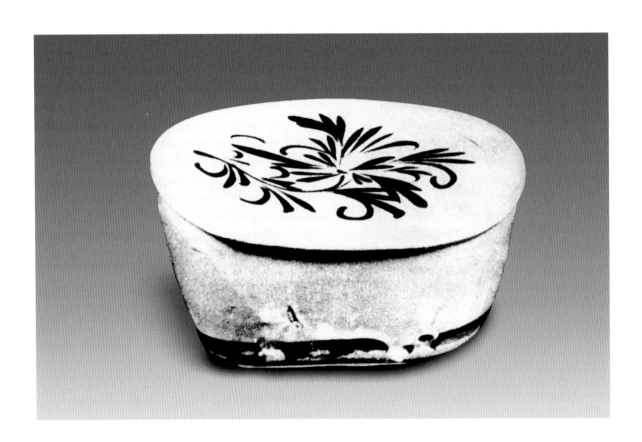

腰圆形白地褐花枕

金

瓷质

长 24.5 厘米，宽 20 厘米，高 12.5 厘米

Bean-shaped Pillow with Brown Floral Patterns on a White Ground

Jin Dynasty

Porcelain

Length 24.5 cm/ Width 20 cm/ Height 12.5 cm

胎质细而坚，呈灰白色，施化妆土、透明釉，
底部无釉，背面有气孔。枕面绘折枝花，周
壁白釉无饰。

杨永德藏

The greyish white body of the pillow is of fine
and hard texture and coated with engobe and
transparent glaze except the bottom. There are
pores on the upper edge of the back. On the
pillow face is painted a flowering branch, while
the white-glazed peripheral walls are plain
without decoration.

Collected by Yang Yongde

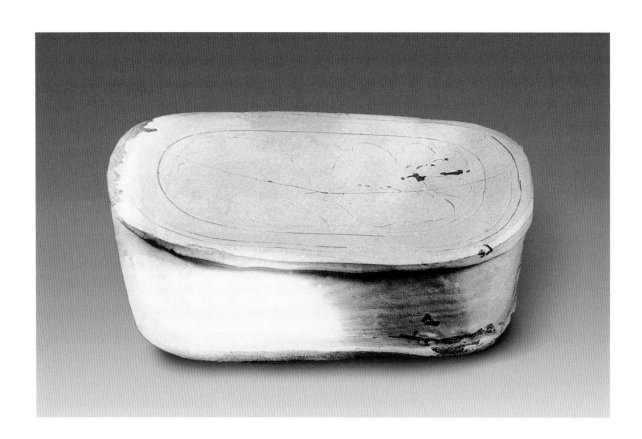

腰圆形白地刻花枕

金

瓷质

长 27.7 厘米，宽 18.7 厘米，高 11 厘米

Bean-shaped Pillow with Floral Patterns on a White Ground

Jin Dynasty

Porcelain

Length 27.7 cm/ Width 18.7 cm/ Height 11 cm

胎质灰白坚硬,施化妆土、透明釉,底部无釉,背面上有气孔。枕面刻画折枝花,周壁白釉无饰。底部印有横式单栏"张家造"戳记。磁县出土。

中国磁州窑博物馆藏

The greyish white body of the pillow is hard and coated with engobe and transparent glaze except the bottom. There are pores on the upper edge of the back. On the pillow face is painted a flowering branch, while the peripheral walls are white-glazed with no decoration. The bottom is stamped with a single-horizontal-column inscription of "Zhang Jia Zao" (Made by Zhang's). It was unearthed in Ci County, Hebei Province.

Preserved in China Cizhou Kiln Museum

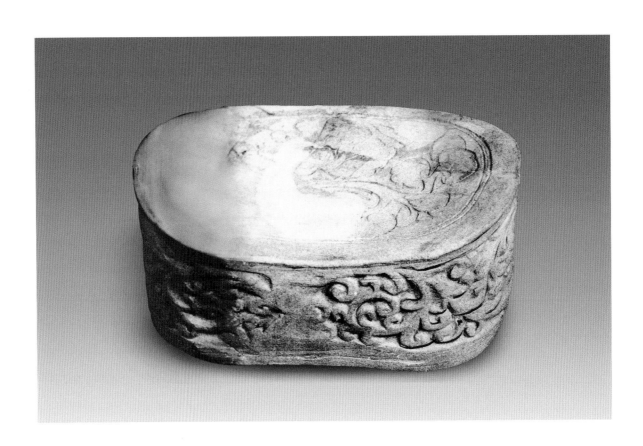

腰圆形无釉刻花枕

金

瓷质

长 26 厘米，宽 19 厘米，高 8 厘米

Unglazed Bean-shaped Pillow with Floral Patterns

Jin Dynasty

Porcelain

Length 26 cm/ Width 19 cm/ Height 8 cm

胎质灰白坚硬，无化妆土、无釉，为素烧品。

枕面有刻画花卉一枝，周壁为压印成的缠枝

花纹饰。磁县观台镇出土。

中国磁州窑博物馆藏

The greyish white body of the pillow is hard,
and with no engobe or transparent glaze, the
pillow belongs to unglazed pottery. On the
pillow face is painted a flowering branch, with
a interlocking floral design embossed on the
peripheral walls. It was unearthed in Guantai
Township, Ci County, Hebei Province.

Preserved in China Cizhou Kiln Museum

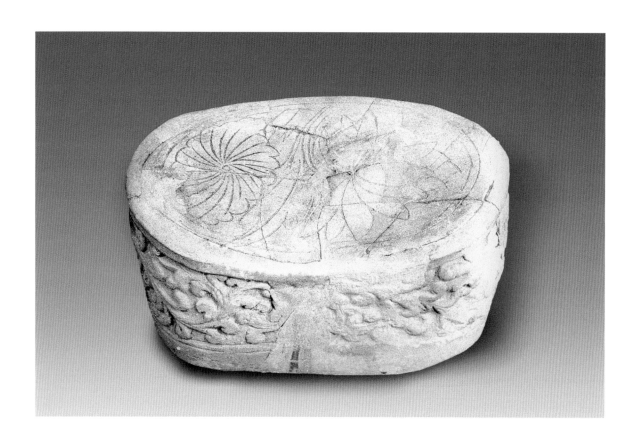

腰圆形素胎刻花枕

金

瓷质

长 26 厘米，宽 19.5 厘米，高 8.5 厘米

Unglazed Bean-shaped Pillow with Floral Patterns

Jin Dynasty

Porcelain

Length 26 cm/ Width 19.5 cm/ Height 8.5 cm

胎质灰白坚硬，施化妆土、透明釉，底部无釉，背面上缘有气孔。枕面有刻画荷花纹，周壁是模具压印成的缠枝花纹。磁县观台镇出土。

中国磁州窑博物馆藏

The greyish white body of the pillow is hard and coated with engobe and transparent glaze except the bottom. There are pores on the upper edge of the back. On the pillow face is painted a lotus, with a interlocking floral design embossed on the peripheral walls. It was unearthed in Guantai Township, Ci County, Hebei Province. Preserved in China Cizhou Kiln Museum

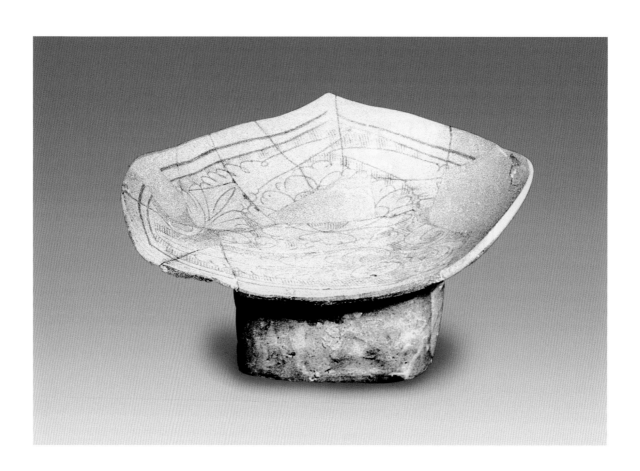

叶形白釉刻花枕

金

瓷质

长 29.3 厘米，宽 28.5 厘米，高 18.5 厘米

White-glazed Foiled Leaf-shaped Pillow with Floral Design

Jin Dynasty

Porcelain

Length 29.3 cm/ Width 28.5 cm/ Height 18.5 cm

胎质灰白坚硬，施化妆土、透明釉，底部无釉。枕面刻画折枝牡丹，花间有篦纹，背面白釉无饰。磁县观台镇出土。

中国磁州窑博物馆藏

The greyish white body of the pillow is hard and coated with engobe and transparent glaze except the bottom. On the pillow face are incised peony patterns decorated with comb marks. There is no decoration on the white-glazed back wall. It was unearthed in Guantai Township, Ci County, Hebei Province.

Preserved in China Cizhou Kiln Museum

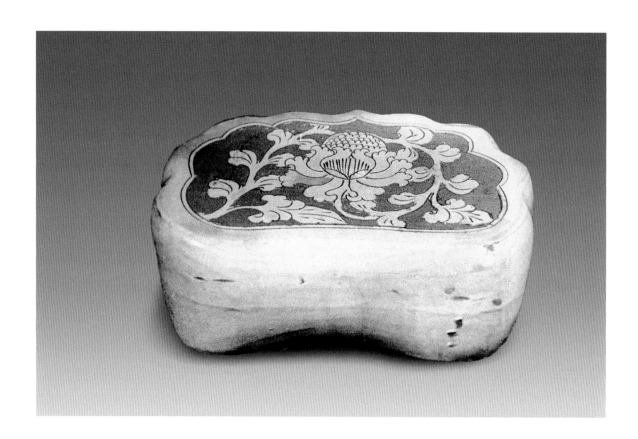

如意形白釉刻花枕

金

瓷质

长 25 厘米，宽 17 厘米，高 10.5 厘米

White-glazed Ruyi-shaped Pillow with Floral Potterns

Jin Dynasty

Porcelain

Length 25 cm/ Width 17 cm/ Height 10.5 cm

胎质灰白坚硬，施化妆土、透明釉，底部无釉，背面上缘有气孔。枕面剔刻折枝花，周壁白釉无饰。山西省长治市出土。

长治市博物馆藏

The greyish white body of the pillow is hard and coated with engobe and transparent glaze except the bottom. On the pillow face are scraped and carved peony patterns, while the peripheral walls are white-glazed with no decoration. It was unearthed in Changzhi City, Shanxi Province.

Preserved in Changzhi Museum

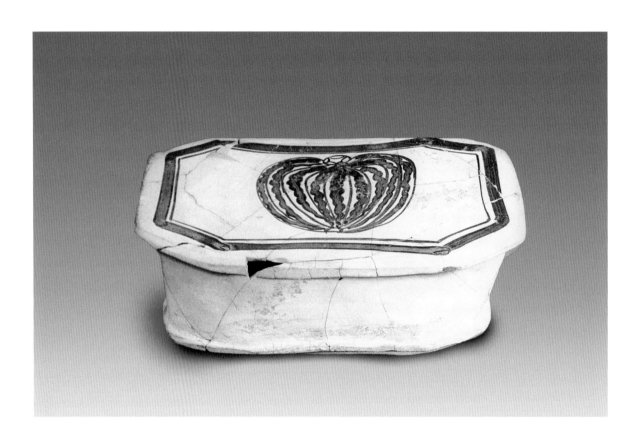

八角形白地黑花瓜纹枕

金

瓷质

长 29.5 厘米，宽 17.5 厘米，高 10.7 厘米

Octagonal Pillow with Black Melon Pattern on a White Ground

Jin Dynasty

Porcelain

Length 29.5 cm/ Width 17.5 cm/ Height 10.7 cm

胎质灰白坚硬，施化妆土、透明釉，底部无釉，背面上缘有气孔。枕面绘瓜一个，周壁白釉无饰。底部印有竖式单栏"张家造"戳记。磁县观台镇东艾口村出土。

中国磁州窑博物馆藏

The greyish white body of the pillow is hard and coated with engobe and transparent glaze except the bottom. There are pores on the upper edge of the back. A melon motif is painted on the pillow face, while no decoration is found on the white-glazed peripheral walls. The bottom is stamped with a single-horizontal-column inscription of "Zhang Jia Zao" (Made by Zhang's). It was unearthed in Dong'aikou Village, Guantai Township, Ci County, Hebei Province.

Preserved in China Cizhou Kiln Museum

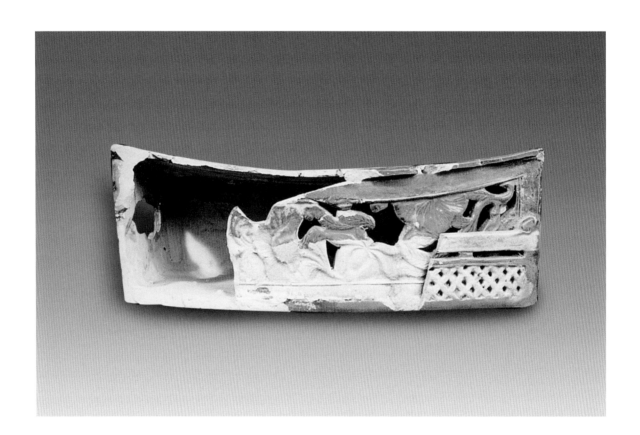

长方形黄绿釉背面镂空枕

金

瓷质

长 34 厘米，宽 18.55 厘米，前高 8.7 厘米，后高 11.3 厘米

Yellowish-green-glazed Rectangular Pillow with Hollowed Back

Jin Dynasty

Porcelain

Length 34 cm/ Width 18.55 cm/ Front Height 8.7 cm/ Rack Height 11.3 cm

胎质灰白坚硬，枕面绿釉水波纹。前立面、两端面为绿釉，无饰。背立面为浮雕镂空，施黄、绿、白三色釉。磁县观台镇出土。

中国磁州窑博物馆藏

The greyish white body of the pillow is hard, and the pillow face is decorated with green-glazed water ripple patterns. The front wall and the faces of the two side walls are all covered with green glaze with no decoration. The back wall, incised with hollowed out relief, is covered with yellow, green and white glazes. It was unearthed in Guantai Township, Ci County, Hebei Province.

Preserved in China Cizhou Kiln Museum

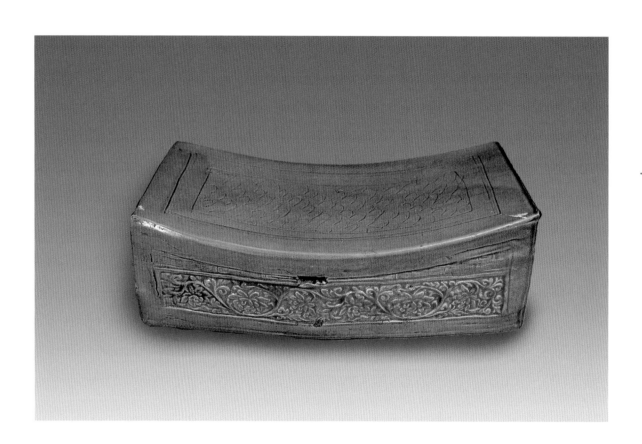

长方形黄绿釉水纹枕

金

瓷质

长 32 厘米，宽 17.5 厘米，高 11 厘米

Yellowish-green-glazed Rectangular Pillow with Water Ripple Patterns

Jin Dynasty

Porcelain

Length 32 cm/ Width 17.5 cm/ Height 11 cm

胎质灰白，施绿釉，背面有浮雕黄釉缠枝花纹。枕面刻有三条线，内画水波纹。磁县都党乡冶子村出土。

王凤龙藏

The greyish white body of the pillow is hard and green-glazed. The back wall is decorated with a yellow glazed relief of an interlocking floral pattern. On the pillow face is carved a pattern of water ripples enclosed by three strings. It was unearthed in Yezi Village, Dudang Township, in Ci County, Hebei Province.

Collected by Wang Fenglong

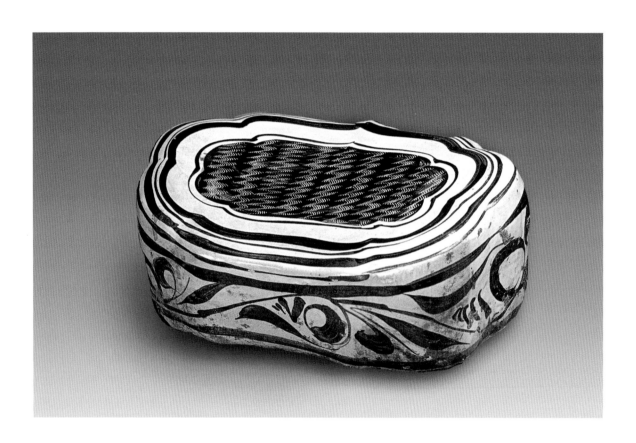

如意形白地黑花水纹枕

金

瓷质

长 31 厘米，宽 23 厘米，高 13.2 厘米

Ruyi-shaped Pillow with Black Water Ripple Patterns on a White Ground

Jin Dynasty

Porcelain

Length 31 cm/ Width 23 cm/ Height 13.2 cm

胎质灰白坚硬，施化妆土、透明釉，底部无釉，
背面上缘有气孔。枕面水纹，周壁有卷草纹
饰。磁县都党乡冶子村出土。

中国磁州窑博物馆藏

The greyish white body of the pillow is hard
and coated with engobe and transparent glaze
except the bottom. There are pores on the upper
edge of the back. A water ripple motif is painted
on the pillow face, with floral scroll design
around the peripheral walls. It was unearthed
in Yezi Village, Dudang Township, Ci County,
Hebei Province.

Preserved in China Cizhou Kiln Museum

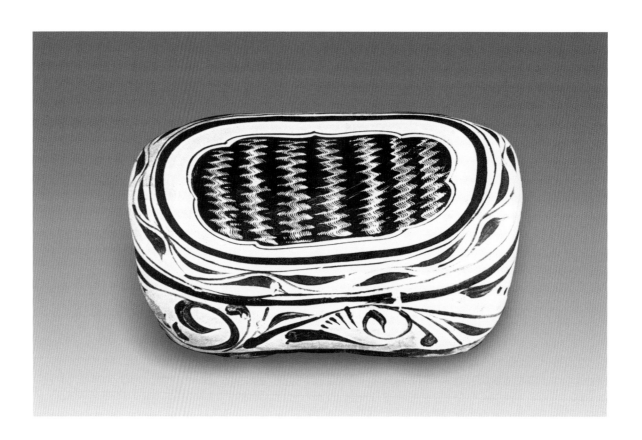

腰圆形白地黑花水纹枕

金

瓷质

长 31 厘米，宽 20.5 厘米，高 13.5 厘米

Bean-shaped Pillow with Black Water Ripple Patterns on a White Ground

Jin Dynasty

Porcelain

Length 31 cm/ Width 20.5 cm/ Height 13.5 cm

胎质灰白坚硬，施化妆土、透明釉，底部无釉，背面上缘有气孔。枕面绘水纹，周壁饰卷草纹。底部印有"张家造"戳记。磁县观台镇出土。

安阳博物馆藏

The greyish white body of the pillow is hard and coated with engobe and transparent glaze except the bottom. There are pores on the upper edge of the back. On the pillow face is painted a water ripple motif, with floral scroll designs around the peripheral walls. The bottom is stamped with a seal of "Zhang Jia Zao" (Made by Zhang's). It was unearthed in Guantai Township, Ci County, Hebei Province.

Preserved in Anyang Municipal Museum

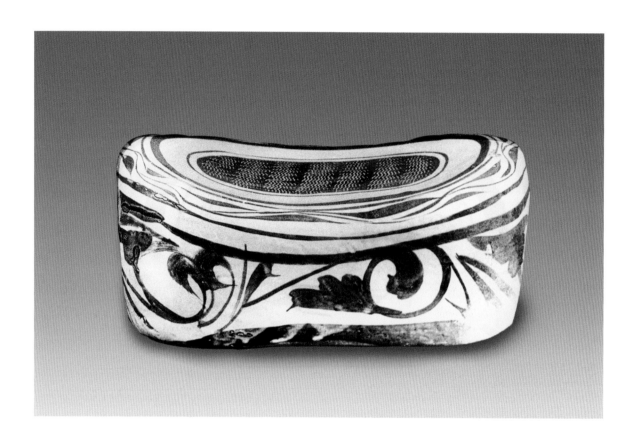

腰圆形白地黑花水纹枕

金

瓷质

长 30 厘米，宽 21 厘米，高 12.9 厘米

Bean-shaped Pillow with Black Water Ripple Patterns on a White Ground

Jin Dynasty

Porcelain

Length 30 cm/ Width 21 cm/ Height 12.9 cm

胎质灰白坚硬，施化妆土、透明釉，底部无釉，背面有气孔。枕面绘水波纹，周壁饰卷草纹。底部印有横式"张家造"戳记。磁县观台镇东艾口村出土。

中国磁州窑博物馆藏

The greyish white body of the pillow is hard and coated with engobe and transparent glaze except the bottom. There are pores on the upper edge of the back. On the pillow face is painted a water ripple motif, with floral scroll designs around the peripheral walls. The bottom is stamped with a horizontal seal of "Zhang Jia Zao" (Made by Zhang's). It was unearthed in Dong'aikou Village, Guantai Township, Ci County, Hebei Province.

Preserved in China Cizhou Kiln Museum

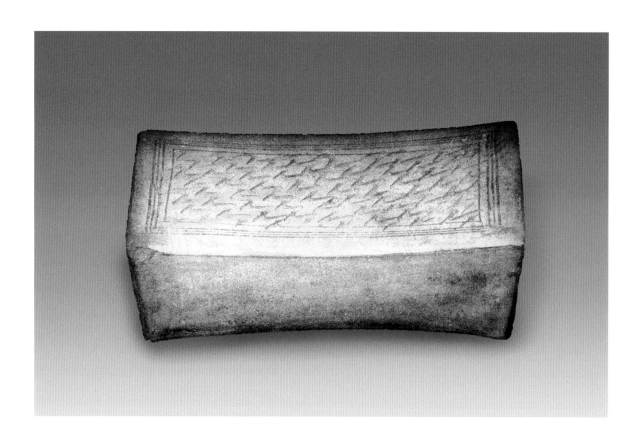

扇形白釉水纹枕

金

瓷质

长 34.6 厘米，宽 20 厘米，高 13 厘米

White-glazed and Fan-shaped Pillow with Water Ripple Design

Jin Dynasty

Porcelain

Length 34.6 cm/ Width 20 cm/ Height 13 cm

胎质灰白坚硬，无化妆土和透明釉，背面上
缘有气孔。枕面刻画水波纹，后立面有印成
的缠枝花卉图案，前立面和两端面无饰。

邯郸市博物馆藏

The greyish white body of the pillow is hard
without engobe or transparent glaze. There are
pores on the upper edge of the back. On the
pillow face is incised a water ripple motif, while
on the rear wall an interlocking floral scroll
designs. No decoration is found on the front
wall and the two side walls.

Preserved in Handan Museum

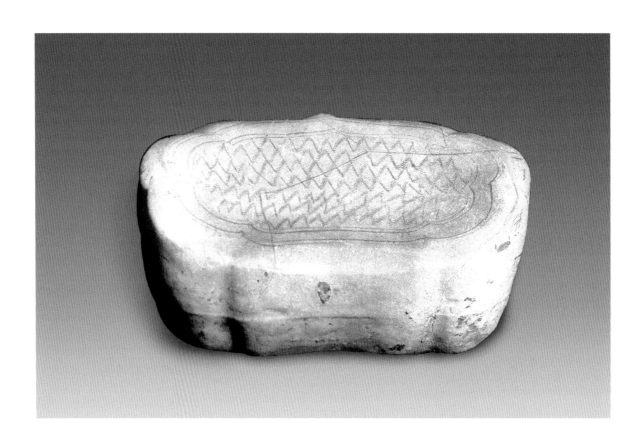

如意形白地水波纹枕

金

瓷质

长 30.7 厘米，宽 22.5 厘米，高 13.7 厘米

Ruyi-shaped Pillow with Water Ripple Patterns on a White Ground

Jin Dynasty

Porcelain

Length 30.7 cm/ Width 22.5 cm/ Height 13.7 cm

胎质灰白坚硬，施化妆土、透明釉，底部无釉，背面上缘有气孔。枕面刻画有水波纹，周壁白釉无饰。磁县岳城水库出土。

峰峰矿区文物保管所藏

The greyish white body of the pillow is hard and coated with engobe and transparent glaze except the bottom. There are pores on the upper edge of the back. On the pillow face is incised a water ripple motif, while the peripheral walls are white-glazed without any decoration. It was unearthed in Yuecheng Reservoir in Ci County, Hebei Province.

Preserved in Department of Cultural Relics Conservation of Fengfeng Mine

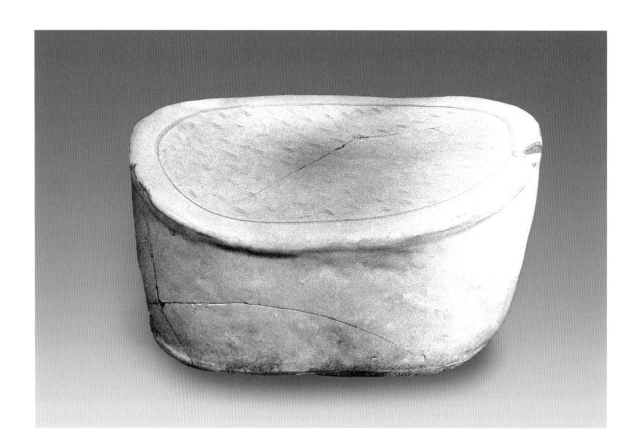

腰圆形白地水波纹枕

金

瓷质

长 25 厘米，宽 18.7 厘米，高 11 厘米

Bean-shaped Pillow with Water Ripple Patterns on a White Ground

Jin Dynasty

Porcelain

Length 25 cm/ Width 18.7 cm/ Height 11 cm

胎质灰白坚硬，施化妆土、透明釉，底部无釉。枕面刻画有水波纹，周壁白釉无饰。磁县都党乡冶子村出土。

中国磁州窑博物馆藏

The greyish white body of the pillow is hard and coated with engobe and transparent glaze except the bottom. On the pillow face is incised a water ripple motif, while the peripheral walls are white-glazed without any decoration. It was unearthed in Yezi Village, Dudang Township, Ci County, Hebei province.

Preserved in China Cizhou Kiln Museum

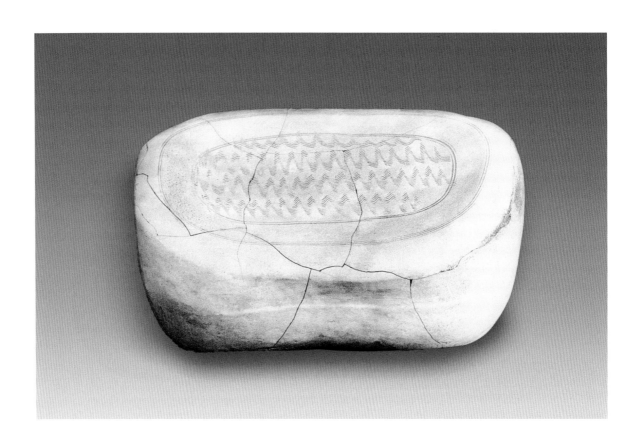

腰圆形白地水波纹枕

金

瓷质

长 30.5 厘米，宽 22 厘米，高 12 厘米

Bean-shaped Pillow with Water Ripple Patterns on a White Ground

Jin Dynasty

Porcelain

Length 30.5 cm/ Width 22 cm/ Height 12 cm

胎质灰白坚硬，施化妆土、透明釉，底部无釉。
枕面刻画有水波纹，周壁白釉无饰。磁县都
党乡冶子村出土。

中国磁州窑博物馆藏

The greyish white body of the pillow is hard
and coated with engobe and transparent glaze
except the bottom. On the pillow face is incised
a water ripple motif, while the peripheral walls
are white-glazed without any decoration. It was
unearthed in Yezi Village, Dudang Township,
Ci County, Hebei province.

Preserved in China Cizhou Kiln Museum

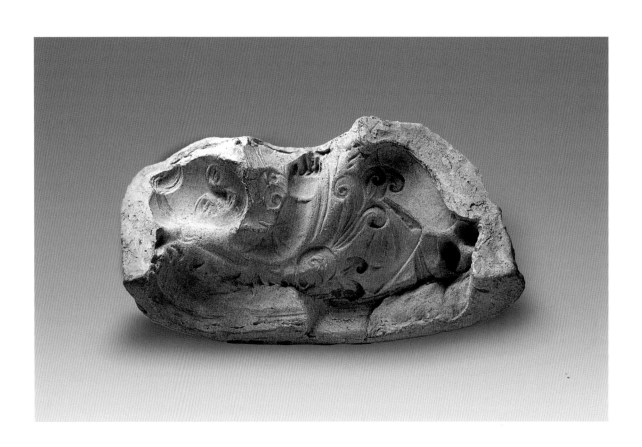

孩儿瓷枕模具

金

瓷质

长 21.7 厘米，高 10.3 厘米

用瓷泥制成，胎质灰白坚硬，为瓷模具的一半。

磁县观台镇出土。

中国磁州窑博物馆藏

Child-shaped Pillow Mould

Jin Dynasty

Porcelain

Length 21.7 cm/ Height 10.3 cm

The object is half of a pillow mould. The greyish white pillow body, made of petuntse, is of hard texture. It was unearthed in Guantai Township, Ci County, Hebei Province.

Preserved in China Cizhou Kiln Museum

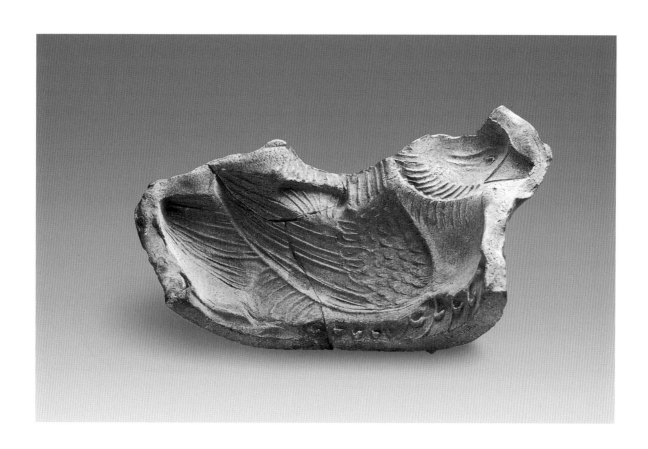

鸳鸯瓷枕模具

金

瓷质

长 29.7 厘米，高 15 厘米

用瓷泥制成，胎质灰白坚硬，为瓷枕模具的一半。

磁县观台镇出土。

中国磁州窑博物馆藏

Mandarin-duck-shaped Pillow Mould

Jin Dynasty

Porcelain

Length 29.7 cm/ Height 15 cm

The object is half of a pillow mould. The greyish white pillow body, made of petuntse, is of hard texture. It was unearthed in Guantai Township, Ci Count y, Hebei Province.

Preserved in China Cizhou Kiln Museum

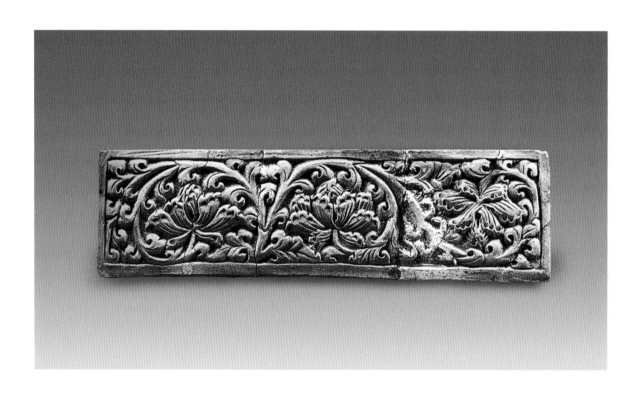

瓷枕模具（模）

金

瓷质

长 49.5 厘米，宽 14.5 厘米，厚 2.7 厘米

用瓷泥制成，胎质灰白坚硬，雕花精细。磁县观台镇出土。

中国磁州窑博物馆藏

Pillow Mould (Male Die)

Jin Dynasty

Porcelain

Length 49.5 cm/ Width 14.5 cm/ Height 2.7 cm

The greyish white body of the pillow mould, made of petuntse, is of hard texture, with delicately carved patterns. It was unearthed in Guantai Township, Ci County, Hebei Province.

Preserved in China Cizhou Kiln Museum

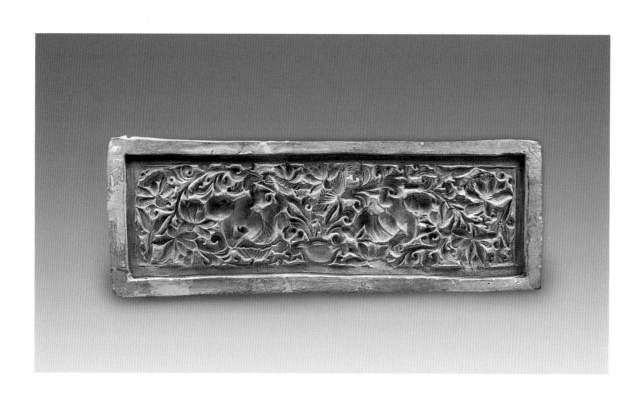

瓷枕模具（范）

金

瓷质

长 46 厘米，宽 16.5 厘米，厚 1.7 厘米

用瓷泥制成，胎质灰白坚硬，雕花精细。磁县观台镇出土。

中国磁州窑博物馆藏

Pillow Mould (Female Die)

Jin Dynasty

Porcelain

Length 46 cm/ Width 16.5 cm/ Height 1.7 cm

The greyish white body of the pillow mould, made of petuntse, is of hard texture, with delicately carved patterns. It was unearthed in Guantai Township, Ci County, Hebei Province.

Preserved in China Cizhou Kiln Museum

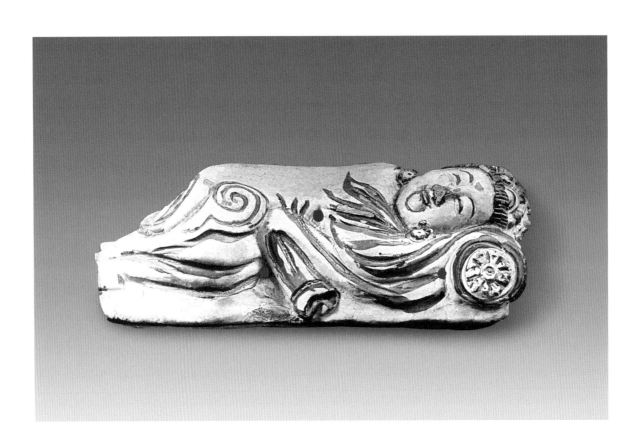

白釉黑彩人物纪年枕

元

瓷质

长 39 厘米，宽 10 厘米，高 12.8 厘米

White-glazed Commemorative Pillow with Black Figure Design

Yuan Dynasty

Porcelain

Length 39 cm/ Width 10 cm/ Height 12.8 cm

胎质灰白坚硬，施化妆土、透明釉，底部无
釉。卧睡人物上绘有黑彩纹。底部有墨书"至
正贰年六月初四日陆仕安索申家庄窑"。磁
县岳城水库出土。

峰峰矿区文物保管所藏

The greyish white body of the pillow is hard
and coated with engobe and transparent glaze
except the bottom. On the surface of the lying
figure are painted black lines. The bottom
is stamped with an ink inscription of "Made
in Shen jiazhuang Kiln on June 4th (lunar
calendar) in 1342". It was unearthed in the
reservoir of Yuecheng in Ci County, Hebei
Province.

Preserved in Department of Cultural Relics
Conservation of Fengfeng Mining District

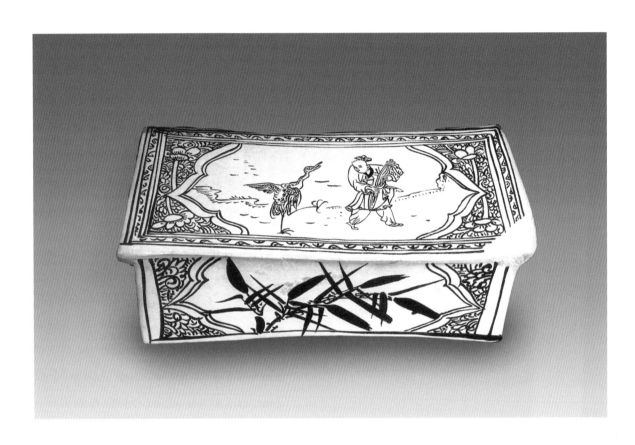

长方形白地黑花人物故事枕

元

瓷质

长 30.5 厘米，宽 16 厘米，高 13.5 厘米

Rectangular Pillow with Black Figure and Floral Design on a White Ground

Yuan Dynasty

Porcelain

Length 30.5 cm/ Width 16 cm/ Height 13.5 cm

胎质灰白坚硬，施化妆土、透明釉，底部无
釉。卧睡人物上绘有黑彩纹。底部有墨书"至
正贰年六月初四日陆仕安索申家庄窑"。磁
县岳城水库出土。

峰峰矿区文物保管所藏

The greyish white body of the pillow is hard
and coated with engobe and transparent glaze
except the bottom. On the surface of the lying
figure are painted black lines. The bottom
is stamped with an ink inscription of "Made
in Shen jiazhuang Kiln on June 4th (lunar
calendar) in 1342". It was unearthed in the
reservoir of Yuecheng in Ci County, Hebei
Province.

Preserved in Department of Cultural Relics
Conservation of Fengfeng Mining District

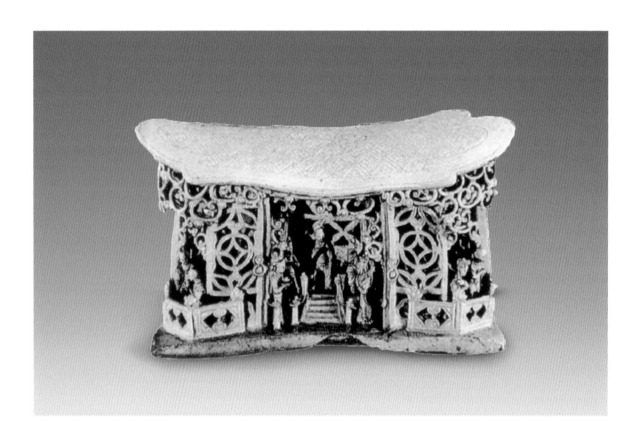

影青透雕人物枕

元

瓷质

长 31.5 厘米，宽 16.5 厘米，高 18 厘米

Engraved Misty Blue Pillow with Figure Designs

Yuan Dynasty

Porcelain

Length 31.5 cm/ Width 16.5 cm/ Height 18 cm

通体施钴蓝釉，饰云纹及折枝花叶纹。蓝釉晶莹润泽。枕面为花瓣形，上装饰刻画"卍"字纹。枕体四面为人物故事图，正面为"广寒宫"的神话故事，殿门敞开，楼梯清晰可见，嫦娥端坐中间。两旁有女侍两人。1981 年安徽岳西出土。

岳西文物局藏

The pillow is zaffre-glazed, and decorated with cloud patterns and branches of flora patterns. The zaffre glaze is bright and smooth. On the petal-shaped pillow face are carved " 卍 " patterns. Figures and scenes are painted on the four sides of this pillow. On the front side is painted the fairy tale of "the Moon Palace", whose gate is open. The palace stairs can be seen clearly. Chang'e, the goddess in the moon, is sitting in the middle, served by two maids on the sides of her.It was unearthed in Yuexi, Anhui Province,in 1981.

Preserved in Bureau of Cultural Heritage of Yuexi county

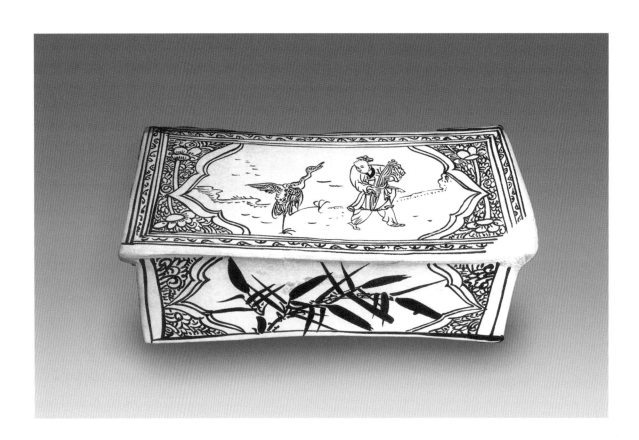

长方形白地黑花人物故事枕

元

瓷质

长 30.5 厘米，宽 16 厘米，高 13.5 厘米

Rectangular Pillow with Black Figure and Floral Design on a White Ground

Yuan Dynasty

Porcelain

Length 30.5 cm/ Width 16 cm/ Height 13.5 cm

胎质灰白坚硬，施化妆土、透明釉，底部无釉，背面上缘有气孔。枕面绘一人抱琴，一只仙鹤起舞。前立面绘竹，后立面绘折枝牡丹，两端面绘花卉。底部印有竖式双栏上莲叶、下荷花"古相张家造"戳记。磁县观台镇东艾口村出土。

中国磁州窑博物馆藏

The greyish white body of the pillow is hard and coated with engobe and transparent glaze except the bottom. There are pores on the upper edge of the back wall. On the pillow face are painted a dancing crane and a man holding the harp, on the front wall bamboos, on the back wall a peony pattern, and on the faces of the two side walls floral patterns. The bottom is stamped with a single-vertical-column seal of "Gu Xiang Zhang Jia Zao" (Made by Zhang's in ancient Xiangzhou), with decorations of a lotus leaf motif on the upper edge and a lotus blossom motif on the lower edge. It was excavated in Dong'aikou village, Guantai Township, Ci County, Hebei Province.

Preserved in China Cizhou Kiln Museum

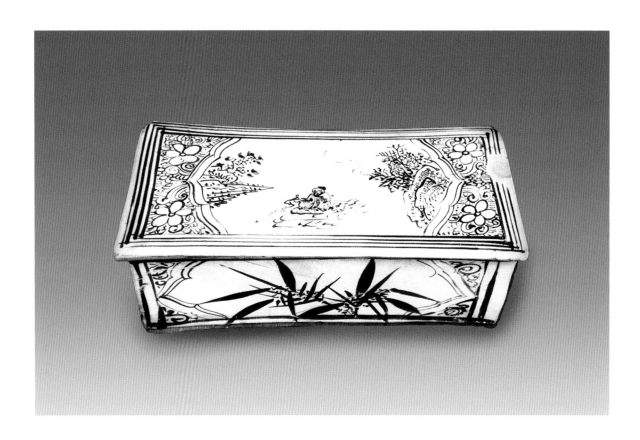

长方形白地黑花人物故事枕

元

瓷质

长 31 厘米，宽 15 厘米，高 13 厘米

Rectangular Pillow with Black Figure and Floral Design on a White Ground

Yuan Dynasty

Porcelain

Length 31 cm/ Width 15 cm/ Height 13 cm

胎质灰白坚硬，施化妆土、透明釉，底部无釉，背面上缘有气孔。枕面绘有人物故事，前立面绘竹，后立面绘折枝牡丹，两端面绘花卉。磁县岳城水库出土。

峰峰矿区文物保管所藏

The greyish white body of the pillow is hard and coated with engobe and transparent glaze except the bottom. There are pores on the upper edge of the back wall. On the pillow face is painted a story scene, on the front wall bamboos, on the back wall a peony pattern, and on the faces of the two side walls floral patterns. It was excavated from the reservoir of Yuecheng in Ci County, Hebei Province.
Preserved in Department of Cultural Relics Conservation in Fengfeng Mining District

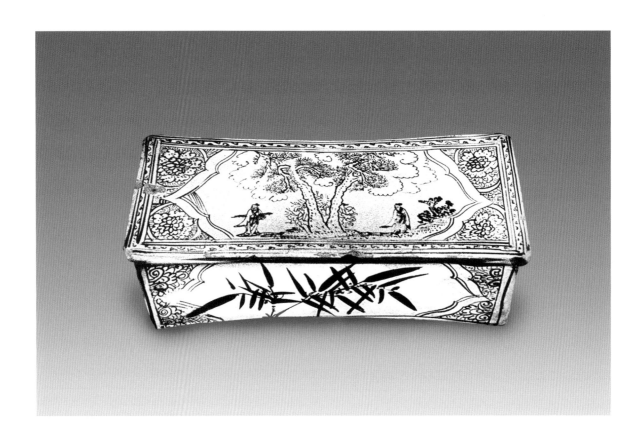

长方形白地黑花人物故事枕

元

瓷质

长 44 厘米，宽 18 厘米，高 15.5 厘米

Rectangular Pillow with Black Figure and Floral Design on a White Ground

Yuan Dynasty

Porcelain

Length 44 cm/ Width 18 cm/ Height 15.5 cm

胎质灰白坚硬，施化妆土、透明釉，底部无釉，背面上缘有气孔。枕面绘人物故事，前立面绘竹，后立面绘牡丹，两端面绘花卉，背面两边有墨书文字"古相张家造，艾山枕用功"。底部印有竖式上莲叶、下荷花"张家造"戳记。磁县观台镇出土。

安阳博物馆藏

The greyish white body of the pillow is hard and coated with engobe and transparent glaze except the bottom. There are pores on the upper edge of the back wall. On the pillow face is painted a story scene, on the front wall bamboos, on the back wall a peony pattern, and on the faces of the two side walls floral patterns. On the two edges of the back wall are found ink inscriptions "Made by Zhang's in ancient Xiangzhou" and "Made at the foot of Ai Mountain". The bottom has a vertical seal of "Zhang Jia Zao" (Made by Zhang's), with the decoration of a lotus leaf motif on the upper edge and a lotus blossom motif on the lower edge. It was excavated in Guantai Township, Ci County, Hebei Province.

Preserved in Anyang Municipal Museum

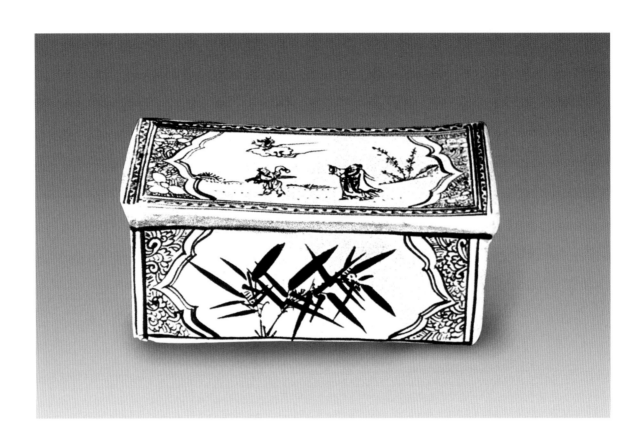

长方形白地黑花人物故事枕

元

瓷质

长 30.2 厘米，宽 16 厘米，高 13.2 厘米

Rectangular Pillow with Black Figure and Floral Design on a White Ground

Yuan Dynasty

Porcelain

Length 30.2 cm/ Width 16 cm/ Height 13.2 cm

胎质细而坚，呈灰白色，部分有开片，施化妆土、透明釉，背面上缘有气孔。枕面绘一老一少人物，指看天空中的飞龙，前立面绘竹，后立面绘牡丹，两端面绘花卉。底部印有竖式双栏上莲叶、下荷花"古相张家造"戳记。

杨永德藏

The greyish white body of the pillow is of fine and hard texture and coated with engobe and transparent glaze, on parts of which crackles can be seen. There are pores on the upper edge of the back. On the pillow face are painted an old figure and a young one pointing at the dragon in the air, on the front wall bamboos, on the back wall a peony pattern, and on the faces of the two side walls floral patterns. The bottom is stamped with a double-vertical-column seal of "Gu Xiang Zhang Jia Zao" (Made by Zhang's in ancient Xiangzhou), with the decoration of a lotus leaf motif on the upper edge and a lotus blossom motif on the lower edge.

Collected by Yang Yongde

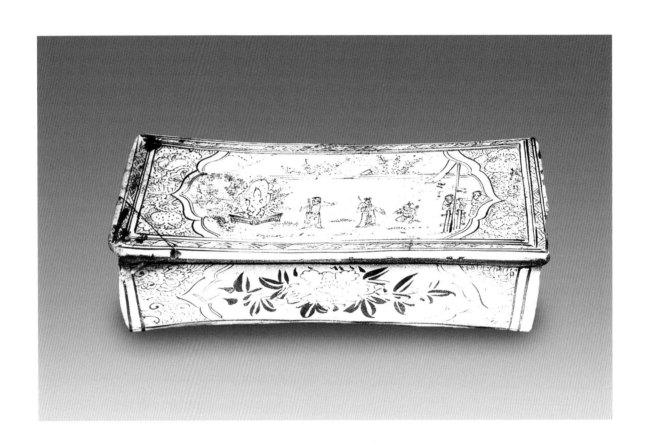

长方形白地黑花人物故事枕

元

瓷质

长 41 厘米，宽 17.6 厘米，高 14.3 厘米

Rectangular Pillow with Black Figure and Floral Design on a White Ground

Yuan Dynasty

Porcelain

Length 41 cm/ Width 17.6 cm/ Height 14.3 cm

胎质灰白坚硬，施化妆土、透明釉，底部无釉，背面上缘有气孔。枕面绘人物故事。前立面绘折枝牡丹，后立面绘三个人物一棵树，左右两边书"相地张家造，艾山枕用功"。底部印有竖式双栏上莲叶、下荷花"古相张家造"戳记。磁县岳城水库出土。

峰峰矿区文物保管所藏

The greyish white body of the pillow is hard and coated with engobe and transparent glaze except the bottom. There are pores on the upper edge of the back wall. On the pillow face is painted a story scene, on the front wall a peony pattern, and on the back wall three people and a tree with ink inscriptions on both edges, "Made by Zhang's in ancient Xiangzhou" and "Made at the foot of Ai Mountain". The bottom is stamped with a vertical double column seal of "Gu Xiang Zhang Jia Zao" (Made by Zhang's in ancient Xiangzhou), with decorations of a lotus leaf motif on the upper edge and a lotus blossom motif on the lower edge. It was excavated from the reservoir of Yuecheng in Ci County, Hebei Province.

Preserved in Department of Cultural Relics Conservation in Fengfeng Mining District

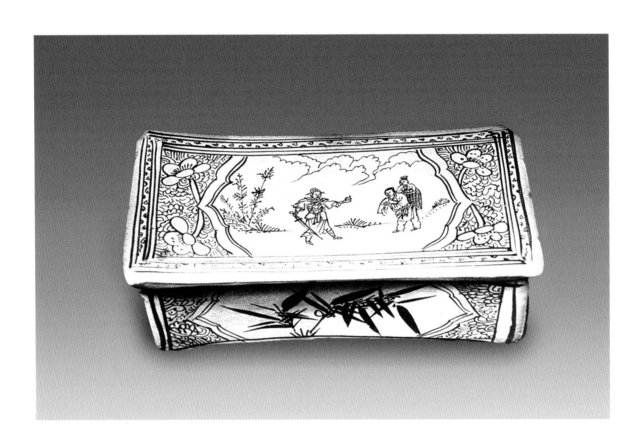

长方形白地黑花人物故事枕

元

瓷质

长 31.8 厘米，宽 15.1 厘米，高 11.7 厘米

Rectangular Pillow with Black Figure and Floral Design on a White Ground

Yuan Dynasty

Porcelain

Length 31.8 cm/ Width 15.1 cm/ Height 11.7 cm

胎质灰白坚硬，施化妆土、透明釉，底部无釉，背面上缘有气孔。枕面绘人物故事，前立面绘竹，后立面绘折枝牡丹，两端面绘花卉。底部印有竖式双栏上莲叶、下荷花"古相张家造"戳记。磁县岳城水库出土。

峰峰矿区文物保管所藏

The greyish white body of the pillow is hard and coated with engobe and transparent glaze except the bottom. There are pores on the upper edge of the back wall. On the pillow face is painted a story scene, and on the front wall bamboos, with a peony pattern on the back wall and floral motifs on the faces of the two side walls. The bottom is stamped with a vertical double column seal of "Gu Xiang Zhang Jia Zao" (Made by Zhang's in ancient Xiangzhou), with decorations of a lotus leaf motif on the upper edge and a lotus blossom motif on the lower edge. It was excavated from the reservoir of Yuecheng in Ci County, Hebei Province.

Preserved in Department of Cultural Relics Conservation in Fengfeng Mining District

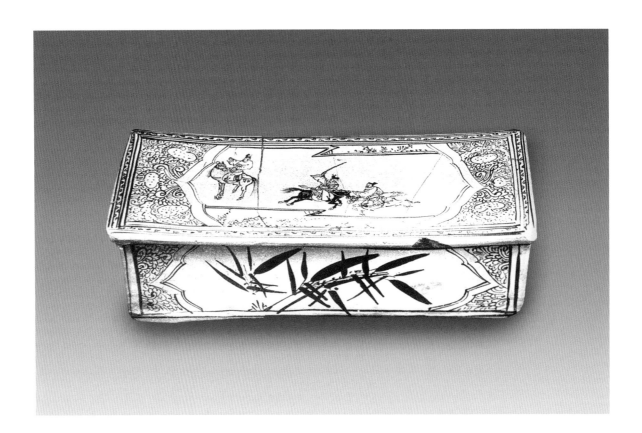

长方形白地黑花人物故事枕

元

瓷质

长 39.8 厘米，宽 17.4 厘米，高 14.2 厘米

Rectangular Pillow with Black Figure and Floral Design on a White Ground

Yuan Dynasty

Porcelain

Length 39.8 cm/ Width 17.4 cm/ Height 14.2 cm

胎质灰白坚硬，施化妆土、透明釉，底部无釉，背面上缘有气孔。枕面绘人物故事，前立面绘竹，后立面绘折枝牡丹，两端面绘花卉。底部印有竖式双栏上莲叶、下荷花"古相张家造"戳记。磁县岳城水库出土。

峰峰矿区文物保管所藏

The greyish white body of the pillow is hard and coated with engobe and transparent glaze except the bottom. There are pores on the upper edge of the back wall. On the pillow face is painted a story scene, and on the front wall bamboos, with a peony pattern on the back wall and floral motifs on the faces of the two side walls. The bottom is stamped with a vertical double column seal of "Gu Xiang Zhang Jia Zao" (Made by Zhang's in ancient Xiangzhou), with decorations of a lotus leaf motif on the upper edge and a lotus blossom motif on the lower edge. It was excavated from the reservoir of Yuecheng in Ci County, Hebei Province.
Preserved in Department of Cultural Relics Conservation in Fengfeng Mining District

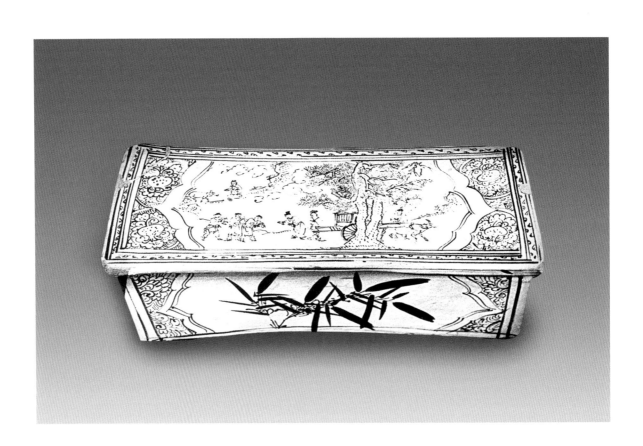

长方形白地黑花人物故事枕

元

瓷质

长 39.1 厘米，宽 17.6 厘米，高 13.8 厘米

Rectangular Pillow with Black Figure and Floral Design on a White Ground

Yuan Dynasty

Porcelain

Length 39.1 cm/ Width 17.6 cm/ Height 13.8 cm

胎质灰白坚硬，施化妆土、透明釉，底部无釉，背面上缘有气孔。枕面绘有人物故事，前立面绘竹，后立面绘折枝牡丹，两端面绘花卉。印有竖式双栏上莲叶、下荷花"古相张家造"戳记。磁县岳城水库出土。

峰峰矿区文物保管所藏

The greyish white body of the pillow is hard and coated with engobe and transparent glaze except the bottom. There are pores on the upper edge of the back wall. On the pillow face is painted a story scene, and on the front wall bamboos, with a peony pattern on the back wall and floral motifs on the faces of the two side walls. The bottom is stamped with a vertical double column seal of "Gu Xiang Zhang Jia Zao" (Made by Zhang's in ancient Xiangzhou), with decorations of a lotus leaf motif on the upper edge and a lotus blossom motif on the lower edge. It was excavated from the reservoir of Yuecheng in Ci County, Hebei Province.

Preserved in Department of Cultural Relics Conservation in Fengfeng Mining District

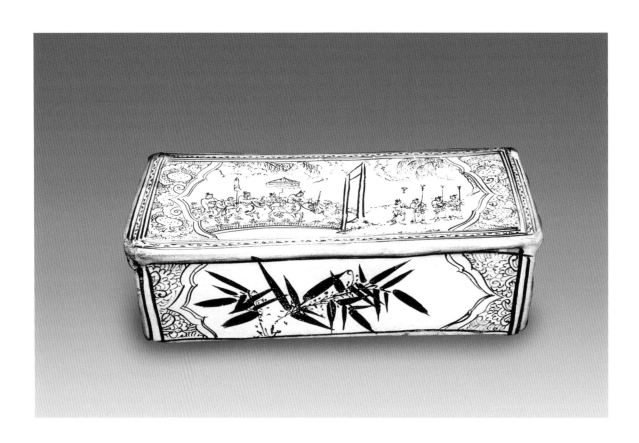

长方形白地黑花人物故事枕

元

瓷质

长 38.5 厘米，宽 17.7 厘米，高 14.5 厘米

Rectangular Pillow with Black Figure and Floral Design on a White Ground

Yuan Dynasty

Porcelain

Length 38.5 cm/ Width 17.7 cm/ Height 14.5 cm

胎质灰白坚硬，施化妆土、透明釉，底部无釉，背面上缘有气孔。枕面绘有人物故事，前立面绘竹，后立面绘折枝牡丹，两端面绘花卉。底部印有竖式双栏上莲叶、下荷花"古相张家造"戳记。磁县出土。

中国磁州窑博物馆藏

The greyish white body of the pillow is hard and coated with engobe and transparent glaze except the bottom. There are pores on the upper edge of the back wall. On the pillow face is painted a story scene, and on the front wall bamboos, with a peony pattern on the back wall and floral motifs on the faces of the two side walls. The bottom is stamped with a vertical double column seal of "Gu Xiang Zhang Jia Zao" (Made by Zhang's in ancient Xiangzhou), with decorations of a lotus leaf motif on the upper edge and a lotus blossom motif on the lower edge. It was excavated in Ci County, Hebei Province.

Preserved in China Cizhou Kiln Museum

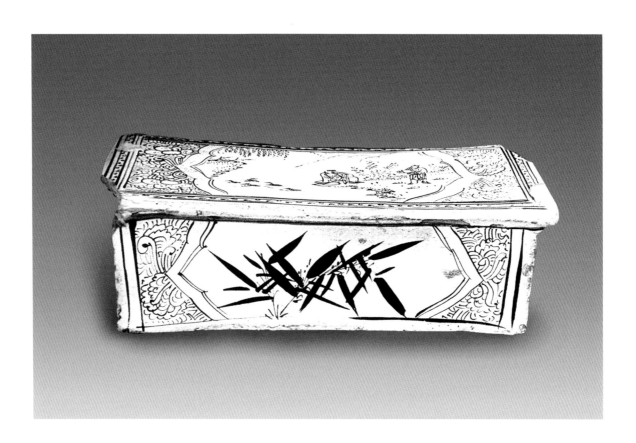

长方形白地黑花放鸭纹枕

元

瓷质

长 31.8 厘米，宽 15.1 厘米，高 11.7 厘米

Rectangular Pillow with Black Duck and Floral Design on a White Ground

Yuan Dynasty

Porcelain

Length 31.8 cm/ Width 15.1 cm/ Height 11.7 cm

胎质灰白坚硬，施化妆土、透明釉，底部无釉，背面上缘有气孔，角残。枕面绘两个人物，一人坐在河边，观河里的五只鸭子戏水。前立面绘竹，后立面绘折枝牡丹，两端面绘花卉。底部印有竖式双栏上莲叶，下荷花"古相张家造"戳记。磁县岳城水库出土。

峰峰矿区文物保管所藏

The greyish white body of the pillow is hard and coated with engobe and transparent glaze except the bottom. There are pores on the upper edge of the back wall. One corner of the pillow is broken. On the pillow face are painted two figures, one of whom is sitting on the river bank watching five ducks playing with water. A bamboo design is drawn on the front wall, with a peony pattern on the back wall and floral motifs on the faces of the two side walls. The bottom is stamped with a double-vertical-column seal of "Gu Xiang Zhang Jia Zhao" (Made by Zhang's in ancient Xiangzhou), with decorations of a lotus leaf motif on the upper edge and a lotus blossom motif on the lower edge. It was excavated from the reservoir of Yuecheng in Ci County, Hebei Province.

Preserved in Department of Cultural Relics Conservation in Fengfeng Mining District

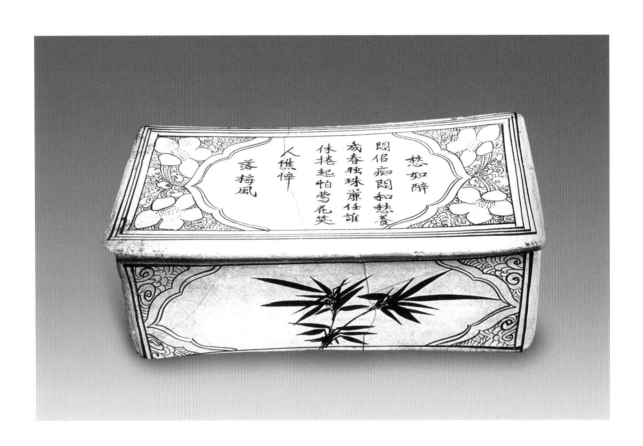

长方形白地黑花文字枕

元

瓷质

长 31 厘米，宽 16.7 厘米，高 14.5 厘米

Rectangular Pillow with Black Inscription and Floral Design on a White Ground

Yuan Dynasty

Porcelain

Length 31 cm/ Width 16.7 cm/ Height 14.5 cm

胎质灰白坚硬，施化妆土、透明釉，底部无釉，背面上缘有气孔。枕面墨书《落梅风》曲一首。前、立面绘竹，后立面绘折枝牡丹，两端面绘荷花。底部印有竖式单栏上莲叶、下荷花"李家造"戳记。磁县岳城出土。

The greyish white body of the pillow is hard and coated with engobe and transparent glaze except the bottom. There are pores on the upper edge of the back wall. On the pillow face is found an ink inscription of a poem. On the front wall is painted a bamboo design, with a peony pattern on the back wall and lotus motifs on the faces of the two side walls. The bottom is stamped with a single-vertical-column seal of "Li Jia Zhao" (Made by Li's), with decorations of a lotus leaf motif on the upper edge and a lotus blossom motif on the lower edge. It was excavated in Yuecheng of Ci County, Hebei Province.

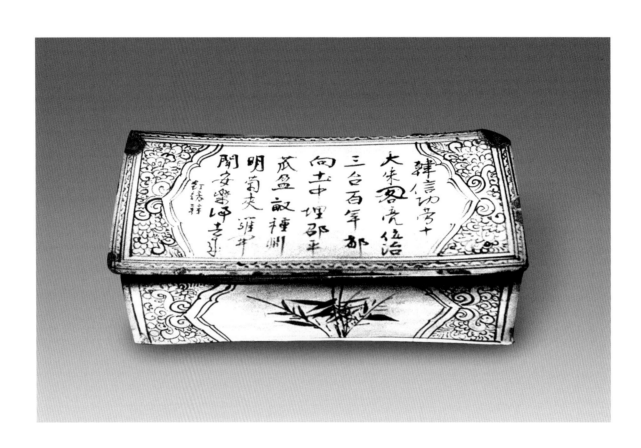

长方形白地黑花文字枕

元

瓷质

长 31 厘米，宽 15 厘米，高 12.5 厘米

Rectangular Pillow with Black Inscription and Floral Design on a White Ground

Yuan Dynasty

Porcelain

Length 31 cm/ Width 15 cm/ Height 12.5 cm

胎质灰白坚硬，施化妆土、透明釉，底部无
釉，背面上缘有气孔。枕面有墨书《红绣鞋》
曲一首。前立面绘竹，后立面绘荷、鸟，两
端面绘花卉。磁县岳城水库出土。

邯郸市博物馆藏

The greyish white body of the pillow is hard
and coated with engobe and transparent glaze
except the bottom. There are pores on the upper
edge of the back wall. On the pillow face is
found an ink inscription of a poem. On the front
wall is painted a bamboo design, with peony
and bird patterns on the back wall and lotus
motifs on the faces of the two side walls. It was
excavated from the reservoir of Yuecheng in Ci
County, Hebei Province.

Preserved in Handan Museum

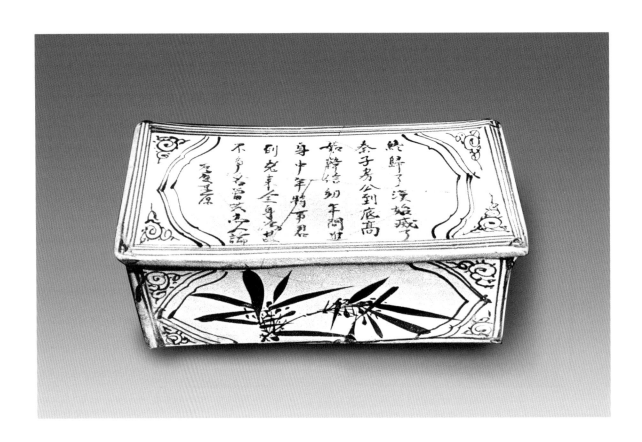

长方形白地黑花文字枕

元

瓷质

长 30.8 厘米，宽 15.9 厘米，高 14.7 厘米

Rectangular Pillow with Black Inscription and Floral Design on a White Ground

Yuan Dynasty

Porcelain

Length 30.8 cm/ Width 15.9 cm/ Height 14.7 cm

胎质灰白坚硬，施化妆土、透明釉，底部无釉，背面上缘有气孔。枕面墨书《庆东原》曲一首。前立面绘竹，后立面绘折枝牡丹，两端面绘花卉。底部印有竖式双栏上莲叶、下荷花"张家造"戳记。磁县南关兴礼西街出土。

中国磁州窑博物馆藏

The greyish white body of the pillow is hard and coated with engobe and transparent glaze except the bottom. There are pores on the upper edge of the back wall. On the pillow face is found an ink inscription of a poem. On the front wall is painted a bamboo design, with a peony pattern on the back wall and lotus motifs on the faces of the two side walls. The bottom is stamped with a vertical double column seal of "Zhang Jia Zhao" (Made by Zhang's), with the decoration of a lotus leaf motif on the upper edge and a lotus blossom motif on the lower edge. It was excavated from West Xingli Street of Nanguan in Ci County, Hebei Province. Preserved in China Cizhou Kiln Museum

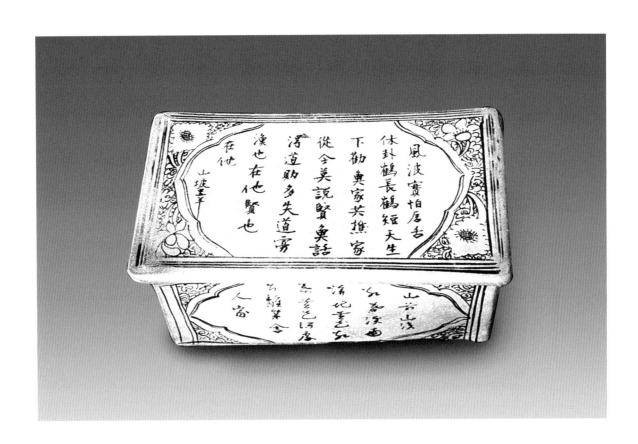

长方形白地黑花文字枕

元

瓷质

长 28.5 厘米，宽 16 厘米，高 14 厘米

Rectangular Pillow with Black Inscription and Floral Design on a White Ground

Yuan Dynasty

Porcelain

Length 28.5 cm/ Width 16 cm/ Height 14 cm

胎质灰白坚硬，施化妆土、透明釉，底部无釉，背面上缘有气孔。枕面书陈草庵《山坡羊》曲一首，前后立面也书有文字。底部印有竖式双栏上莲叶、下荷花"王家造"戳记。磁县城南出土。

中国磁州窑博物馆藏

The greyish white body of the pillow is hard and coated with engobe and transparent glaze except the bottom. There are pores on the upper edge of the back wall. On the pillow face is found an ink inscription of a poem, with inscriptions on the front and the back walls as well. The bottom is stamped with a vertical double column seal of "Wang Jia Zao" (Made by Wang's), with decorations of a lotus leaf motif on the upper edge and a lotus blossom motif on the lower edge. It was excavated in the southern suburbs of Ci County, Hebei Province. Preserved in China Cizhou Kiln Museum

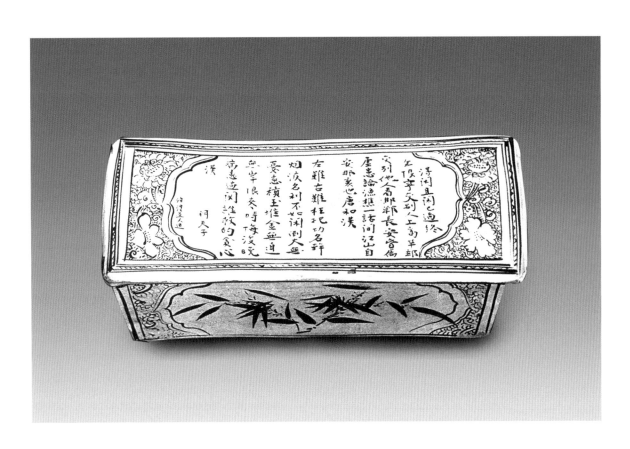

长方形白地黑花文字枕

元

瓷质

长 46.7 厘米，宽 17.7 厘米，高 15.5 厘米

Rectangular Pillow with Black Inscription and Floral Design on a White Ground

Yuan Dynasty

Porcelain

Length 46.7 cm/ Width 17.7 cm/ Height 15.5 cm

胎质灰白坚硬，施化妆土、透明釉，底部无釉，背面上缘有气孔。枕面有墨书《朝天子》曲两首。前立面绘竹，后立面绘折枝牡丹，两端面绘荷花。枕面左边刻画有"漳滨逸人造"五字。磁县都党乡冶子村出土。

中国磁州窑博物馆藏

The greyish white body of the pillow is hard and coated with engobe and transparent glaze except the bottom. There are pores on the upper edge of the back wall. On the pillow face is found an ink inscription of one verse. On the front wall is painted a bamboo design, with a peony pattern on the back wall and lotus motifs on the faces of the two side walls. On the left side of the pillow face are carved five Chinese characters "Zhang Bin Yi Ren Zao". It was excavated in Yezi Village, Dudang Township, Ci County, Hebei Province.

Preserved in China Cizhou Kiln Museum

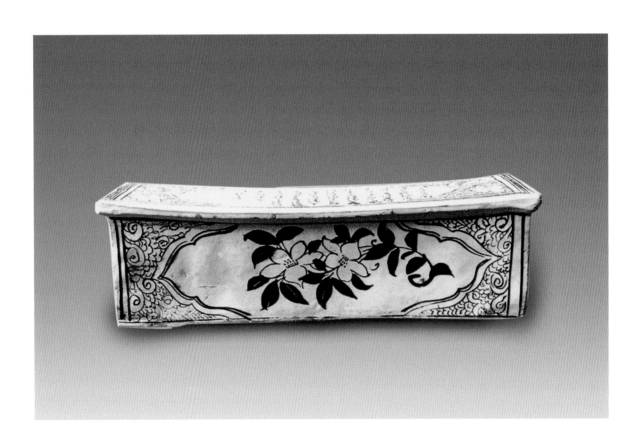

长方形白地黑花文字枕

元

瓷质

长 42 厘米，宽 17 厘米，前高 10.5 厘米，后高 14 厘米

Rectangular Pillow with Black Inscription and Floral Design on a White Ground

Yuan Dynasty

Porcelain

Length 42 cm/ Width 17 cm/ Front Height 10.5 cm/ Backs Height 14 cm

胎质灰白坚硬，施化妆土、透明釉，底部无釉，背上缘有气孔。枕面抄录词一首，前立面绘折枝花，后立面绘牡丹，右边竖式墨书"滏源王家造"五字。端面绘荷花。磁县观台镇东艾口村出土。

The greyish white body of the pillow is hard and coated with engobe and transparent glaze except the bottom. There are pores on the upper edge of the back wall. On the pillow face is found an ink inscription of one poem. On the front wall is painted a flowering branch design, with a peony pattern on the back wall. On the right side of the pillow face are carved five Chinese characters "Fu Yuan Wang Jia Zao" (Made by Wang's in Fuyuan). It was excavated in Dong'aikou Village, Guantai Township, Ci County, Hebei Province.

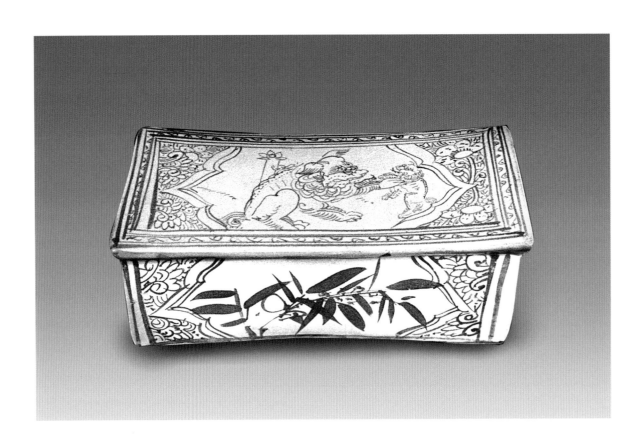

长方形白地黑花狮纹枕

元

瓷质

长 29.2 厘米，宽 14.2 厘米，高 12.5 厘米

Rectangular Pillow with Black Lion Pattern on a White Ground

Yuan Dynasty

Porcelain

Length 29.2 cm/ Width 14.2 cm/ Height 12.5 cm

胎质灰白坚硬，施化妆土、透明釉，底部无釉，背面上缘有气孔。枕面绘有大、小狮子两个。前立面绘竹，后立面绘折枝花，两端面绘花卉。底部印有竖式双栏"张家造"戳记。磁县观台镇出土。

安阳博物馆藏

The greyish white body of the pillow is hard and coated with engobe and transparent glaze except the bottom. There are pores on the upper edge of the back wall. On the pillow face are painted a big and a small lions. On the front wall is painted a bamboo design, with a flowering branch pattern on the back wall and lotus motifs on the faces of the two side walls. The bottom is stamped with a vertical double column seal of "Zhang Jia Zhao" (Made by Zhang's). It was excavated in Guantai Township, Ci County, Hebei Province.

Preserved in Anyang Municipal Museum

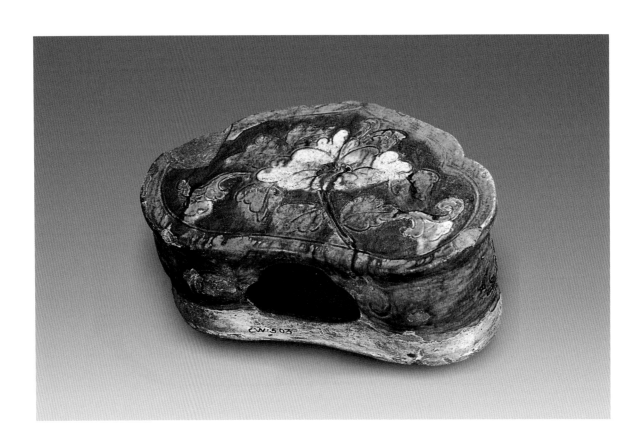

如意形三彩纹枕

元

瓷质

长 26 厘米，宽 16.4 厘米，高 12.5 厘米

Tri-colour Ruyi-shaped Pillow

Yuan Dynasty

Porcelain

Length 26 cm/ Width 16.4 cm/ Height 12.5 cm

胎质灰白坚硬，施化妆土、绿黄釉，周壁有
纹饰。枕面为三彩花卉图纹。磁县出土。

中国磁州窑博物馆藏

The greyish white body of the pillow is hard
and coated with engobe and greenish-yellow
glaze. The peripheral walls are incised with
stripe patterns. On the pillow face are painted
tri-colour floral motifs. It was unearthed in Ci
County.

Preserved in China Cizhou Kiln Museum

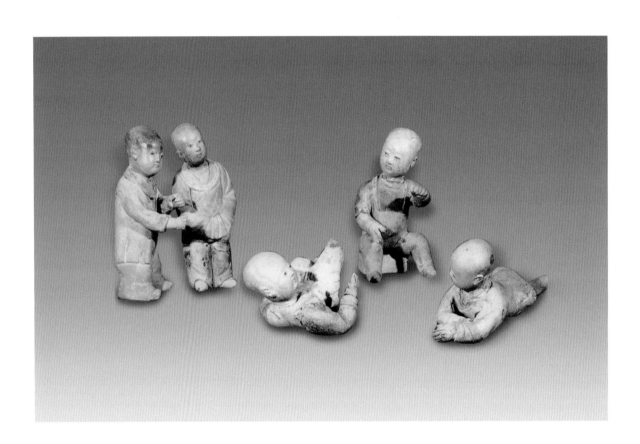

捏像相扑泥孩儿

宋

泥质

均高约 10 厘米

Clay Figurines of Sumo-wrestling Children

Song Dynasty

Clay

Average Height 10 cm

这是一组5个反映宋代相扑场面的捏像泥孩儿，均经过烧制，有的略施彩绘。其中，两个嬉玩的儿童互相相扑而倒，笑态可掬；三个旁观的小儿，一个似为"裁判"，另两个在坦然观望。整组塑像各具神态，生活气息浓厚。1980年江苏省镇江市大市口出土。

镇江博物馆藏

This set of clay figurines, which portrays the scene of five children practising sumo, was all fired with some paintings. Two of the kids, with smiles on their faces, fall on the ground after practicing sumo wrestling. A third one resembles a judge, and the other two are watching at ease. Featuring different postures and expressions, the clay figurines are imbued with a strong smack of genuine life. It was unearthed in Dashikou, Zhenjiang City, Jiangsu Province in 1980.

Preserved in Zhenjiang Museum

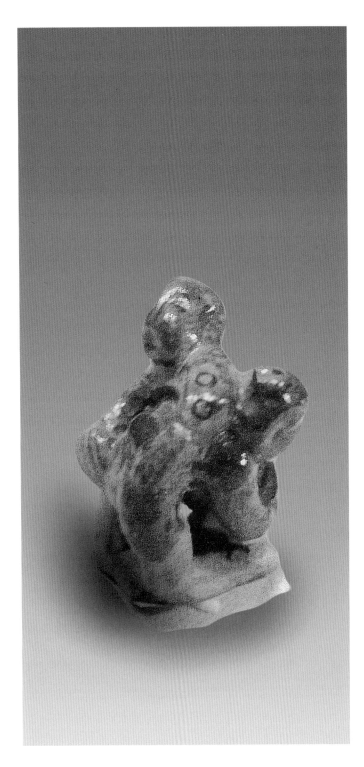

绿釉相扑陶俑

宋

瓷质

高 6.4 厘米

Green-glazed Pottery Figurines of Sumo-wrestlers

Song Dynasty

Porcelain

Height 6.4 cm

胎呈白色，施绿釉。两相扑俑皆赤足，头系发髻，身束腰带，胯间绷护裆带，互相搂抱，并备以双手抱着对方臀部，全身用力，奋力抗争，设法摔倒对方，呈现了一幅难解难分的动人形象。

河南博物院藏

The white body is glazed green. The two bare-footed figurines, with buns on their heads, belts at their wrests, and jockstraps at their lower bodies, are clasping each other, hands on the hips of their adversary. They are trying very hard to tumble their adversary. This set of pottery figurines vividly portrays the scene of two wrestlers grappling with each other.

Preserved in Henan Museum

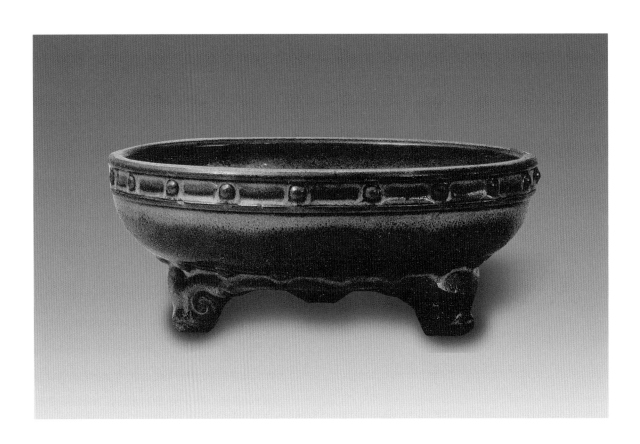

紫红釉鼓钉洗

北宋

瓷质

口径 23.8 厘米，高 9.1 厘米

Purplish-red-glazed Washer with Drum-nail Design

Northern Song Dynasty

Porcelain

Mouth Diameter 23.8 cm/ Height 9.1 cm

胎体厚重，深灰色。器作鼓形，直口，鼓腹，平底，附兽面形足。器底施酱色釉，内壁施天蓝釉，外表施釉较厚，呈紫红色。钧窑（今河南省禹县）产品，釉色独特，多为天蓝色乳光釉，紫红色釉更为突出，是红釉与蓝釉相互熔合的结果，釉色凝厚，绚丽多彩，属宫廷陈设用品。

青岛市博物馆藏

With a thick and heavy body in dark grey, the drum-shaped washer has a straight mouth, a plump stomach, and a flat bottom with animal-face-shaped feet. The bottom is coated with dark-reddish-purple glaze, with sky-blue glaze on the interior and thick purplish-red glaze on the exterior. It belongs to Jun ware (porcelain fired in Jun Kiln which is currently located in Yu County in Henan Province), which is characterized by unique glaze colour. Jun ware mostly features sky-blue glaze with an opalescent shine, but the products are more outstanding with purplish red glaze which results from the fusion of red and blue glazes. This washer is covered with bright and colourful glaze. It was used as an ornament at the imperial palace.

Preserved in Qingdao Municipal Museum

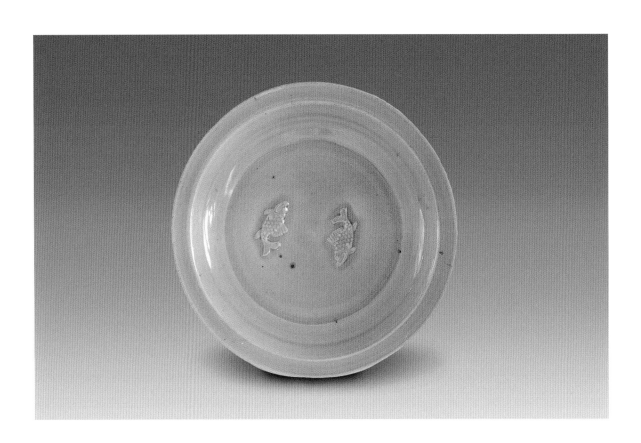

龙泉窑双鱼洗

南宋

瓷质

口径 18 厘米

Washer with Double Fishes Pattern, Longquan Ware

Southern Song Dynasty

Porcelain

Mouth Diameter 18 cm

板沿口，弧形腹，圈足较规整，盘内底心印双鱼纹凸起，里外满施豆绿色釉，釉开细纹片，边棱釉薄处呈白色，圈足内有釉，露胎处呈火石红色。双鱼洗是南宋和元代较常见的器型。

林存义藏

The washer has a flanged mouth rim, a bow-shaped body, and an ordered ring foot. Decorated with convex double fishes pattern on the interior bottom, the washer is glazed pea green with tiny crackles both on the interior and the exterior, but the rim is thinly glazed white. The interior of the ring foot is glazed. Its flint red body is exposed on the unglazed part. The washer with double fishes pattern is commonly found in the wares of the Southern Song Dynasty and the Yuan Dynasty.

Collected by Lin Cunyi

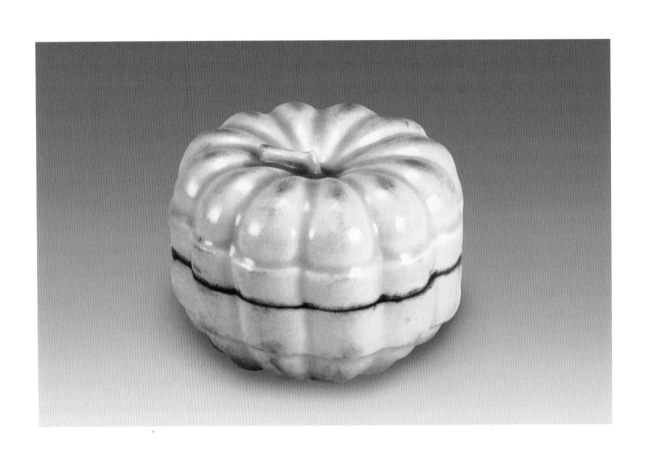

青白釉瓜楞盒

北宋

瓷质

口径 7.4 厘米，通高 5 厘米

Blue-and-white-glazed Box in the Shape of Pumpkin

Northern Song Dynasty

Porcelain

Mouth Diameter 7.4 cm/ Height 5 cm

盒作上下对合的 12 南瓜楞，盖顶有瓜藤装饰，平底。满施青白釉，胎体坚密细腻，釉色莹润如玉，造型优美逼真，是景德镇典型器。1978 年泰县洪林公社尤南大队出土。

扬州博物馆藏

The lid and the body of the box are perfectly matched and shaped into a twelve-lobed pumpkin with a flat bottom. The lid is decorated with melon vine. The solid and fine body is coated with smooth jade-like blue-and-white glaze. This box, characterized by its vivid shape and beautiful glaze colour, is typical of porcelain ware made in Jingdezhen. It was unearthed from Younan Team of Honglin Commune, in Tai County, Jiangsu Province, in 1978.

Preserved in Yangzhou Museum

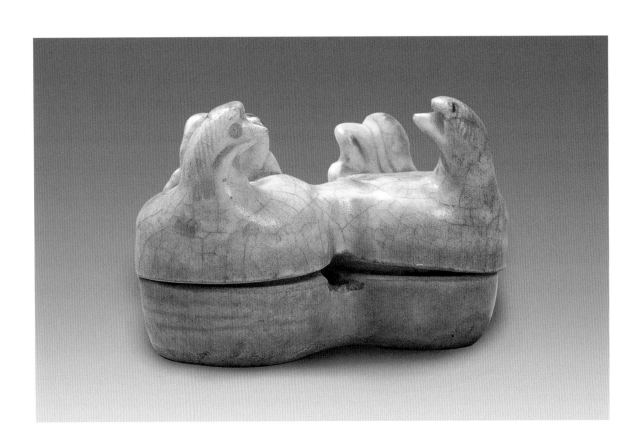

青白釉鸟形瓷粉盒

宋

瓷质

宽 8 厘米，盒高 5 厘米，盖高 3.5 厘米

Greenish-white Porcelain Compact with Bird Design

Song Dynasty

Porcelain

Width 8 cm/ Box Height 5 cm/ Lid Height 3.5 cm

粉盒盖由两只飞鸟堆塑而成,飞鸟昂首对视,似作鸳鸯嬉水状，造型生动别致。釉面白中泛青，发色纯正自然，是宋代青白釉瓷器之精品。

南京六合区文物保管所藏

Two flying birds, moulded on the lid, cast their eyes at each other with heads up, looking like a pair of mandarin ducks dabbling in the water. With vivid shape and natural glaze, the compact is considered a masterpiece of greenish-white porcelain ware of the Song Dynasty.

Preserved in the Department of Cultural Relics Conservation of Liuhe County, Nanjing

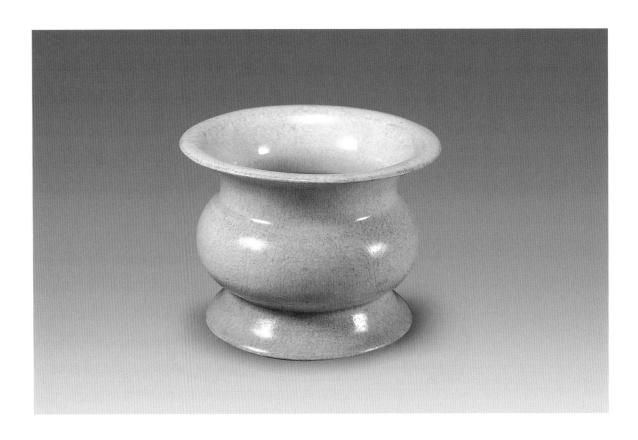

青白釉暗花缠枝牡丹纹渣斗

北宋

瓷质

口径 15.2 厘米，底径 12.4 厘米，高 10.8 厘米

Greenish-white Spittoon Incised with Interlocking Peony Pattern

Northern Song Dynasty

Porcelain

Mouth Diameter 15.2 cm/ Bottom Diameter 12.4 cm/ Height 10.8 cm

口沿外翻，束颈，扁圆腹，喇叭状圈足。胎体坚致，釉色白中泛青，釉质光润。器物内外施釉，砂底，可见细密旋胎纹及粘砂。腹部划暗花缠枝牡丹纹，划纹纤细。

常州博物馆藏

The spittoon has an everted mouth rim, a narrow neck, a melon-shaped belly and a trumpet-shaped ring foot. The fine and hard body is smoothly coated with greenish-white glaze. The ware, glazed both on the interior and the exterior, has a sand bottom on which can be seen fine and dense rotatory patterns and adhering sand. Around the belly are incised slender and delicate interlocking peony patterns. Preserved in Changzhou Museum

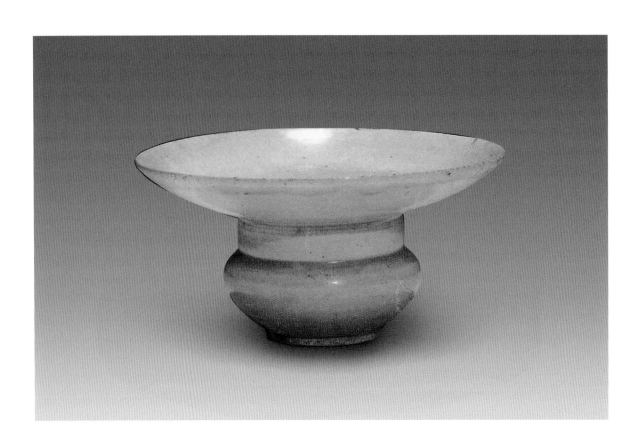

影青瓷唾盂

宋

瓷质

口径 18 厘米，高 9 厘米

Misty-blue-glazed Spittoon

Song Dynasty

Porcelain

Mouth Diameter 18 cm/ Height 9 cm

敞口，短颈，鼓腹，浅圈足。造型生动。四川简阳宋墓出土。

四川博物院藏

The vividly designed spittoon has a flared mouth, a short neck, a drum belly and a shallow ring foot. It was unearthed from a tomb of the Song Dynasty in Jianyang, Sichuan Province.

Preserved in Sichuan Museum

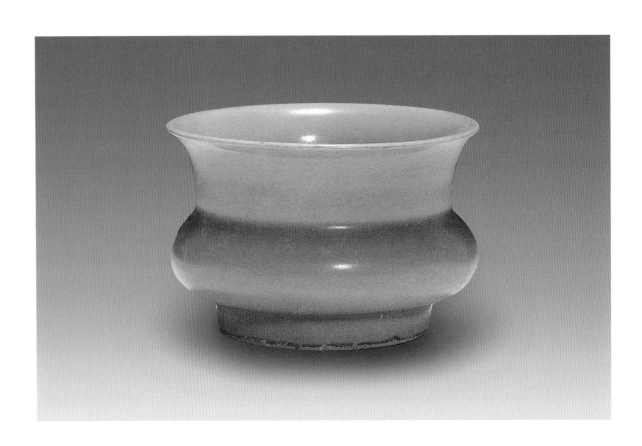

豆青瓷唾盂

宋

瓷质

口径 12.8 厘米，高 8.3 厘米

Pea-green-glazed Spittoon

Song Dynasty

Porcelain

Mouth Diameter 12.8 cm/ Height 8.3 cm

口沿外撇，直颈，鼓腹，圈足。瓷色莹润素雅。
四川简阳宋墓出土。

四川博物院藏

The spittoon has an everted mouth rim, a
straight neck, a drum belly and a foot rim.
The glaze colour is smooth and elegant. It was
unearthed from a tomb of the Song Dynasty in
Jianyang, Sichuan Province.

Preserved in Sichuan Museum

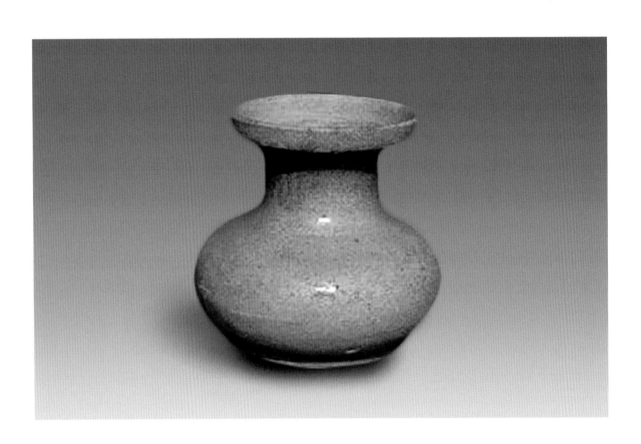

青釉唾壶

宋

瓷质

口外径 9 厘米，脖径 5.1 厘米，腹径 11.9 厘米，底径 9 厘米，通高 13.8 厘米，腹深 9.9 厘米，重 635 克

Celadon Spittoon

Song Dynasty

Porcelain

Mouth Outer Diameter 9 cm/ Neck Diameter 5.1 cm/ Belly Diameter11.9 cm/ Bottom Diameter 9 cm/ Height 13.8 cm/ Depth 9.9 cm/ Weight 635 g

壶束颈，盘口，口唇上卷，腹鼓，圈足。卫
生用品。

广东中医药博物馆藏

This spittoon has a constricted neck, a dish-
shaped mouth with the lip scrolled upward,
a drum belly and a ring foot. It was used as a
sanitary article.

Preserved in Guangdong Chinese Medicine
Museum

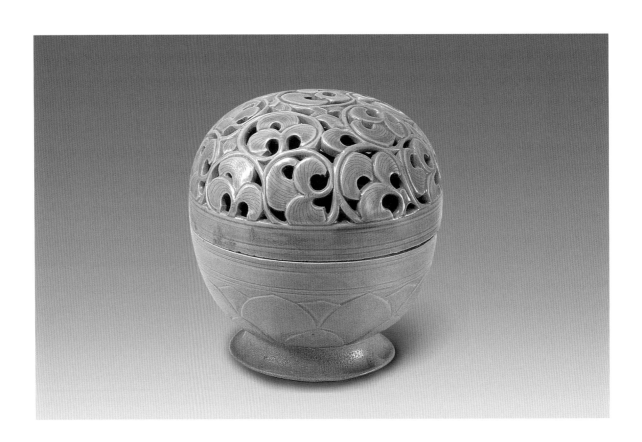

青瓷熏炉

北宋

瓷质

口径 17.5 厘米，底径 12.6 厘米，通高 19.5 厘米

Celadon Incense Burner

Northern Song Dynasty

Porcelain

Mouth Diameter 17.5 cm/ Bottom Diameter 12.6 cm/ Height 19.5 cm

炉盖缠枝花卉镂孔，炉身下腹重瓣仰莲，造型奇特别致，装饰构图庄重严谨，内外施薄釉，釉色青绿，滋润光泽如凝脂。

黄岩博物馆藏

The top of the lid is decorated with openwork design of interlocking flowers, while the lower abdomen with double-petalled lotus patterns. The design of the burner is of delicacy and uniqueness, and the adorning composition is of precision. Both the exterior and interior are covered with thin bluish-green glaze which looks as smooth as cream.

Preserved in Huangyan Museum

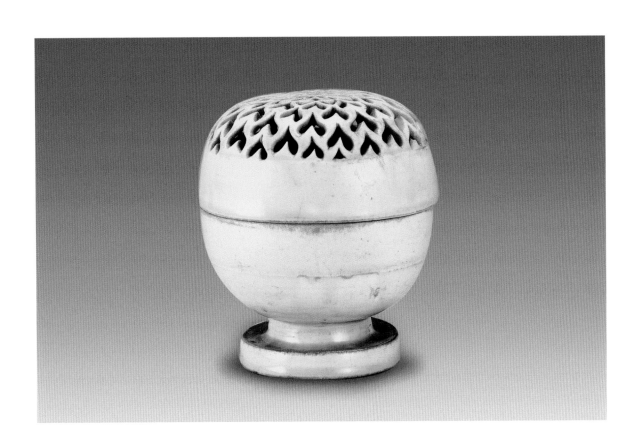

青白釉香薰

北宋

瓷质

腹径 15.3 厘米，底径 10.5 厘米，通高 16.5 厘米

Bluish-white-glazed Incense Burner

Northern Song Dynasty

Porcelain

Abdomen Diameter 15.3 cm/ Bottom Diameter 10.5 cm/ Height 16.5 cm

该器为传世之物。薰为上下对合的球形，薰盖布满"火焰状"镂孔，以子母口与薰体结合，薰体中腹有一道凹状弦纹。底座束胫，高圈足，平底。胎质坚密白细，器内无釉，器外满施青白色釉，釉色莹润如玉。器型美观敦实，为实用器。

扬州博物馆藏

The incense burner is a masterpiece handed down from the ancient times. It is in the shape of a globe composed of two hemisphere-shaped parts. The top of the lid, decorated with flame-shaped openwork design, joins the lower body as a snap lid. Around the middle part of the stomach is incised a concave string. The base has a constricted neck, a high ring foot and a flat bottom. The exterior of the fine and white body is coated with bluish-white glaze, which is as smooth and bright as jade, while the interior is unglazed. With the elegant and solid shape, the burner was used as an object of daily use.

Preserved in Yangzhou Museum

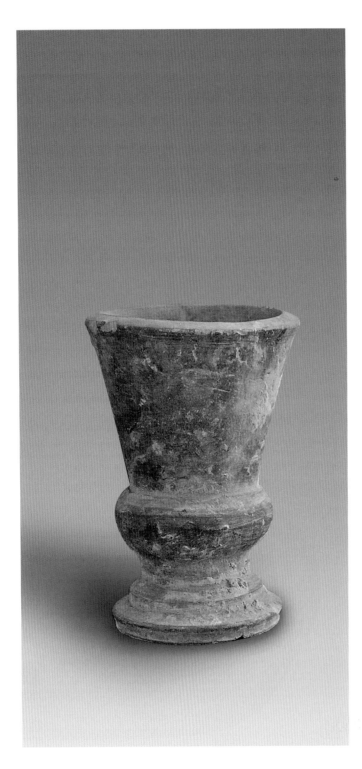

陶香筒

元

陶质

口径10厘米，底径8厘米，通高14厘米。

重500克

Incense Burner

Yuan Dynasty

Pottery

Mouth Diameter 10 cm/ Bottom Diameter

8 cm/ Height 14 cm/ Weight 500 g

喇叭口，鼓腹，平底，接近底部有台棱纹。

宗教用器，祭祀用具。完整无损。

陕西医史博物馆藏

The incense burner has a trumpet-shaped mouth, a drum-shaped belly, a flat bottom with tiers of ribbings carved close to the bottom. The well-preserved burner was used as a ritual article.

Preserved in Shaanxi Museum of Medical History

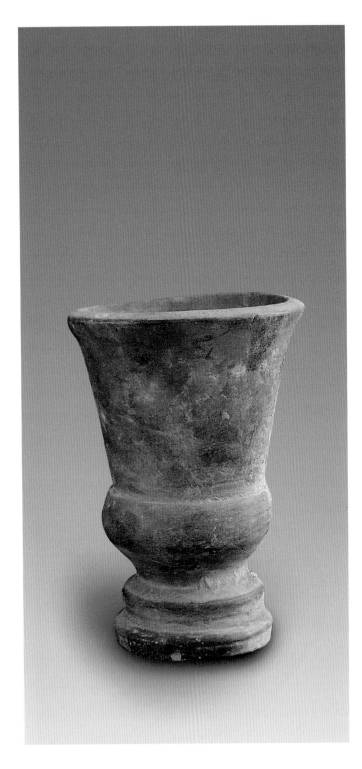

陶香筒

元

陶质

口径 10 厘米，底径 8 厘米，通高 14 厘米，
重 500 克

Incense Burner

Yuan Dynasty

Pottery

Mouth Diameter 10 cm/ Bottom Diameter
8 cm/ Height 14 cm/ Weight 500 g

喇叭口，鼓腹，平底，接近底部有台棱纹。
宗教用器，祭祀用具。完整无损。

陕西医史博物馆藏

The incense burner has a trumpet-shaped mouth, a drum-shaped belly, a flat bottom with tiers of ribbings carved close to the bottom. The well-preserved burner was used as a ritual article.

Preserved in Shaanxi Museum of Medical History

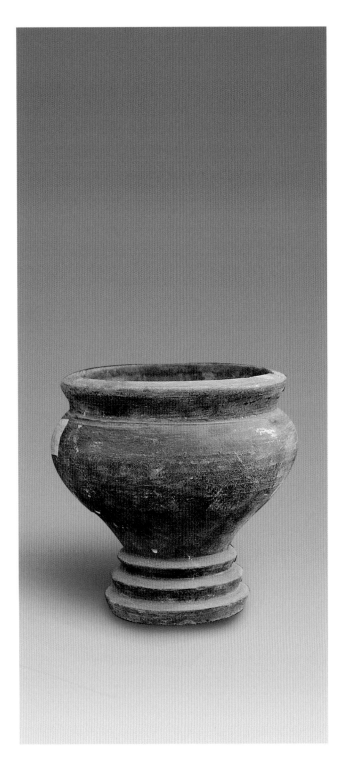

陶香炉

元

陶质

口径 14.5 厘米，底径 9.5 厘米，通高 15 厘
米，重 1000 克

Incense Burner

Yuan Dynasty

Pottery

Mouth Diameter 14.5 cm/ Bottom Diameter
9.5 cm/ Height 15 cm/ Weight 1,000 g

敛口，圆腹，腹斜收，平底，接近底部有三层台棱纹。宗教用器，祭祀用具。完整无损。

陕西医史博物馆藏

The incense burner has a contracted mouth, a swelling body, a contracting belly and a flat bottom with three tiers of ribbings carved close to the bottom. The well-preserved burner was used as a ritual article.

Preserved in Shaanxi Museum of Medical History

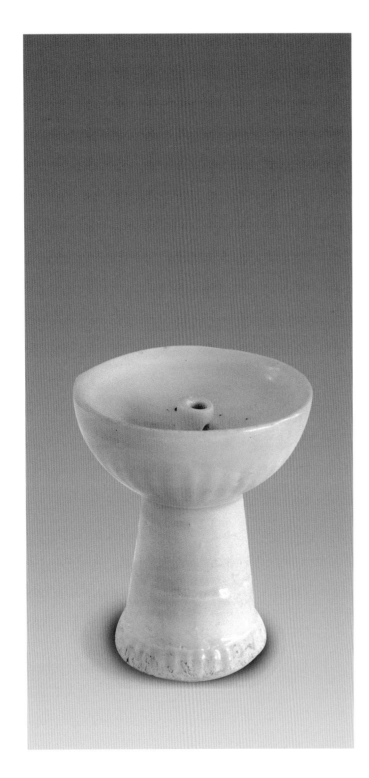

白釉高足油灯

元

瓷质

口径 7.2 厘米，高 9 厘米

White-glazed Stem Oil Lamp

Yuan Dynasty

Porcelain

Mouth Diameter 7.2 cm/ Height 9 cm

敛口，深腹，高圈足外撇。盏内装一圆筒形心，近底处一边有一小孔，与空心相通，为穿灯之用。灯外壁腹下饰凸菊瓣纹，中部饰凸双弦纹一周。施卵白色釉，是元代景德镇创烧的一种新品种。

周振武藏

The lamp has a contracted mouth, a deep belly and a flaring high ring foot. Inside the lamp is designed a hollow tube, functioning as the wick and connected to a vent hole near the bottom. Below the exterior stomach are adorned chrysanthemum petal patterns in relief, while around the middle section is incised a tier of convex double string lines. This lamp, coated with opalescent glaze, was a new type created in Jingdezhen in the Yuan Dynasty.

Collected by Zhou Zhenwu

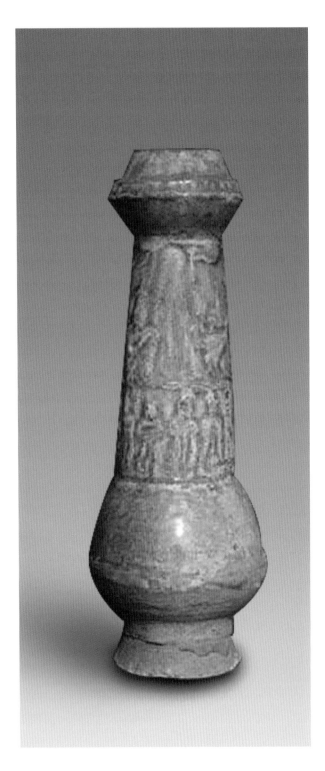

神仙瓶

宋

瓷质

口外径 4.8 厘米，腹径 9.1 厘米，底径 6.7 厘米，

通高 26.3 厘米，腹深 24.1 厘米，重 510 克

Bottle with Immortal Figurines

Song Dynasty

Porcelain

Mouth Outer Diameter 4.8 cm/ Belly Diameter

9.1 cm/ Bottom Diameter 6.7 cm/ Height 26.3 cm/

Depth 24.1 cm/ Weight 510 g

长颈，颈上堆人物等花纹，口部呈罐状，口沿平，鼓腹，圈足。随葬品。

广东中医药博物馆藏

The bottle has a long neck decorated with figurine and floral patterns, a pot-shaped mouth with a flat rim, a drum belly and a ring foot. It was a burial object.

Preserved in Guangdong Chinese Medicine Museum

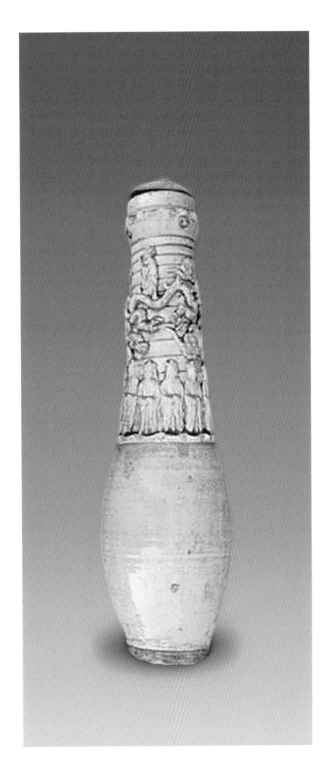

神仙瓶

宋

瓷质

口外径 9.6 厘米，腹径 17.8 厘米，底径 12.7 厘米，通高 63 厘米，腹深 55 厘米，重 5000 克

Bottle with Immortal Figurines

Song Dynasty

Porcelain

Mouth Outer Diameter 9.6 cm/ Belly Diameter 17.8 cm/ Bottom Diameter 12.7 cm/ Height 63 cm/ Depth 55 cm/ Weight 5,000 g

带盖，盖顶有纽，平口，长颈，颈部堆龙纹，

颈下部栽人物花纹，腹稍鼓，圈足。随葬品。

广东中医药博物馆藏

The bottle has a lid topped with a knob, a flat
mouth, a long neck, a slightly plump belly and
a ring foot. Around the neck is carved a coiled
dragon pattern and below the neck is a tier of
figurine patterns. It was a burial object.

Preserved in Guangdong Chinese Medicine
Museum

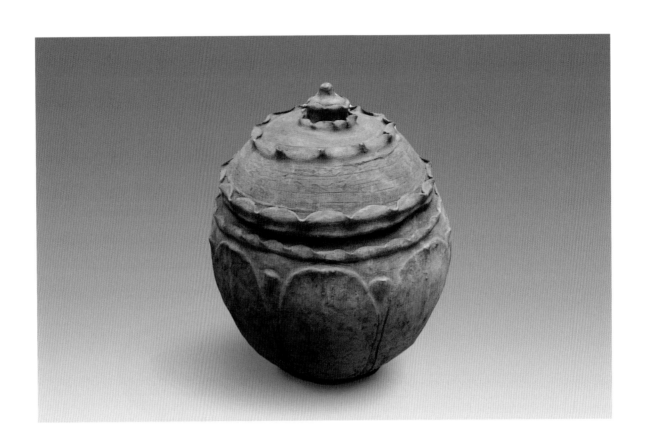

骨灰罐

宋

陶质

口径 27 厘米，底径 19.5 厘米，高 28 厘米

Funeral Urn

Song Dynasty

Pottery

Mouth Diameter 27 cm/ Bottom Diameter 19.5 cm/ Height 28 cm

敛口，鼓腹，饼形足，饰莲瓣纹，罐口塑荷叶纹，钵形盖，盖沿塑荷叶纹，塔形纽，器形完好。古代火葬骨灰装敛器。唐宋为我国火葬较为流行时期，迄至元明，云南及四川西昌火葬墓较多。墓中陶质骨灰罐是最常用葬具，并有用套罐盛装骨灰，本器即为套罐之外罐，其内再放置一种小陶罐。1985 年于四川西昌北山大理国火葬墓出土。

成都中医药大学中医药传统文化博物馆藏

The well-preserved funeral urn has a contracted mouth, a swelling belly, and a pie-shaped bottom. Lotus petal patterns are carved on the exterior, while lotus leaf patterns are moulded around the mouth rim as well as the rim of the bowl-shaped lid. On the top of the lid is a pagoda-shaped knob. The urn was used as a container for the ashes of cremators in the ancient times. Cremation flourished during the Tang Dynasty and Song Dynasty, and was mostly seen in the cremation tomb in Yunnan and Sichuan provinces till the Yuan Dynasty and Ming Dynasty. In the tomb, pottery funeral urn, as part of a whole set, is most commonly used as the funeral ware to keep ashes. This ware is an outer urn, inside which is placed a smaller one. It was unearthed in Daliguo Cremation Tomb in Beishan, Xichang, Sichuan Province, in 1985.

Preserved in Museum of Traditional Chinese Medicine Culture, Chengdu University of Traditional Chinese Medicine

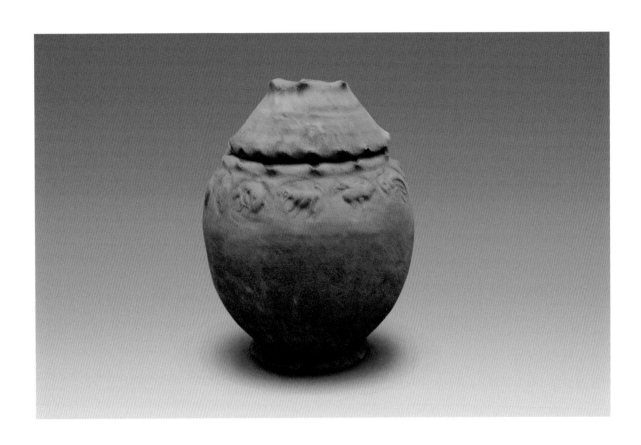

骨灰罐

宋

陶质

口径 14 厘米，底径 12.8 厘米，高 22.5 厘米，盖高 16 厘米

Funeral Urn

Song Dynasty

Pottery

Mouth Diameter 14 cm/ Bottom Diameter 12.8 cm/ Urn Height 22.5 cm/ Lid Height 16 cm

敛口，鼓腹，饼形足，肩部贴塑饰有十二生肖，腹部有刻
画纹，碗形盖，盖口为荷叶纹，器形完好，内部残存骨殖，
表面常饰有金箔，并有贝壳、佛教纹饰铜片等，为骨灰套
罐之内罐，置于外罐之内，直接盛装骨灰，是宋代火葬
墓中最常见的葬具。1985 年于四川西昌北山大理国火葬
墓出土。

成都中医药大学中医药传统文化博物馆藏

The funeral urn has a contracted mouth, a convex body, a
pie-shaped foot and a bowl-shaped lid with a lotus-leaf-
shaped rim. The shoulder is decorated with twelve Chinese
zodiac signs in relief, under which carved decoration can be
found around the belly. Inside the well-preserved urn are the
skeleton remains usually decorated with gold foil, shells and
copper sheets with Buddhist patterns adorned on its surface.
This ware, commonly seen in the cremation tombs in the
Song Dynasty as a funeral article to keep ashes, is an inner
funeral urn of a set, often placed within a bigger urn. It is
one of the most common funerary articles. It was unearthed
in Daliguo Cremation Tomb in Beishan, Xichang, Sichuan
Province, in 1985.

Preserved in Museum of Traditional Chinese Medicine
Culture, Chengdu University of Traditional Chinese Medicine

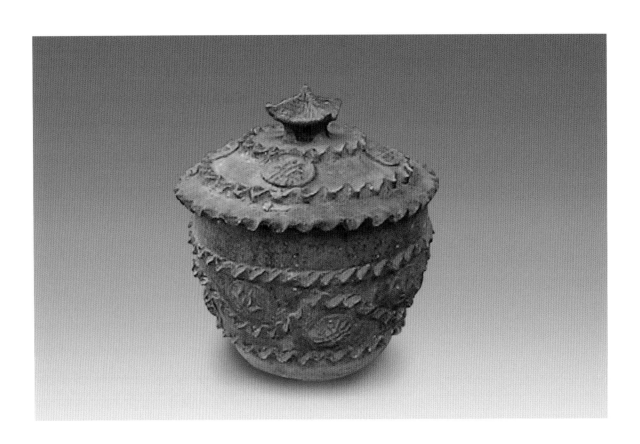

陶骨灰罐

宋

陶质

口外径 19 厘米，腹径 20.7 厘米，通高 23.2 厘米

Funeral Urn

Song Dynasty

Pottery

Mouth Outer Diameter 19 cm/ Belly Diameter 20.7 cm/ Height 23.2 cm

圆罐形，平底，敞口，有盖，饰附加堆纹，

工艺较佳。盛装骨灰的容器。保存基本完好。

1978 年入藏。

中华医学会 / 上海中医药大学医史博物馆藏

The funeral urn, made of greyish black pottery,
has a globular body, a flat bottom, an open
mouth, and a lid. This delicate handcraft is
decorated with additional convex pattern. This
well-preserved urn was used as a bone ash
container. It was collected in 1978.

Preserved in Chinese Medical Association/
Museum of Chinese Medicine, Shanghai
University of Traditional Chinese Medicine

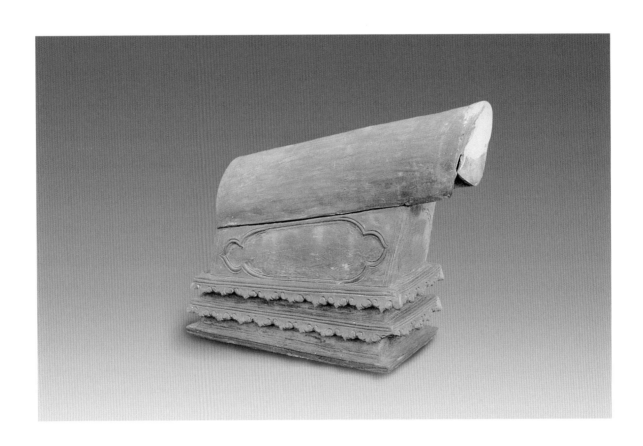

陶棺

金

陶质

总长 57 厘米，最宽处 26.5 厘米，通高 50 厘米

Coffin

Jin Dynasty

Pottery

Length 57 cm/ Width (at the widest point) 26.5 cm/ Height 50 cm

由棺盖、棺体、须弥座三部分构成。盖可取下，盖内有墨书"大定十八年"铭文。1989 年于陕西澄城善化采集。

陕西医史博物馆藏

This coffin comprises of three parts: lid, body and high base with decorating mouldings. There is an inscription on the detachable lid, reading "Da Ding Shi Ba Nian" (The Eighteenth year of Dading Reign). It was collected in Shanhua of the Chengcheng County, Shaanxi Province.

Preserved in Shaanxi Museum of Medical History

索 引
（馆藏地按拼音字母排序）

Index

参考文献

[1] 李经纬 . 中国古代医史图录 [M]. 北京：人民卫生出版社，1992.

[2] 傅维康，李经纬，林昭庚 . 中国医学通史：文物图谱卷 [M]. 北京：人民卫生出版社，2000.

[3] 和中浚，吴鸿洲 . 中华医学文物图集 [M]. 成都：四川人民出版社，2001.

[4] 上海中医药博物馆 . 上海中医药博物馆馆藏珍品 [M]. 上海：上海科学技术出版社，2013.

[5] 西藏自治区博物馆 . 西藏博物馆 [M]. 北京：五洲传播出版社，2005.

[6] 崔乐泉 . 中国古代体育文物图录：中英文本 [M]. 北京：中华书局，2000.

[7] 张金明，陆雪春 . 中国古铜镜鉴赏图录 [M]. 北京：中国民族摄影艺术出版社，2002.

[8] 文物精华编辑委员会 . 文物精华 [M]. 北京：文物出版社，1964.

[9] 谭维四 . 湖北出土文物精华 [M]. 武汉：湖北教育出版社，2001.

[10] 常州市博物馆 . 常州文物精华 [M]. 北京：文物出版社，1998.

[11] 镇江博物馆 . 镇江文物精华 [M]. 合肥：黄山书社，1997.

[12] 贵州省文化厅，贵州省博物馆 . 贵州文物精华 [M]. 贵阳：贵州人民出版社，2005.

[13] 徐良玉 . 扬州馆藏文物精华 [M]. 南京：江苏古籍出版社，2001.

[14] 昭陵博物馆，陕西历史博物馆 . 昭陵文物精华 [M]. 西安：陕西人民美术出版社，1991.

[15] 南通博物苑 . 南通博物苑文物精华 [M]. 北京：文物出版社，2005.

[16] 邯郸市文物研究所 . 邯郸文物精华 [M]. 北京：文物出版社，2005.

[17] 张秀生，刘友恒，聂连顺，等 . 中国河北正定文物精华 [M]. 北京：文化艺术出版社，1998.

[18] 陕西省咸阳市文物局 . 咸阳文物精华 [M]. 北京：文物出版社，2002.

[19] 安阳市文物管理局 . 安阳文物精华 [M]. 北京：文物出版社，2004.

[20] 深圳市博物馆 . 深圳市博物馆文物精华 [M]. 北京：文物出版社，1998.

[21]《中国文物精华》编辑委员会 . 中国文物精华（1993）[M]. 北京：文物出版社，1993.

[22] 夏路，刘永生.山西省博物馆馆藏文物精华 [M].太原：山西人民出版社，1999.

[23] 文物精华编辑委员会.文物精华 [M].文物出版社，1957.

[24] 山西博物院，湖北省博物馆.荆楚长歌：九连墩楚墓出土文物精华 [M].太原：山西人民出版社，2011.

[25] 刘广堂，石金鸣，宋建忠.晋国雄风：山西出土两周文物精华 [M].沈阳：万卷出版公司，2009.

[26] 沈君山，王国平，单迎红.滦平博物馆馆藏文物精华 [M].北京：中国文联出版社，2012.

[27] 张家口市博物馆.张家口市博物馆馆藏文物精华 [M].北京：科学出版社，2011.

[28] 浙江省文物考古研究所.浙江考古精华 [M].北京：文物出版社，1999.

[29] 故宫博物院.故宫雕刻珍萃 [M].北京：紫禁城出版社，2004.

[30] 故宫博物院紫禁城出版社.故宫博物院藏宝录 [M].上海：上海文艺出版社，1986.

[31] 首都博物馆.大元三都 [M].北京：科学出版社，2016.

[32] 新疆维吾尔自治区博物馆.新疆出土文物 [M].北京：文物出版社，1975.

[33] 王兴伊，段逸山.新疆出土涉医文书辑校 [M].上海：上海科学技术出版社，2016.

[34] 刘学春.刍议医药卫生文物的概念与分类标准 [J].中华中医药杂志，2016，31（11）:4406-4409.

[35] 上海古籍出版社.中国艺海 [M].上海：上海古籍出版社，1994.

[36] 紫都，岳鑫.一生必知的 200 件国宝 [M].呼和浩特：远方出版社，2005.

[37] 谭维四.湖北出土文物精华 [M].武汉：湖北教育出版社，2001.

[38] 张建青.青海彩陶收藏与鉴赏 [M].北京：中国文史出版社，2007.

[39] 银景琦.仡佬族文物 [M].南宁：广西人民出版社，2014.

[40] 廖果，梁峻，李经纬.东西方医学的反思与前瞻 [M].北京：中医古籍出版社，2002.

[41] 梁峻，张志斌，廖果，等.中华医药文明史集论 [M].北京：中医古籍出版社，2003.

[42] 郑蓉，庄乾竹，刘聪，等.中国医药文化遗产考论 [M].北京：中医古籍出版社，2005.